Diagnosis as Cultural Practice

# Language, Power and Social Process 16

*Editors*

Monica Heller
Richard J. Watts

Mouton de Gruyter
Berlin · New York

# Diagnosis as Cultural Practice

*edited by*

Judith Felson Duchan
Dana Kovarsky

Mouton de Gruyter
Berlin · New York

Mouton de Gruyter (formerly Mouton, The Hague)
is a Division of Walter de Gruyter GmbH & Co. KG, Berlin.

*Library of Congress Cataloging-in-Publication Data*

Diagnosis as cultural practice / edited by Judith Felson Duchan, Dana Kovarsky.
p. cm. – (Language, power and social process ; 16)
Includes bibliographical references and index.
ISBN 3-11-018466-4 (hardcover : alk. paper) – ISBN 3-11-018467-2 (pbk. : alk. paper)
1. Diagnosis. 2. Diagnosis – Cross-cultural studies. I. Duchan, Judith F. II. Kovarsky, Dana. III. Series.
[DNLM: 1. Diagnosis. 2. Cross-Cultural Comparison. WB 141 D53637 2005]
RC71.D522 2005
616.07'5–dc22
2005023837

⊗ Printed on acid-free paper which falls within the guidelines of the ANSI to ensure permanence and durability.

ISBN-13: 978-3-11-018466-2 hb
ISBN-10: 3-11-018466-4 hb
ISBN-13: 978-3-11-018467-9 pb
ISBN-10: 3-11-018467-2 pb

*Bibliographic information published by Die Deutsche Bibliothek*

Die Deutsche Bibliothek lists this publication in the Deutsche Nationalbibliografie; detailed bibliographic data is available in the Internet at <http://dnb.ddb.de>.


Cover design: Christopher Schneider.
Printed in Germany.

# Acknowledgments

The editors would like to thank the individual authors for their patience and perseverance in bringing this book to fruition, and Madeline Maxwell for conceiving of this book in the first place.

# Contents

# Contributing authors

*Wayne Beach*
Department of Speech Communication
San Diego State University, CA
wbeach@mail.sdsu.edu

*Barbara Bokhour*
Boston University School of Public Health
Boston, MA
bokhour@bu.edu

*Donal Carbaugh*
Department of Anthropology
Wayne State University, Detroit, MI
carbaugh@comm.umass.edu

*Judith Duchan*
State University of New York at Buffalo
Buffalo, NY
duchan@buffalo.edu

*Mary L. Foster-Galasso*
Director of the Evangeline Parish Library
Ville Platte, LA
Mary.Galasso@worldnet.att.net

*Philip Glenn*
Department of Communication
Emerson College, Boston, MA
Phillip_Glenn@emerson.edu

*John Heritage*
Department of Sociology, UCLA
Los Angeles, CA
heritage@ucla.edu

*Charlotte Jones*
Department of Communication Studies
Carroll College, Helena, MT
cjones@carroll.edu

*Timothy Koschmann*
Department of Medical Education
Southern Illinois University, Carbondale, IL
tkoschmann@siumed.edu

*Dana Kovarsky*
Department of Communicative Disorders
University of Rhode Island
Kingston, RI
dko7137u@postoffice.uri.edu

*Elaine Meyer*
Harvard Medical School and Brown University
Boston, MA and Providence, RI
Elaine.Meyer@childrens.harvard.edu

*G. H. Morris*
California State University
San Marcos, CA
bmorris@csusm.edu

*Christian Nelson*
Department of Marketing and Health Communication
Emerson College, Boston, MA
xianknelson@mac.com

*Laura Polich*
Department of Communication Disorders and Deaf Education
Lamar University, Beaumont, TX
laura.polich@earthlink.net

*Linda Snelling*
Department of Pediatrics and Anesthesiology
Brown University, Providence, RI
Linda_Snelling@brown.edu

*Cindy Suopis*
Department of Communication
University of Massachusetts at Amherst,
Amherst, MA
csuopis@uww.umass.edu

*Frances Trix*
Department of Anthropology
Wayne State University, Detroit, MI
ftrix@umich.edu

*Ozum Ucok*
Department of Speech Communication
and Rhetorical Studies
Hofstra University, Hempstead, NY
sphiou@hofstra.edu

# Chapter 1
# Introduction

*Judith Felson Duchan and Dana Kovarsky*

*We begin this book with an overview of the issues and practices associated with diagnosis that are raised by the authors of the chapters. Some of the ideas expressed in the chapters and reviewed in this introduction are that diagnosis:*

- *is a way of experiencing, doing, and thinking that is pervasive in western culture.*
- *is constructed by lay people as well as professional experts.*
- *is socially situated and culturally sensitive.*
- *is a process and product of social interaction and social discourse.*
- *can have a life altering impact on those diagnosed.*

This book is about diagnosis, an activity that we associate with professional experts, but one that is practiced by lay people as well. People, whether trained as diagnosticians or not, frequently engage in diagnostic reasoning as they come to grips with their own ailments or the symptoms of others, and even when they write letters of reference, or evaluate a "sick media."

The authors in this volume show how diagnoses are fundamental to western culture. They demonstrate this in various ways. One of the most powerful statements made by the authors has to do with the impact of diagnoses on themselves or their families. Yet another focus of the volume is on how professional diagnoses are formulated in relation to their historical, institutional and discursive contexts. The pervasiveness of diagnosis is further underlined by other authors who show how diagnostic thinking is used to create meaning in everyday life contexts. The breadth and scope of the studies, when taken together, make the overwhelming case for the omnipresence and powerfulness of diagnostic thinking in all aspects of the culture.

We begin with authors who are concerned with ways people experience diagnoses. Members of the culture who are recipients of a diagnosis interact with professionals during the diagnostic process. Various chapters explore how individuals may redefine themselves according to their diagnostic classification, and how they interact with others when dealing with the diagnosis as an event in their lives. The enabling and disabling aspects of diagnostic practices are treated by the authors of this volume in relation to behavioral and communication disorders (Galasso, chapter 2), Alzheimer's disease (Bokhour, chapter 3), and cancer (Ucok, chapter 4).

The authors in the second section of this book analyze cultural practices involved in doing diagnoses. They examine diagnostic situations involving professional experts such as physicians (e.g., Heritage, chapter 5, and Kovarsky, Snelling, and Meyer, chapter 9), speech-language pathologists (Duchan, chapter 10), psychotherapists (Morris, chapter 7), and medical students (Glenn and Koschmann, chapter 8). Some chapters talk about the processes of arriving at a diagnosis (Glenn and Koschmann and Kovarsky, Snelling, and Meyer), while others describe the interactional or historical contexts in which the diagnoses are constructed (Duchan and Heritage), and still others treat diagnosis in a more general way, as a means for formulating a problem (Morris).

In a third section of this volume, the authors show how diagnostic thinking can extend to situations that are not ordinarily thought of as involving diagnoses. The authors in section three examine the use of a diagnostic logic in the construal of everyday contexts such as the interpretation of letters of recommendation (Trix, chapter 12), the structuring lay group discussion about menopause (Suopis and Carbaugh, chapter 13), and in diagnostic talk about communication itself (Nelson, chapter 14).

The book contains several themes that hinge on the idea that diagnoses and diagnostic thinking are cultural constructions that pervade today's society. The authors in all three sections of the book show that these diagnoses do not exist as a piece of objective, decontextualized, problem solving done only by health professionals, but are deeply embedded in cultural practices of everyday life.

## 1. Cultural ideas and assumptions underpinning diagnoses

Diagnosis, as typically defined, is the process of determining the nature and cause of a disease by its symptoms. The result of the process is also called a diagnosis. The acts of doing and receiving a diagnosis carry with them a number of cultural practices, described in detail in this book. Among them are the assigning and enacting of expert roles involving the professional diagnostician, the stigma associated with being diagnosed, the importance of diagnosis for entitlements to goods and services, the powerful effects of diagnosis on one's personal identity, the role of interaction in accomplishing a diagnosis, and the general spread of diagnostic reasoning practices into a variety of aspects of social life. In short, the chapters in this volume reveal the pervasiveness of diagnosis as a communicative practice across a variety of culturally situated activities.

### *1.1. Diagnosis as a culturally constructed practice*

From going to church to visiting the doctor's office to using the Internet, culture comes to life through the situated communicative practices of those who experience it (Carbaugh 1996; Duranti 1997). In this view, "culture can be seen as a constructed reality that is inherited and built from symbols that shape our actions, identities, thoughts, and sentiments" (Maxwell, Poeppelmeyer, and Polich 1999: 145). Those communicative practices that help constitute culture are grounded in what Bourdieu (1985) refers to as the *habitus* or the "inclination of agents to evaluate and act upon the world in typical ways" (Hanks 1996: 239). Rooted in previous experiences, values, expectancies, and ideas, the habitus can be thought of as a generative system of perceptual and action schemes (ibid.: 239–240) that interactants draw upon and modify as they participate in social activities like diagnosis.

The ideas associated with diagnosis are flexible and are likely to change with the context. For example, as will be seen in the chapters in this volume, the enactment of diagnosis will differ depending upon whether diagnosis is viewed from the perspective of the diagnostician, the person diagnosed, or caregivers. What is common to all of these diagnostic situations is that a problem exists, that it has a physical or psychological cause (usually the source of the diagnostic name), and that receiving a diagnosis can serve to explain the problem as well as predict its course. Further, members of the culture see many diagnoses as socially stigmatizing (Kovarsky, Duchan, and Maxwell 1999). These common features are what those carrying out diagnostic practices draw upon as they construct and seek to make sense of their actions and interactions.

### *1.2. Stigma and entitlement associated with diagnosis*

Diagnosis, whether lay or expert, often carries with it a stigma as is evidenced by the conflict that some individuals experience between getting treatment and hiding their condition. Polich discusses the terrible stigma in Nicaragua that arises from the pervasive belief that deafness is caused by God's vengeance on a family for its sins (Polich, chapter 11).

In the US there is also considerable concern when children are "labeled" as "emotionally disturbed" or "mentally retarded" or "learning disabled" for the purposes of special education because of the stigmatizing consequences. Parents in many cases fight to remove their children from special education in favor of placing them unassisted in regular classrooms. That is, the damage arising from a label is perceived by some as greater than the benefit obtained from specialized services.

Certain categories, such as "learning disability" and "attention deficit disorder," are quite politicized to the point where critics argue that they have no medical or behavioral basis and are used to discriminate against some children for sociopolitical reasons. Under the heading of *Disproportionate Placement in Special Education*, records from the federal Office for Civil Rights show that African American students have been enrolled in special education in disproportionately high numbers in more than half the nation's school districts (Eig 1991).

Diagnoses also serve as entitlements. They are required to obtain insurance money, social security payments, or other public funds for medical treatment. In addition, diagnoses are needed to receive such social benefits as services from professional specialists, medical equipment, home remodeling, or income tax deductions. A psychiatrist's diagnosis in a courtroom can lead to psychiatric treatment instead of the death penalty. Galasso (chapter 2) describes how diagnostic labels applied to a child may be changed strategically by a parent in an effort to obtain needed educational and medical treatments and resources.

## *1.3. The everyday nature of diagnosis*

Ordinary individuals, including some of the authors in this volume, find themselves trying to make sense of expert diagnoses as they go about understanding events in their own lives. As a parent and an author, Galasso searches for appropriate diagnostic terms that will explain her son's behavior as she continuously seeks to cope with the nature and consequences of his developmental disability. Tied to her own expectations for motherhood and marriage, her own responses to professional evaluation become a place for self-recrimination. She describes having to learn how to turn off professional diagnoses in order to leave time for other family concerns.

In the diagnostic process, authentic behavior that is tied to motivation or emotion can become reconstructed as a symptom. For example, his alcoholism caused him to hit his son, or his madness caused him to murder his friend. Such diagnostic explanations of an individual's behavior can have both positive and negative effects. Treating behavior as a symptom can be dehumanizing – it's not her fault, we say, it's her disease that caused her to do it. On the other hand, diagnostic reconstruction of behavior can also be humanizing and liberating – he isn't bad after all, he's autistic.

Antaki (1994: 1) characterizes such diagnostic explanations as a type of everyday social reasoning "as people make sense of their worlds and (perhaps) impose that sense on other people". What counts as evidence (symptoms, for example) and what counts as appropriate reasoning thus become keys to an understanding of how diagnosis works as a cultural practice. For example, it is impaired speech rather than impaired hearing that historically has counted as evidence of deafness in Nicaragua (see Polich, chapter 11)

In chapter 12, Trix examines the appropriateness of the everyday use of diagnostic reasoning practices as they are manifested in letters of recommendation. Perhaps more telling is that the understanding of diagnostic practice can help illuminate what does count as an explanation of a state or a behavior and what can be ignored and rejected. That is, diagnosis as a situated, cultural reasoning practice privileges certain explanations over others.

Bokhour (chapter 3) adds yet another domain to be considered when examining the everyday nature of diagnosis – that of the "ward world." She analyzes the talk of professionals working in an inpatient Alzheimer's unit by recording meetings where they discuss the needs of a patient, Mr. Weinberg. Bokhour concludes that the primary "world" driving the discourse is that having to do with the exigencies of everyday caregiving on the ward.

## *1.4. Diagnosis and identity*

A diagnosis represents a crucial moment in the construction of identity because it invokes cultural premises about who we are and our potential relationships with others (see Suopis and Carbaugh, chapter 13). In some instances, the impact of a diagnosis on an individual's sense of self is positive. In a case study of a transgendered individual, one woman described her sense of relief at receiving a formal, medical diagnosis of Gender Identity Disorder (Nichols and Kovarsky 2003). Ucok, in this volume (chapter 5), presents a case of positive identity reconstruction in her description of an artist who, through interactions with others, transforms her diagnosis of breast cancer into a new "aesthetic" self.

## *1.5. The talk and interactional dynamics of diagnosis*

Conversation analysts, with their emphasis on the sequential, turn-by-turn organization of talk-in-interaction (Drew and Heritage 1992; Sacks, Schegloff, and Jefferson 1974; Schegloff 1992), have examined the discourse that takes place between diagnosticians and those being diagnosed (Frankel 1983; Gill and Maynard 1995; Heath 1992; Heritage and Stivers 1999; Maynard 1992, 2003; Peräkylä 1998; Stivers 1998). Conversation analysis has been used to study discourse associated with the delivery of a diagnosis (Gill and Maynard 1995; Peräkylä 1998), the interactional work done to prepare the patient for the upcoming diagnosis (Heritage and Stivers 1999; Maynard 1992; Stivers 1998), and the manner in which participants display moral authority and accountability to one another (Peräkylä 1998).

In this volume, conversation analytic methods and philosophical underpinnings have informed the work of various authors, as they examine the talk associated with doing diagnosis. For example, Heritage (chapter 5) uses conversation analysis to show how physicians go about negotiating their authority and accountability in their discussions with their patients and Glenn and Koschmann (chapter 8) use conversation analysis to examine how members of a diagnostic team negotiate a diagnosis.

Past studies of the interactional dynamics of medical interactions have shown the many ways that doctors control the content and structure of medical interviews (Heath 1982; Mishler 1984; West 1984). In this book, Jones and Beach (chapter 6) examine the ways that patients, operating in this authoritative discourse, manage to solicit information from their physicians, Morris (chapter 7) reveals what happens in interactions when patients do not do what is expected, and Suopis and Carbaugh (chapter 13) show the interactional dynamics between lay diagnosticians in informal chat rooms.

### *1.6. The role of the expert*

In the United States professional experts are the ones who are granted institutional authority to make official diagnoses. The selection and dispensation of treatments are also typically seen as the responsibility of experts. The expert professionals' reign over diagnosis and treatment is a complex political issue related to the apportionment of autonomy and control over oneself and others. The abrogation of autonomy among the diagnosed is especially profound in the US, a culture that places particular value on self-determination. This view of professionals as experts is not true in other countries. For example, Laura Polich (chapter 11) describes the role of the hearing expert in Nicaragua as having little influence on the cultural view of deafness.

The idea of diagnosis is based on a premise that there must be something behind (or underlying) the symptoms that one is suffering and that one needs specialized knowledge to find it (Duchan, chapter 10). The process of doing a diagnosis has been treated naively as involving a one-step logical inference, going from symptoms to cause. However, as Glenn and Koschmann show in their analysis of the talk from a group of student diagnosticians who are working together to diagnose a client (chapter 9), the act of diagnosing is not a straightforward process. Rather, it involves weighing a number of factors; and in the case of team diagnoses, it involves working with others to create and evaluate diagnostic hypotheses. The various diagnostic hypotheses of Glenn and Koschmann's students resulted in highlighting some symptoms over others, with different symptoms being better accounted for by different diagnoses.

Selecting and carrying out treatments is also in the purview of the expert, whose training and experience is regarded by some as a necessary requisite for making informed treatment decisions. Expert diagnosis is closely associated with treatment in that the existence of a treatment actually can locate the disease. Many conditions become classified by experts as a disease once there is treatment for them. That is, the treatment drives the diagnosis. The medicalization of conditions such as hyperactivity and even the natural process of aging (Suopis and Carbaugh, chapter 13) has occurred partly because there are now treatments for it. Finally, as is seen in the chapter by G. H. Morris (chapter 7), an expert's reformulation of a problem in a psychotherapeutic context can serve both as a diagnosis, in that it gets at the cause underlying the symptoms, and as a treatment, in that understanding problems in a new way can offer new directions for solving them.

Nuances in the expert role are revealed by John Heritage (chapter 5), in his examination of the ways physicians assume authority and are made accountable for their diagnoses and prescribed treatments. He shows from his detailed analysis of medically-based interactions between physicians and their patients, that the physician's authority and accountability are dynamic constructs that are in delicate balance. Similarly, Charlotte Jones and Wayne Beach (chapter 6) show various ways patients violate physician authority during medical interactions by doing things such as offering the doctor their own suggested diagnostic account of their symptoms. They also analyze in detail the physician's attempts to maintain control and their inability to respond to patients' suggestions that occur at the wrong time in the interaction. Together the findings of these authors show the boundaries and interactional conditions of expert authority.

## *1.7. Diagnosis as objective science*

Modern-day diagnosis is closely associated with the scientific method. Diagnoses are regarded as scientific hypotheses that serve to explain disease. In this frame, the best diagnoses are seen as those that are objectively verifiable and measurable, based in objective science. Other diagnoses, ones that must be inferred or that are mere descriptions of symptoms rather than explanations of them are seen as less valid, less believable, and in need of further verification.

Treatments for less objectively verifiable diagnoses may not be covered by medical insurance. Nowadays, therapies given for non-diagnosed conditions are questioned. But this was not always the case. Elocutionists of the 19th century, for example, who worked as private practitioners, did not see their task as one grounded in objective science. Rather, as Judy Duchan points out in her chapter on the history of diagnostic practices in the field of speech-language pathology, therapists of yore carried out their therapies without a diagnosis. Their framework for practice followed an educational or curricular model rather than the biomedical one that governs their practices today.

In the discursive practices of medicine, this scientific objective stance is realized in what Mishler (1984: 122) has termed the "voice of medicine." This voice is characterized by "disinterested" observers who are operating in "objective space and time" according to "the principles of scientific rationality and formal logic". In an effort to facilitate diagnosis and treatment, this voice is revealed through the use of medical terminology, the presentation of objective descriptions of physical symptoms, and the classification of these symptoms within a reductionist biomedical model.

One learns from those authoring the chapters in this book that trying to adhere to scientific objectivism in an effort to explain diagnostic practices distorts both the process and product of diagnosis. Diagnosis, instead, is a situated practice, subject to the exigencies of historical conditions (Duchan and Polich), institutional practices (Bokhour), interactions of those in the diagnostic situation (Jones and Beach), and the intersubjective lifeworlds of those impacted by diagnosis (Galasso; Kovarsky, Snelling, and Meyer; and Ucok).

## 2. Table of contents

This book examines the issues surrounding diagnosis by treating it as a cultural practice that comes to life through a variety of discursive activities. In order to see the various sides of diagnoses, we have selected authors from varying disciplines and life experience. The chapters include professionals who are engaged in the practice of diagnosis, individuals who have personally received such professional diagnoses, and scholars who are neither. The larger cultural sense of making diagnoses and of being diagnosed is treated here as originating and being carried out in particular situations with particular others (Duchan, Maxwell, and Kovarsky 1999).

### *2.1. Section 1: Experiencing diagnoses*

In the first section of the book, the authors turn their attention to how diagnoses are experienced in everyday life contexts. The cultural impact of diagnoses on recipients is brought alive and concretized in the tellings of one individual who is a parent of a child with a diagnosis (Galasso, chapter 2).

Barbara Bokhour also discusses the impact of diagnosis on the life of the person diagnosed in chapter 3. She shows how a person's diagnosed condition becomes the focus of a ward staff as they make decisions about their patient, Mr.

Weinberg. Mr Weinberg has Alzheimer's disease, and it is his disease, rather than his personal concern that govern most of the discourse among professionals involved in his care. It is a classic illustration of how the disease becomes the focus of treatment rather than the person who needs support for his symptoms.

In chapter 4 Ozum Ucok also shows the objectifying nature of diagnosis by examining how the discursive practices of medical diagnosis contribute to a diminished sense of self. However, in this chapter an artist with breast cancer is able to reconstruct her negative sense of self by reformulating a new and positive identity based on her aesthetics as an artist. Ucok traces these changes by analyzing the way the person describes pictures of herself.

### *2.2. Section 2: Doing diagnoses*

In the second section of the book, the authors identify the procedures through which diagnoses are created and negotiated. Although the content of the procedures vary considerably with the professional area, the sequential practices of the interaction are similar. Certain conclusions preside over other possibilities. Interaction between experts and clients involves evaluation of clients' behavior and claims are then challenged or validated by the diagnostic process. This set of procedures, and the ways of thinking that are associated with them, is described by professionals as the "medical model." The experts who operate according to this model include not only medical professionals, but anyone who engages in the practice of doing diagnosis.

The first three chapters of this section point to various ramifications of the authoritarian nature of doing diagnosis according to the culturally defined medical model. John Heritage, in chapter 5, poses the problem of how professional diagnosticians assume and carry out their authority in the diagnostic interview. He illustrates the discourse differences between doctor-centered and patient-centered styles, and shows how patients respond to doctor-centered discourse.

Chapter 6, by Charlotte Jones and Wayne Beach, focuses on various ways patients try to penetrate the authoritarian discourse of physicians. They examine, for example, how and when patients ask questions, offer their own diagnoses, and solicit diagnostic explanations from their physicians. They also identify and compare the communicative dynamics of successful and unsuccessful efforts of patients to achieve their personal agendas as they contend with the authoritarian dictates of diagnostic interactions.

In chapter 7, G. H. Morris shows a rare instance in which the authoritarianism of professional interactions fails. By examining the intricacies of this counterexample, he shows how diagnostic interactions require mutual cooperation between the expert and those being diagnosed. In his analysis Morris examines what happens when the efforts of a psychotherapist run amok as he seeks to formulate a diagnosis with his clients. The husband strenuously disagrees with the therapist's assessment thereby blocking the possibility of the couple working with the therapist to gain insights into possible sources of their difficulties.

In a context once removed from face-to-face, doctor-patient interaction, Phil Glenn and Timothy Koschmann (chapter 8) examine the process of training medical students to achieve diagnosis. They examine the discourse of the medical students as they offer diagnostic hypotheses about a particular patient. The authors then go on to describe what group members do with the offered hypotheses to arrive at a final diagnosis.

Dana Kovarsky, Linda Snelling, and Elaine Meyer in chapter 9 challenge the commonly held notion that diagnosis and treatment requires an objective discourse stance from the physician. They compare the objective and subjective voices of physicians interacting with one another as they evaluate what caused the death of children under their care. These authors conclude that, when supported, physicians readily talk about subjective concerns as well as objective ones, and that each kind of discourse enriches the other.

Chapter 10, by Judy Duchan, steps out of here-and-now time to examine some historical contexts for doing diagnoses. Her focus is on the diagnostic practices of speech therapists in the $19^{th}$ and $20^{th}$ centuries. She shows that early therapies of elocutionists were not based on diagnostic classification and that it was only when the biomedical model was gaining momentum in the US in the late $19^{th}$ and early $20^{th}$ centuries that diagnosis was seen as inimical to speech therapy practices.

Deafness is the topic of Laura Polich's chapter 11. Historically tracing the attitudes and services provided to Nicaraguans who are deaf, Polich reveals the powerful impact of cultural attitudes on formulating and interpreting diagnosis.

### *2.3. Section 3: The spread of diagnostic reasoning*

Diagnostic reasoning is also evidenced in other types of everyday discursive activities. These are discussed in the chapters comprising section three of this volume. Frances Trix (chapter 12) shows how letters of recommendation are structured along the lines of diagnostic thinking. In this chapter she examines the discourse of written letters of recommendation for those seeking medical school faculty positions. Her analysis illustrates how diagnostic thinking is part of the reasoning practices of the authors of these letters.

In chapter 13, Suopis and Carbaugh explore women's everyday ways of speaking about menopause as they seek to formulate their own diagnoses and treatments. The authors document the spread of diagnosis into cultural domains once considered natural conditions of life by analyzing personal impact statements in which women identify themselves and explain their symptoms to one another. Their medicalized view of menopause reflects a cultural change from previous eras when menopause was seen as a natural condition of aging rather than a diagnosable entity.

Finishing off this volume, Christian Nelson (chapter 14) reveals how diagnostic reasoning is attached, through metaphor, to the very fabric of communication itself.

When taken together, the chapters in this book point to the pervasiveness of diagnosis in Western culture. By examining the institutional, historical, discursive, and personal contexts of diagnosis, the authors explore the many cultural practices associated with diagnosis and thereby uncover the central role diagnosis plays in the daily and long-term management of all of our lives and social identities.

The insights of these authors, when taken together, offer potential readers an unusual picture of how diagnoses exert powerful influences on many aspects of society. The information the authors offer will be relevant to readers from a number of disciplines, beginning with academics, professionals, and students in the health care professions who ground their practices in diagnostic outcomes. The material is also central to concerns of researchers of speech communication, language, discourse, social interaction, and disability studies. Finally, the book provides all readers with a glimpse into how they, too, may be unwittingly engaging in diagnostic practices in their everyday lives.

It is our hope that this text will provide its readers from different academic and professional orientations, with a common ground for collaboration, and that those who read this book will continue the interdisciplinary conversations begun by its authors.

## *References*

Antaki, Charles
1994 *Explaining and Arguing: The Social Organizations of Accounts.* Thousand Oaks, CA: Sage Publications.

Bourdieu, Pierre
1985 The genesis of the concepts of habitus and field. *Sociocentrum* 2, 11–24.

Byrne, Patrick and Barrie Long
1976 *Doctors Talking to Patients.* London: Her Majesty's Stationary Office.

Carbaugh, Donal
1996 *Situating Selves: The Communication of Social Identities in American Scenes.* Albany, NY: State University of New York Press.

Drew, Paul and John Heritage (eds.)
1992 *Talk at Work: Interaction in Institutional Settings.* Cambridge: Cambridge University Press.

Duchan, Judith, Madeline Maxwell, and Dana Kovarsky
1999 Evaluating competence in the course of everyday interaction. In Kovarsky, D., J. Duchan, and M. Maxwell (eds.), *Constructing (In) Competence: Disabling Evaluations in Clinical and Social Interaction.* Mahwah, NJ: Erlbaum.

Duranti, Alessandro
1997 *Linguistic Anthropology.* Cambridge: Cambridge University Press.

Eig, Jonathan
1991 Black students likelier to be placed in special ed than whites, data show. *The Dallas Morning News*, 1, September 29.

Frankel, Richard M.
1983 The laying on of hands: Aspects of the organization of gaze, touch, and talk in a medical encounter. In Fisher, S. and A. D. Todd (eds.), *The Social Organization of Doctor-Patient Communication.* Washington, DC: Center for Applied Linguistics, 19–54.

Gill, Virginia T. and Douglas W. Maynard
1995 On 'labeling' in actual interaction: Delivering and receiving diagnoses of developmental disabilities. *Social Problems* 42, 11–37.

Hanks, William F.
1996 *Language and Communicative Practices.* Boulder, CO: Westview Press.

Heath, Christian
1992 Diagnosis and assessment in the medical consultation. In Drew, P. and J. Heritage (eds.), *Talk at Work: Interaction in Institutional Settings.* Cambridge: Cambridge University Press, 235–267.

Heritage, John and Tanya Stivers
1999 Online commentary in acute medical visits: A method of shaping patient expectations. *Social Science and Medicine* 49, 1501–1517.

Kovarsky, Dana, Judith Duchan, and Madeline Maxwell (eds.)
1999 *Constructing (In)competence: Disabling Evaluations in Clinical and Social Interaction.* Mahwah, NJ: Erlbaum.

Lakoff, George
1991 *Women, Fire and Dangerous Things.* Chicago, IL: University of Chicago Press.

Maynard, Douglas W.
1992 On clinicians' co-implicating recipients in the delivery of diagnostic news. In Drew, P. and J. Heritage (eds.), *Talk at Work: Interaction in Institutional Settings.* Cambridge, UK: Cambridge University Press, 331–358.
2003 *Bad News, Good News: Conversational Order in Everyday Talk and Clinical Settings.* Chicago: University of Chicago Press.

Maxwell, Madeline, Diana Poeppelmeyer, and Laura Polich
1999 Deaf members and nonmembers: The creation of culture through communication practices. In Kovarsky, D., J. Duchan, and M. Maxwell (eds.), *Constructing (In)competence: Disabling Evaluations in Clinical and Social Interaction.* Mahwah, NJ: Erlbaum, 111–124.

Mishler, Eliott
1984 *The Discourse of Medicine: Dialectics of Medical Interviews.* Norwood, NJ: Ablex.

Nichols, Laurie and Dana Kovarsky
2003 The emergent self: The case of a transgendered woman. Paper presented at the American Speech-Language-Hearing Association Conference. Chicago, Ill, November, 2003
Peräkylä, Anssi
1998 Authority and accountability: The delivery of diagnosis in primary health care. *Social Psychology Quarterly* 61, 301–320.
Sacks, Harvey, Emmanuel Schegloff, and Gail Jefferson
1974 A simplest systematics for the organization of turn-taking for conversation. *Language* 50, 696–735.
Schegloff, Emmanuel
1992 On talk and its institutional occasions. In Drew, P. and J. Heritage (eds.), *Talk at Work: Interaction in Institutional Settings.* Cambridge, UK: Cambridge University Press, 101–134.
Stivers, Tanya
1998 Pre-diagnostic commentary in veterinarian–client interaction. *Research on Language and Social Interaction* 31, 241–277.
West, Candace
1984 *Routine Complications: Troubles with Talk between Doctors and Patients.* Bloomington, IN: Indiana University Press.

# Section 1. Experiencing diagnosis

# Chapter 2

# Diagnosis as an aid and a curse in dealing with others

*Mary L. Foster-Galasso*

*In this chapter Mary L. Foster-Galasso ruminates over the efforts of her family to cope with her son's diagnosis of a developmental disorder. Galasso explores the differential, strategic use and impact of diagnostic terms like "autism," "PDD-NOS (pervasive developmental disorder, not otherwise specified)," or "seizure disorder." She sees these diagnoses as a gateway for navigating social institutions and everyday interactions: "being used as a gateway, it all depends on what gate we're trying to open, and how rusted the hinges are". For example, she used the label "autism" when securing a classroom aide, and the label "seizure disorder" when negotiating medications with a physician. Finally, Galasso notes how she herself gets diagnosed as a "Bad Mom" in situations where her son does not conform to others' expectations. Her chapter shows that diagnoses, for those living with them, are dynamic, influential, situationally sensitive, and co-created constructs to be fought for and fought against.*

My son Calvin (name changed to protect his privacy) is eleven. Back when he was about seven, we were shaking hands and saying, "Peace be with you" at a key point in the Catholic Mass, when Calvin suddenly shattered our family's peace by asking the older woman beside him – in his too-high-pitched, just slightly off "normal" voice, and of course standing just a tad too close, so he could practically look up her nostrils – "Why do you have that big moustache?"

I tried to hush him and look apologetic, but neither my husband Gary nor I could say more, because the congregation is totally silent in the next part of the Mass. By the end of the service, I thought the incident was all over. But it wasn't. As soon as the final notes of the recessional hymn died away, she was waiting for us, blocking our path to the aisle, her large body a mass of indignation. Displaying her wounded feelings, and just waiting to give us a piece of her mind. "I've been watching you at church. You can't control that little rascal."

I tried to make excuses. "I'm sorry about what Calvin said. He has a problem with what to say, because he's got a type of autism." I knew it wouldn't do any good to force *him* to apologize, since then he'd just get fixated on the moustache and never stop talking about it, either to her or to us.

At that stage I was as annoyed at Calvin as she was, but he hadn't intended to hurt her feelings. Paradoxically, I was pretty annoyed at her, as well, for putting us on the spot. I almost wanted to ask her if she knew anything about hair removal products.

"... he's got a type of autism." I'd used a diagnosis word, offering it up like an appeasement, or perhaps a hope for some shared understanding. Understand us better, maybe even pity us if you want, but step aside and let us get into the aisle and out of here. Now.

The diagnosis word had its effect; one I hadn't intended: "Well, you know, there are places for people like him."

Maybe I had offered up the word as part of a sincere attempt to mend fences and educate my fellow parishioner. Or maybe I had held up the diagnosis as sort of a magic charm or shield to ward off further unpleasant discussion so we could dash out the door and off to lunch. Either way, it hadn't worked. With the weird power of words, my son had turned instantly from a "little rascal" into part of a group: "people like him," "people" who need special separate "places."

The ironic part is that Calvin doesn't have a diagnosis of autism at all, and never has had one. Not technically, anyway. When he was first tentatively diagnosed in Hawaii at age two (tentatively, because everyone we saw at three different medical centers seemed hesitant to label a child this young, especially one who had also had tubes placed in his ears and could have been suffering from the effects of earlier hearing impairment), speech and medical professionals used the terms "autistic-like" or "autistic symptoms" quite a lot – but didn't write them down. We did finally see a written tentative diagnosis of "PDD nos": Pervasive developmental disorder, not otherwise specified. Back at our remote home in the Kwajalein Atoll of the Marshall Islands, we studied photocopied pages of the then-current DSM, underlining key words and comparing diagnostic criteria from one pervasive developmental disorder to another. We grasped the basic point: Calvin showed some of the defining criteria for an autism diagnosis, but not all. We tried to ignore an even more basic point: by whatever name that was used his development was not "normal" at all, and probably never would be.

In our newness to the world of developmental disorders, we, too, quickly breathed a sigh of relief. At least he isn't autistic, my husband Gary and I told ourselves. At least not that. We had yet to learn that a developmental disorder by any name or any amount of severity is a little bit like being just a few seconds pregnant or just a few seconds dead: life had changed, and it wasn't going to change back miraculously.

At least not autistic. At least not that. So how come about five years later in Maryland we were voluntarily using the term "autistic" to an upset stranger? For starters, because "PDD nos" means nothing to people outside of certain fields. People do have at least some ideas about autism. Admittedly, these ideas are usually based on television or movie portrayals of savants or "miracle cures," but at least they're – generally – sympathetic ideas. "PDD nos" generally just invokes a response like "huh?" (I've even received this response from a well-informed parent of a grown autistic child: the term just wasn't current in her area when her son was being diagnosed.) Or, perhaps more often, instead of a "huh?" response, it confuses the hearer because of somewhat sound-alike terms like "ADHD" or "ADD." The hearer then offers some comment such as, "My nephew has that, but he doesn't act this way. Maybe you need to change ..." Into the dots, any number of well-meaning suggestions about diet, bedtime, discipline, and rewards get inserted. One is supposed to stand and listen gratefully to information already known and with very limited relevance (any relevance having already been tested and tried, probably numerous times).

So we said "autism." Not really a lie, in any case, since "PDD nos" is part of the spectrum of pervasive developmental disorders that includes autism. Besides, at that time Calvin was far more like a high-functioning autistic child than he was like one with any other diagnosis we had seen, so it made sense in talking to another layman to use this diagnostic term.

Talking to medical, speech, and educational professionals is another matter, and requires different terminology. It is very much a matter of the situation controlling the choice of words, or at least heavily influencing the choice. It can help level the "me rushed and overworked doctor/you poor ignorant parent of patient who will try to get me further behind in my schedule" playing ground a bit by using "PDD nos" right away with a new pediatrician. On the other hand, it might annoy a new neurologist – that's the neurologist's call to make, not the parents', so it has to be couched a bit differently for the specialist. When dealing with a busy neurologist who is having an initial appointment with Calvin, I've been known to say something like this: "Here's his foot of medical records from overseas, and here's a ten page summary of them that I prepared. The term neurologists and developmental pediatricians have used most to describe him in the past is pervasive developmental disorder."

In other circumstances, when the goal is not a long-term relationship, my husband Gary or I may find it makes more sense to use some of the other terms or labels Calvin has carried with him in the past or still carries: "motor ataxia," "ADHD," "seizure disorder." Particularly back when Calvin was on seizure medication, it was important to emphasize the seizure disorder part if Calvin saw a different pediatrician while we were on vacation. We learned that point very well one time when a different doctor put him on an antibiotic. His seizure medication suddenly got toxic and he panicked because he saw two of everything. (We had told the nurse what medications he was on, and she had written it down, but we hadn't discussed them with the doctor.) Gary became my hero then, as in many other times in the past, when he held Calvin for two hours straight until the double vision had fully worn off and Calvin had drifted to sleep.

Whether to use a diagnosis, and if so, which one? A lot depends on the purpose of the conversation or interrogation. Is it a gateway to something we need, or not? A general school report to keep Calvin's special education services going, for example, may only need the special education catch-all label, "multihandicapped." On the other hand, a request to have the county school system's one and only autism specialist come out and evaluate his classroom situation as part of a desperate effort to get funding for a classroom aide may require at least the "PDD nos," and we may briefly wish for a "code 14," or whatever the current number is, autism label instead.

Discussions with the county science fair coordinator when Calvin was scheduled to participate in the county fair required yet another approach. We wanted Calvin accompanied rather than left alone to possibly panic and wander away in the large, noisy crowd, yet we also did not want the judges to be aware of the situation. Here the label we found most effective in discussing the problem with the coordinator was "high-functioning autism," since many lay people understand that people with autism can have trouble with noise and crowds and unpredictable routines, yet also be gifted in some areas and be able to compete in them.

So, if the diagnosis is being used as a gateway, it all depends on what gate we're trying to open, and how rusted the hinges are. Calvin, for example, was the first child we know of with his level of symptoms to be included at his particular home school, a school his sister attended for six years. When we held our first meeting with the now-retired principal, in preparation for Calvin's move from the wing environment he'd attended for five years at a school further away, the first words out of the principal's mouth were, "Why are you bringing him here?" The goal then in discussing the diagnosis had to be to emphasize the positives, to show how much Calvin had learned and how cooperative he was. Two years later, when Calvin fell apart under the pressures of departmentalization (i.e., having different teachers for all major academic subjects), we had a new goal with a new principal: to show that Calvin could still learn and thrive, but needed a classroom aide to make it possible. There we needed the county's autism specialist to emphasize the negative effects for Calvin of departmentalization and to write the report to help secure funding for an aide. In each case the gates swung open, but it took different approaches, labels, and terms to make it possible.

It also depends on whether the gate is one that we just want to get through, get shut, and leave behind as quickly as possible. For example, when Calvin was four he fell and cut his forehead late one night on the brick fireplace. I was exhausted when I drove him to the Air Force base emergency room. We knew long waits happened, but we weren't prepared for what happened after the long wait.

The emergency room doctor was accompanied by a physician's assistant. He needed to train the young man. To do that, he had to work through the procedure very slowly, explaining each step in excruciating detail as he went along. Strapping my son down to a papoose board. My son who generally hated to be held or hugged. Covering his tactilely sensitive face with a cloth and running iodine solution or something that looked like it, all over his face, so it dripped in places where I knew he couldn't tolerate even a bead of sweat. Taking what seemed all of eternity as he explained the ins and outs of stitching to the trainee.

I kept saying, "Calvin is autistic. He hates what you're doing to him. He thinks you're torturing him. You are torturing him. Please get this over. Please."

They acted as if they didn't hear me, just kept talking to each other as they discussed the fine points of stitching. When days later it was time to get the stitches removed, I snuck into Calvin's bedroom in the dark and, using a small flashlight and small sharp scissors, cut the stitches out myself. I wouldn't have brought him back to them.

The scar is just a little one, but it's something we don't forget. Despite all their fine stitching discussions and the slow work pace, it still left a scar on his forehead. No big problem, but it left an invisible scar for me, as well. And in this case diagnoses – any diagnoses – did us no good at all.

But when I see Calvin thriving with a classroom aide – a classroom aide he struggled without for years – I see the good that proper use of diagnosis can do. Proper use of an appropriate diagnosis by concerned professionals has made successful inclusion possible, and made us eternally grateful to them, although we all regularly continue to irritate each other.

There's no final happy ending, at least none that we can visualize yet. Daily, it's still a matter of pushing open stuck gates, and it's still a complex matter of mixed motivations. When I decide Calvin has done all the math he can do for the night and – invoking his diagnosis and IEP – draw a line halfway down the math page and stop him there, am I doing it for him? Or for me, because I'm sick of the math too, sick of the constant stream of homework, and want to go work on a short story while he plays Nintendo? Or maybe actually talk to my husband or teenage daughter for a change before I completely lose contact with their lives?

And should the choice be there? Should Calvin see that he's doing less math than the others? On the other hand, since some days he's readily able to do it all, would it be self-defeating to have that math sheet halved every day, with only the top part coming home?

Ultimately, I've decided that, mixed motives or not, and mixed effects on Calvin's sense of empowerment or powerlessness or not, the bottom line is that my husband Gary and I know when we've done all we can for the day. I know we're happier and healthier as a family when one of us draws a line, both actually and metaphorically. It need not always be the same one of us drawing the line, just whichever parent is most sane and clear-headed on any given day. But the line has to be drawn, since we turn into a miserable mess of a family when one of us doesn't do it. When we don't draw a line, when we play into others' expectations too much – be they doctors or teachers or grandmothers or church school teachers or piano teachers or karate instructors; or, on a really rotten day, all of the above – that's when I wind up acting like a shrew. For make no mistake: no one can be worse to a child with a diagnosis than his own mother.

Against every standard, every situation, the "mom" gets evaluated right along with her son. Implied diagnoses of "lazy," "disorganized," "failure," "ignorant," "inappropriate," "distracted," "unmotivated," etc. leave their scars, too. Maybe not a scar; instead, maybe a brand across the forehead that says, "BAD MOM."

Does Gary get a "BAD DAD" label, as well? I don't think so, not even if he's the one dealing with a particular school issue. Rightly or wrongly, I feel that more expectations and disappointments are piled on the mom. But maybe I'm wrong. Maybe men just are less ready to shoulder every sack of guilt that's shoved their way. All I know is that I feel the "BAD MOM" label and don't wear it particularly well.

If Calvin doesn't remember how to tell the time for the neurologist (who doesn't need to be doing a form of ad hoc achievement testing on him at the end of a long school day, after he's waited an hour in her waiting room); if he doesn't eat nicely on the meal out with his grandmother (who without warning has changed the outing from one to Burger King to one to a seafood restaurant); if he doesn't graph his x and y coordinates neatly on his math homework (although with motor ataxia he's doing the work as fast and neatly as he can): I get the evaluation. It may be a sigh or sniff of disapproval, or a small undermining glance at the end of an already too-long day. It may be an exhortation to review this or that with him in the car while driving (although the traffic is already more than enough, thank you, without adding distracting drills and new failure opportunities to it, too). It may be a nice but ultimately nonsensical note from a teacher saying that Calvin might want to redo this graph before report card time (although why should he put in more hours doing something no better than he has already done it?).

In any case, I'm the one getting and interpreting the feedback, and then struggling, often unsuccessfully, not to pass along the hurt as sighs, sobs, or cutting words to my son. The diagnosis and evaluation become a bad additional child for me to deal with.

It is easy under the circumstances to lose sight of the fact that the diagnosis is a multi-purpose, artificial, variable, situational, thing: not alive and not my first concern. Once it becomes important in and of itself, then I'm not just the mother who wants to scream "buy some hair removal cream" at a stranger; I'm the person who winds up tearing apart my little boy's sense of competency and his self-image as a loveable person. If this goes on long enough, I can even pick up a few new diagnoses of my own, or at least blow my blood pressure and marriage sky high. At least I always feel in danger of both.

It has taken a long time, but now I choose: what to tell others, what to accept as Calvin's burden and my own, what to discard as not his burden and not my own. I still make mistakes – horrible mistakes – but am determined to no longer keep Calvin up until past eleven p.m. because some medical professional has volunteered that we need to review time-telling. I no longer ruin a weekend because some childless math teacher thinks Calvin might, "if he gets bored," like to plot sixty-seven ordered pairs of x and y coordinates over the weekend. And I no longer even bother to argue with family over why it won't be possible to add more stops or visits to an already overstressed day or visit. When I slip and regress, Gary is there, to step in and save us all. I hope this doesn't change, but I also hope I won't slip and need catching so often, either. Like Calvin's diagnoses, I'm evolving, too.

And the diagnosis does evolve. Lately more and more I hear, "Asperger Syndrome" or "Asperger's Syndrome" applied to Calvin. Like all the others so far, it fits Calvin very well in some ways but not at all in others. Because it is a new one to many people, it doesn't have as many connotations – sympathetic or negative – attached to it by the general population. It won't do as a plea for understanding and tolerance from laymen. But, on the other hand, it won't automatically invoke responses like, "Well, you know, there are places for people like him."

Still generally conversationally neutral, it neither opens or shuts gates, except in very specialized contexts.

But that, like many other things involving diagnosis, is fast changing. Within a week after first writing the words above, I encountered two uses of the diagnosis "Asperger's" around here – and from laymen, not professional diagnosticians.

The first was in the local advertising paper, "The Penny Saver." A community ad there stated that a group was forming locally for parents of children with Asperger's who were being homeschooled (i.e., taught at home). When we first came to Maryland, the only group we knew about that seemed to be dealing with Asperger's was the local Autism Society. Now there is a separate support group, at least for homeschooling.

The second encounter was a personal one that startled me. I need to explain first that Calvin takes the *same* thing to school in his lunchbox almost every day, and has done so for years. One custard style strawberry yogurt (only one brand acceptable to him), one orange juice box (no calcium supplements allowed), one chocolate pudding cup, one apple, one carrot stick. Day after day.

Lately it's a lunch that has been hard to come by. More and more yogurt manufacturers seem to want to go away from plain old strawberry to more fancy flavors with sprinkles and mixed tastes (strawberry banana, watermelon, etc.). My son won't even accept strawberry vanilla, let alone any other changes. And the orange juice box makers seem intent on adding calcium to aid in strong bones and teeth. Which is fine, except that it won't do my son's bones and teeth any good, since he can taste the subtle flavor change and doesn't want to have anything to do with even a sip of the "improved" juice.

There is a store close to my house where I'd loved to shop, but which after a while I had to keep bypassing to venture farther and farther afield in search of the components for Calvin's lunches. One day, while picking up dry cleaning at the shop next door, I made up my mind: why not go see the manager of this closest store and explain what I needed? I was reluctant to face another personal discussion with another stranger, but Calvin really needed to have a lunch he would eat. Besides, I was sick of wandering from store to store! So I put the dry cleaning in the van, went next door, and asked directions to the store manager's office.

The manager listened carefully and wrote down what I wanted. Then he said (quote approximate), "Did you see the special on insulin and autism the other night?"

I braced myself for another discussion of another miracle cure, but then suddenly came the unexpected: "My daughter has Asperger's. They call it pervasive developmental disorder sometimes, and sometimes other names. It can be hard."

I felt like hugging him, and we wound up discussing that television special, and whether karate was good for our kids, and just what our kids' lunches were like. Several days later I came back. The shelves still had nothing but calcium-enriched orange juice boxes, but the dairy cases were now overflowing with strawberry yogurt. The right brand.

One problem: the wrong type. *Not* the custard type. With kids with this diagnosis, product consistency counts, too.

I bought a cart of it, anyway. Will be eating it for lunch and breakfast for a while, myself. And then I'll go see the manager again, and thank him, and this time bring the actual custard type package to show him.

That kind manager soldiers on. He'll contact the supplier again; I'm sure of it. And it is comforting to know that the diagnosis of Asperger's Syndrome means something to him, although I wouldn't wish it on him or anyone to come by his knowledge as he has had to, in trying to understand and help his daughter.

Which brings up one more subject about diagnosis: how do we even begin the process of getting and initially understanding a diagnosis? How do we first take it home and integrate it into our lives, without letting it become that bad additional child who turns family members into monsters and home life into hell? When we open our gate or door, and all the various strange-sounding diagnoses crowd around it, clamoring for admittance like children in costumes out trick or treating at Halloween, how do we judge who gets in initially, and of this admitted group who finally gets invited to stay?

After all, we have our own gateways, too. This element of choice is particularly there for parents of children on the high-functioning end of things. Friends have told me of their own high-functioning child: "I think his cousin has it too, but they never got a diagnosis." Friends have also remarked, especially regarding those ambiguous children who seem to stand on the border between "normal" and "abnormal," on how many different diagnoses they've obtained from different doctors. If each diagnosis is slightly – or more than slightly – different, and if for some rare families even any diagnosis at all seems optional, then is it really necessary to invite any of the available diagnoses to stay and become part of the family? And if you are going to let one through the gate, then how many should you "shop about" for before making a choice?

We *could* have told the woman in church nothing. We *could* have believed there was nothing to tell her. I think we would have been wrong, but this has been done, more times than probably anyone knows. Children with high-functioning autism or Asperger's have been characterized as "odd" or "eccentric." As moving time approaches yet again, I'm facing the temptation to "lose" some of Calvin's records rather than acquire some more. But then I remember our long fight through diagnoses to get the classroom aide that Calvin needed, and imagine life without the help the diagnosis has made possible.

Even if it weren't for that help now, the other problem is the children don't stay children. At some point they become adults who may *not* be able to function on their own and may desperately need the support of others who are not their family members. After all, none of us can shoulder the lives of our children forever. That undiagnosed cousin of a friend's autistic child may wind up with a sad life of problems with the law or drugs or homelessness – preventable problems with the right supports at the right times. Supports perhaps dependent on first obtaining a diagnosis.

But that eccentric child may also wind up surviving, possibly even thriving, without a diagnosis. It's a long-shot, but happens. Besides, any child can also wind up with a sad life in the future, and in the immediacy of the childhood-raising years, it's probably a lot more comforting for a parent to have a "little rascal" rather than one of a group: "people like him." This isn't just a matter of a salve for a parent's feelings: besides the obvious fact that a parent who is less depressed is better able to parent, it can be just generally much more pleasant to be a "little rascal" than one of "people like him." Rascals still get invited to birthday parties, last time I checked, and sleepovers. They may behave badly or strangely and get only invited once, of course. But fear of the unknown may keep the child with a diagnosis from ever being invited at all. Some parents' choices are not so cut and dried as many professionals might believe, and the final decision has, in my opinion, far less to do with a parent's intelligence or level of care for his or her child than it does with previous experiences and the attitude of the community around the family. People open their personal defensive gates to what will aid their family, and try to avoid whatever will lead others to slam gates in their faces, and most especially in the face of their child.

My early experience with opening gates and trying to find a diagnosis for Calvin probably will be of little use to others: it's not something we could reproduce. We were living on a remote island in the Pacific, my husband stationed there as the communications officer, when we realized that Calvin was not developing "normally." He was, however, still within the realm of what our physician or many physicians would see as normal, believing, as one doctor told us, it was "far too early to label" a young child, since each could behave so differently at a medical appointment. Nonetheless, my widowed mother had come to visit us for a few weeks and had convinced me that something must be wrong with Calvin's ears, because he seemed not to pay attention or follow any simple commands. She was used to babysitting my sister's child, who was one year younger; based on differences she saw in the two children's behavior, she was very concerned.

Although the general practice physician on the island found nothing wrong at that time with Calvin's ears, I became determined to get another opinion. There was one problem: the nearest second opinion was two thousand miles across the water away.

At the end of a soldier or civilian employee's first year in the Marshall Islands, he or she gets a trip to Hawaii so that the person (and family, if there is one) can keep from becoming what is locally known as "rock happy": i.e., they need to reconnect with traffic and fast food restaurants and find a place that sells batteries for wrist watches, etc. We wound up in Hawaii expecting to do all these things and much more. But first, we thought, we'll take Calvin for a visit to some pediatricians. They'll find out what's wrong with his ears – why he's not speaking and following directions – and then we'll get this vacation going. We'll see the sights.

We hadn't even thought about the way Calvin spun the wheels on toys, stared into lights and ceiling fans, and kept a pencil flapping in each hand. But the doctors we saw in Honolulu certainly did, although most seemed reluctant to say what they thought. Ultimately, two trips to Hawaii later, they did find a problem with his ears also, but they suspected much more.

We ended up communicating with a lot of soda machines and cafeterias in three different hospitals and clinics, and taking turns spending time with our five-year-old daughter either in a small park near some of the hospitals, watching her swing on the banyan tree vines, or in the little cemetery across from Straub Clinic, walking with her among the gravestones. One would stay with our daughter while the other stayed with Calvin. And that was it for our vacation, and for several follow up trips back to Hawaii as well. We got a lot of sympathy and paperwork out of these trips, but not an actual diagnosis or a plan, other than to get back to the mainland, find Calvin a neurologist, and get Calvin into special education. Which actually wasn't such a bad plan at all, come to think of it.

Sometimes I think back to those days when we were stumbling around Hawaii, searching for that first diagnosis, desperately wanting to know what was wrong. The concept of "diagnosis" didn't create the problem; we were searching for a "diagnosis" because there was an underlying problem. We needed to know what it was, we thought, so that we could eradicate it. We thought we could cure it if we could just first name it. Names have power.

But we didn't see the full shape of what we were trying to name. For example, we saw Calvin's lack of consistent interaction with us and others, but we didn't see the flapping pencils constantly clutched in his hands. To us, they didn't matter.

The pencils still don't matter all that much. We know if we're missing pencils and need one, to go check in Calvin's room. The last time a doctor ever asked us about them was nearly eight years ago, when a military developmental pediatrician noted the flapping pencils and asked how we dealt with the "stimming" (stimulation), which is the technical term for it.

Just a few days before, our new Brittany puppy had dealt with it herself. Rosemary was walking with Calvin in the backyard and decided to leap for the enticingly whirring pencils. They were quite near his face (of course), and before we realized what was happening she suddenly lunged upward and nailed his ear with her sharp puppy teeth, neatly piercing the lobe. We spent the next few hours at the emergency room.

That day soon afterward, when the developmental pediatrician was watching the pencils flutter and asking about the "stimming," Gary and I were worn out. We'd also been waiting about two hours to see this new doctor, after an hour's early morning drive to get to the clinic. We laughed and said almost together that we dealt with the stimming by "siccing" the family dog on him.

Then we saw the look on the doctor's face and realized we'd better amend that statement quickly, before we wound up as clients of social services.

The point here is not as sharp as the puppy's teeth, but it's just as basic: some symptoms matter in one context but not in another. (It's not a good idea to flap things about your face around a hyperactive puppy, for example, but flapping a couple of pencils in one's bedroom may not be a big deal.)

Some symptoms are just part of the overall package. Sometimes the diagnosis matters, and sometimes it's just part of the overall package, too. Portions of both get outgrown and changed, and others stay constant – although the interpretation and significance of them to ourselves and others may change through the years.

Back when Calvin was two and three and we were stumbling around Honolulu, even the best and most sympathetic doctors we saw gave us lengthy reports about symptoms observed, but didn't give us much information to take home and use – neither about diagnosis, nor about any other facet of what to expect, and what to do about it. The communication disorder clinic gave us practical speech help ideas, but nobody else actually said, "Here's what you can do to help, and here's why." As for searching out information on our own, nobody at that stage would actually say a diagnosis, at least not on paper. But without a name, how does one begin to search for information, especially when you live on an island that is about two miles long?

What happened next is not something that can be duplicated. A crew member on our military flight back to the island recognized the symptoms of Calvin and of another child going to and from Hawaii for evaluation. He recognized them because his nine-year-old son with autism had had the same symptoms at the same age. To protect his privacy, I'll call him Jeff, rather than his real name.

From then on, we'd get a call, or the mother of the other child would. An airman on the other end of the line, someone neither of us had ever met: "Jeff sent a package for you." We'd go to the island's gathering center, the tiny snack bar, and there it would be: books and magazines. We read and discussed and learned. Because of Jeff, who lived in California and had not wanted to be on that particular flight at all. Being a religious man, he saw in us a reason why he had needed to be there on that day. Being a very humane and wonderful man, he never stopped caring. And we read and read and read some more, returned the books and waited for the next call from the snack bar, the next stranger's voice saying, "Jeff sent a package for you."

The first book the other mom and I read as we tried to come to grips with it was *Son Rise* by Barry Kaufman (Kaufman 1995), his account of how he and his wife developed a successful program that perhaps cured his son's autistic symptoms. Thank goodness it wasn't the last, or we'd still be stuck on the absolute need for a "cure." Both of our families all but locked ourselves in our respective houses with our respective kids for weeks. We all got stranger and stranger, and soon realized that we couldn't intensively work with our children the way the author's wife had. We didn't question the author's sincerity and success, but soon realized we weren't going to share that success, at least not through following the same method.

Fortunately, the second book we read was *Emergence: Labeled Autistic* (Grandin & Scariano 1996). We needed to learn, and did from its high-functioning autistic author, Temple Grandin, that a diagnosis didn't mean eradicating a problem, but rather as much as possible, adapting a way around it. Temple's descriptions of her childhood and of what treatments had been valuable to her and which had been less helpful or perhaps useless helped us learn how to evaluate choices. Her book also led us to many other helpful sources. Today I am in awe of her later book, *Thinking in Pictures* (Grandin 1996), which I see as true literature that reaches far beyond the interests of the communication disordered community alone.

More and more, we started to learn to adapt rather than try to "cure," but the actual process of doing that never completely ends. And part of us still wants desperately to be able to write our own sequel to *Son Rise*, report our own miracle cure. Because none of this is really linear. Some changes are straight-line, of course: skills mastered, new developmental stages reached. But at each stage the same issues are broached over and over. At each stage the problems are, after all, still pervasive. They pervade everything, locking into speech patterns and understanding of conversations and school lectures, infiltrating body language, motor skills, food choices, and sensitivities or lack of them. *Pervasive*. That is a large part of what the diagnosis means, whatever the technical wording preference of the day. When I first read the term, "Pervasive Developmental Disorder," the word "Pervasive" seemed the least important word in the name. Now I know better.

Remarks still come out at church at times – the latest victim a five-year-old who had his hand up his nostril right before extending his little hand to Calvin in the sign of peace. Calvin was blunt, and loudly determined not to shake a "dirty" hand. Fortunately, the other child's mother just laughed. We didn't; instead, we came down on our eleven-year-old for his insensitivity. Did it help? Who knows? We made ourselves and our son feel terrible, and embarrassed his teenage sister no end, but to what purpose if the behavior doesn't change? And many an adult avoids shaking hands at times, also. After all, when is the last time anyone really wanted to shake hands with someone who had just been picking his nose?

Behaviors do change: some of Calvin's get better. As we get older and more tired, some of ours, especially mine, get worse. And some things never change. Underlying love. Underlying differences. They're still locked together, sometimes battling for control, sometimes peacefully coexisting.

Recently Calvin's neurologist remarked that his hand tremors and motor overflow are as bad as ever, yet his drawing is getting lovely and detailed. She's right. Calvin is still Calvin, but he rises to the occasion – in his own tactless way, and often against the prevailing odds. With his family and friends and the professionals who care about him functioning as both his best allies and his own worst enemies, he soldiers on, ready to face more mismatched diagnoses and achieve small and large miracles along the way.

## Postscript, three years later

Calvin is fourteen now. Two years ago we moved back to the family farm where I was raised in Louisiana. No one packs a lunch to school here, so Calvin has learned gradually to eat what he can stand from the school lunch, just as his sister does. No more yogurts and orange juice boxes. After some initial struggles to get an aide, Calvin has one again, and he continues to make progress in school.

"Asperger's Syndrome" or "Asperger Syndrome" has become much more widely known, and at a conference last fall in Washington, D.C., I was able to buy four books specifically about this diagnosis. I also heard one speaker at the conference say that Asperger has become the new "buzzword" diagnosis for parents who don't want to say that their children have mental problems. I can't address that issue, but I do know that the Asperger diagnosis probably fits Calvin better than any other he has carried.

We still face the same issues but now with two added complications: Calvin's puberty and our own sense of rapidly dwindling free and appropriate education time for Calvin. What will happen when he turns twenty-one? What will his adult life be like? Those issues loom larger and larger now.

As for me, I need the facial hair removal products almost as much and get irritated just as easily as that woman at church did seven years ago. I count on Gary more and more to be the one who provides balance and stability to our lives. I look at our whole family – daughter a year away from high school graduation and college, Gary and I forty-nine and fifty, and Calvin, with his future so uncertain. I fear for us all, especially Calvin. He is so desperate to achieve his dream of being a scientist and still so incapable of managing any form of research and analysis without support.

During math Calvin turns intently to his resource teacher and asks her, in a voice that tears at her heart, "Am I doing good?" The honest answer she doesn't give him is both yes and no: yes because he's come so very far; no because he still has to have one on one support to continue learning at all.

The days continue to be a roller coaster of events and emotions. On one day, Calvin may play the piano at a school assembly; on the next, bullies may lock him in a room, causing him to fall apart while his classmates listen from the other side of the door and make no move to get an adult.

But there are triumphs, too. As I finish this last paragraph, it's a beautiful May Saturday afternoon on the farm. Gary and Calvin just returned yesterday from a student Junior Beta Club (honor society) state convention. Calvin spent Thursday night in a strange motel room with Gary and four other boys. At the dance he danced along with eleven thousand other teenagers in a coliseum he had never stepped into before. And in that crowded coliseum, where once he would have broken out in a sweat and kept his hands clamped over his ears while he screamed, only the dozen children from his own school knew he had any diagnosis at all.

## *References*

Grandin, Temple
1996 *Thinking in Pictures: And other Reports from My Life with Autism.* New York: Vintage Books.
Grandin, Temple and Margaret Scariano
1996 *Emergence: Labeled Autistic.* New York: Warner Books.
Kaufman, Barry
1995 *Son Rise: The Miracle Continues.* Tiburon, CA: H. J. Kramer.

# Chapter 3

# A diagnosed life in an institutional setting: Can the dancer walk?

*Barbara G. Bokhour*

*Adding to Galasso's experiences is this second depiction of the profound impact of diagnosis on those diagnosed and on those who interact with them. Here Bokhour shows how staff in an institution lose sight of an individual, and treat him as a generic patient with a particular diagnosis. The recipient of a diagnosis is Mr. Weinberg, a man with Alzheimer's disease. Bokhour's discourse analysis of staff discussions depicts how treatment of Mr. Weinberg was related more to what they felt should be done with a person with his diagnosis, ignoring their patient's life world. That is, the professionals did not fully address such factors as Mr. Weinberg's concern about swelling in his feet and his anger at having been restrained from walking independently. Rather they focused on his inability to walk safely, and most of their talk about the patient had to do with their execution of typical treatment practices for patients with Alzheimer's disease.*

Individuals who are diagnosed with Alzheimer's disease enter into a life that is largely defined by inevitable decline and eventually death. Those living with the disease experience ongoing assessment and treatment from a variety of professionals, often in constrained institutional settings. The professionals in these settings are influenced by bureaucratic and biomedical frameworks, and consequently the framework of individual lives is often neglected. Institutions, Foucault (1977) argues, are central in the discursive construction of their objects and in the case of medicine those objects are the patients. That is, the organization of the institution – its space, professional staff and bureaucracy – places or "disciplines" bodies into categories most relevant to the functioning of the institution. For medical institutions, the biomedical model, rooted in the scientific approach to the human body, provides a driving objective framework for categorizing those who are ill. In constructing the individual as "patient," medicine subsequently transforms people into objects of medical practice (Cassell 1991; Mishler et al. 1981). Cecil Helman (Helman 1991), depicting his experience as a medical student, poignantly marks the obscuration of the individual in favor of emphasis on the patient as an object of medical practice and the institution.

> The intern in a medical ward takes me aside, and points. "There's an interesting spleen over there," he says, "third bed on the left." I walk along the ward among the rows of beds, and follow his finger. And there it is, just as he said, lying in the third bed on the left – an enormous, black and gelatinous thing, five foot long or more, moist, oozing off the sides of the bed. Nothing but a huge black spleen lying on a hospital bed. But then you blink and rub your eyes, and look again, and the spleen has gone, buried beneath the striped pajamas of a little worn grocer of a man, sleeping in the bed. A small, sighing man with a sore stomach, and an ominous zig-zag chart, like a range of high mountain peaks, pinned to the foot of his bed. (Helman 1991: 120)

Helman's story reflects three models of patients: one as a medical object – the diseased body part; another as a person who is a patient – the body as a self with a social history of a "grocer man"; and yet a third as an institutional object inscribed on a chart. The intern clearly directed Helman toward the diseased body part, thus focusing on only the medical aspect of the patient. The chart, a way for the institution to hold the medical staff accountable, is the graphic inscription of the medical work that was constituted by doing the proper tests, diagnosing disease, and curing patients. The individual, a grocer man with a sore stomach, is edited out of any official account and is evident only in the observation of the individual intern. The objective data remains, pointing toward a diagnosis of something wrong with an "interesting spleen."

In realizing the culture of medicine, professionals construct patients as different types of objects that correspond with different aspects of the world of medical practice. Mishler (Mishler 1984) identified two worlds that physicians and patients attend to in medical consultations: 1) the medical world, in which the relevant information is related to the biomedical aspects of the work that physicians do with their patients, and 2) the lifeworld, in which the relevant information is related to the meaning of illness in the lives of those patients. Thus patients may be constructed as objects in the following ways: 1) the patient as a diseased object – the diagnosis itself – existing as part of the medical world; and 2) the patient as an individual who may be understood in relation to a broadly conceived lifeworld. Patients, however, may also be constructed as institutional objects: part of both the larger framework of the medical institution and the more constrained context of the "ward world" (Bokhour 1998).

Individuals suffering from diseases such as Alzheimer's may subsequently be defined as the diagnosis itself, thereby limiting the ways in which others interact with them, view their potential and make decisions on their behalf. Using a discourse analytic framework, this chapter examines the ways in which a group of professionals negotiates the assessment of such a diagnosed patient living on an inpatient Alzheimer's unit and in doing so redefines his life. More specifically, it will examine the ways in which the institutional framework and shared cultural models of patients as objects influence the manner by which patients are constructed linguistically in communication between team members. In the discourse of the team members we will begin to see how one patient, Mr. Weinberg,[1] disappears and the diagnosis takes his place as the team assesses his changing ability to walk independently as Alzheimer's disease progresses through his body and his mind.

Mr. Weinberg was one patient among many on a specialized treatment unit at a Veterans' Administration Hospital. This chapter closely examines the discourse of an interdisciplinary team of professionals as they discuss Mr. Weinberg's care in bi-weekly meetings. A more exhaustive description of these meetings will follow. The present analysis distinguishes between talk that constructs individuals who are suffering from Alzheimer's disease as medical and institutional objects and talk that constructs patients as individuals. Throughout the team's discussions, their concerns about Mr. Weinberg as an institutional object manifested themselves in two ways: first, in terms of the bureaucratic responsibility of the team to account for his care according to the rules and regulations of the institution; and second, with respect to the everyday pragmatic management of patients in the ward world of the unit. Constructions of the patient as an individual did enter into the discourse at times, but these were most often silenced by the other, more dominant framings of the patient. Constructions of Mr. Weinberg as an individual and as an object of the institution were often in tension with one another, a tension that was reflected both in the discourse of the meetings and in follow-up interviews.

## 1. Theoretical framework for discourse analysis

In this chapter I rely on a broad conceptualization of discourse analysis in which the construction of meaning through language is best understood in the discursive context of institutional practice. According to Gee (Gee 1992, 1996) individuals' language use is constrained and facilitated by the cultural models shared by participants in a particular institutional context. These models are part of what Gee calls "Discourses" (Gee 1992, 1999) with a capital "D": the elements encompassing a community of practice that contribute to both the linguistic and non-linguistic activities of its members:

> Discourses ... are ways of behaving, interacting, valuing, thinking, believing, speaking, and often reading and writing that are accepted as instantiation of particular roles (or "types of people") by specific *groups of people,* whether families of a certain sort, lawyers of a certain sort, bikers of a certain sort, African-Americans of a certain sort, women or men of a certain sort, and so on through a very long list. Discourses are ways of being "people like us". They are "ways of

> being in the world"; they are "forms of life". They are, thus, always and everywhere *social* and products of social histories. (Gee 1996)

In other words, the ways in which we use language and interact in our lives always occur in relationship to the Discourses of which we are members at any given time. The Discourse in which the professionals and Mr. Weinberg were located was the practice of medical professionals in the context of a long-term care facility for persons suffering from Alzheimer's disease. The Discourse includes all of the physical space: the units in which the patients live, their rooms, the living space, and the nurses' stations. It encompasses the activities of the doctors, nurses, therapists, patients and families, and even the maintenance staff. It is also comprised of the written documents, manuals and records of patient care, and clearly, the explicitly discursive activities: the language used in interactions between professionals and patients, professionals and families, patients and families, and amongst professionals. In other words, to understand these discursive interactions, one must consider the entire situation; discourse with a small "d" can only be understood as fully situated in Discourses.

This approach to discourse focuses on what Hanks (Hanks 1996) calls communicative practices extending the focus of analysis beyond the linguistic systems used by individuals to communicate with others to the participants' shared orientation to the social world and their shared categories. Groups of individuals in institutions such as hospitals can then be understood as an interpretive community, in which members share meanings and values to varying degrees. No single individual in the community holds all the pieces of these interpretive schemes in his or her head. Rather these schemes, or cultural models (D'Andrade and Strauss 1992; Holland and Quinn 1987), are socially distributed; different members have different bits and pieces of the models and the overall or master model is composed of all these pieces in concert (Gee 1999).

The following analysis explores how the different cultural models of patients are displayed and negotiated in semiotic activities in the discourse of team meetings. Though primarily concerned with the linguistic aspects of the discourse, it interprets their meaning in the context of ethnographic observation, knowledge of the institutional framework of the interactions, and the participants' reflections upon their own communicative practices.

## 2. The data

### *2.1. The setting*

The case discussed is drawn from a larger study of communication in health care teams conducted at a long-term care center at a Veterans Affairs Hospital. The Department of Veterans Affairs fully funds this center, which specializes in serving aging veterans who suffer from Alzheimer's disease or progressive dementia and serves as a center for research as well. During the study, the patients on four in-patient units (of approximately 25 beds each) were treated and cared for by comprehensive interdisciplinary teams, each comprised of a physician, a nurse manager, a nurse practitioner, several staff nurses, an occupational therapist, a kinesiotherapist, a dietitian, a pharmacist, a social worker, a dentist, and a recreational therapist. These health care providers were involved in both routine care and efforts to maintain patient quality of life. Communication between professionals is central for achieving a goal of acting in concert for the benefit of the patients, and this occurred formally in interdisciplinary team meetings.

### *2.2. Team meetings*

Team members participated in bi-weekly interdisciplinary team meetings, in which they evaluated patients' problems and goals and established treatment plans. During these meetings professionals discussed the treatment they were providing patients and also assessed the status of individuals as they progressed through the course of the disease. Such meetings are mandated by both the Veterans Administration and the Joint Commission on Accreditation of Healthcare Organizations, which is the agency responsible for regulating and monitoring all health care facilities in the country (JCAHO 1996).

The team members met on a bi-weekly basis in a conference room. Sitting around a table, the team members reviewed the treatment plans of four to five patients in a forty-five minute period. Each patient was discussed in the meetings on a quarterly basis, although patients who had been recently admitted were discussed once a month. The meetings proceeded in a standardized format with either the nurse manager or nurse practitioner acting as the team leader. The discussions were largely focused on writing an initial treatment plan or revising a printed out copy of an existing Interdisciplinary Treatment Plan (ITP). These written plans noted the patient's name, social security number, date of admission and religion and provided an identifying ward number. Listed below this orienting information were the "problems-needs-concerns" related to the patient. Associated with each inscribed problem was a "goal" and an "intervention" with a record of the staff person responsible for implementing the intervention. Prior to the meeting, each team member was supposed to review the ITPs for the patients who were to be discussed, and they were also to have these ITPs in front of them throughout the meeting.

### *2.3. Data collection*

Team meetings were audio and videotaped and then transcribed verbatim. Pseudonyms were substituted for the names of all the participants and patients. Team members were interviewed twice: the first time they were asked about general practices in team meetings; and the second time they reflected on specific discussions in team meetings while reviewing them on videotape. In addition, the investigator conducted ethnographic observations of Mr. Weinberg's Alzheimer unit over a period of three months. The data I discuss here comes from a number of sources: one review of Mr. Weinberg's case in a team meeting, my interactions with Mr. Weinberg, and team members' comments in follow-up interviews.

## 3. Who was Mr. Weinberg?

At the time of data collection Mr. Weinberg had just been admitted to the unit.[2] His wife no longer felt able to care for him on her own. I had several interactions with Mr. Weinberg in his first few days at the Alzheimer's unit. Unlike many of the other patients, Mr. Weinberg was still able to walk independently and to hold conversations, although he was often confused during these interactions. On one occasion, Mr. Weinberg began a conversation by telling me how he and his wife were supposed to go dancing that evening. He said that they were excellent dancers and had even won some competitions. He spoke in animated tones as he related his escapades on the dance floor. Dancing had apparently been a very meaningful activity for him in his life and an important aspect of his marriage. He asked me if I knew where his wife was and how to get to the dance hall. He did not know who I was, nor did he seem to realize that he was in the hospital and not on his way to a dance competition. Throughout the conversation I listened and tried to respond to his questions: I did not know where his wife was or when she was coming. I did not know where the dance hall was. As he recounted his stories about dancing, I nodded and said "wow" and "that's great."

Another day, I found him amongst most of the other patients in the day room, sitting in a large chair, restrained from getting up independently by a tray table (imagine an oversized child's high chair). He was banging on the table, angry that he was unable to move around on his own. His frustration was evident and yet the nursing staff, busy with other patients, was unable to attend to him. This incident and others like it made it clear that Mr. Weinberg was searching for ways to make sense of a confusing situation in a new place. He sought assistance to go to the bathroom, even though he wore adult diapers. He tried to figure out how to leave this "place," which he was unable to remember was a hospital.

Based on these brief interactions with Mr. Weinberg, I began to form a picture of an individual whose life had been quite full. He was married to a woman whom he apparently loved very much. They had always danced together. He had been a very independent individual and was now searching for a way to maintain his dignity. His attempts to attain some level of independence and control in his environment were evident in his search for the exits so that he could leave, and in his attempt to locate a bathroom so that he could take care of his most basic needs. As the forthcoming analysis reveals, the discourse of the team meetings even more distinctly omits a view of Mr. Weinberg as an agentive individual.

## 4. Constructing mobility

Being unable to walk is a difficult issue for anyone with a chronic disease. It truly sets the afflicted individual apart from others and distances the self from the person one was before the onset of disease. For Mr. Weinberg this was a particularly troubling circumstance because he could no longer participate in an important lifeworld activity, dancing with his wife. The issue of whether or not a patient could walk was central to much of the assessment and care of the patients on the units. As Alzheimer's patients decline, they gradually lose their abilities to do many things and the loss of the ability to walk is an important marker in this decline. Patients like Mr. Weinberg were viewed in the light of this prognosis of inevitable decline. As we will see below, the discourse reflects this view of each individual as the diagnosis, the generic Alzheimer's patient, and decisions about care, assessments of abilities are often driven by this overall generic perspective.

Two contradictory constructions of Mr. Weinberg's mobility were reflected in the discourse of the team meetings. First, from an institutional perspective, some team members – and particularly the physician – were concerned about the extent to which Mr. Weinberg needed to be restrained with a "posey"[3] or a tray table on the geri-chair to avoid injury. In this framework, Mr. Weinberg is an institutional object; he fits generically into a category of Alzheimer's patients who characteristically lose the ability to walk. Unaware of their limitations, these patients often attempt to walk on their own, creating a situation that is unsafe. Consequently, the institution must protect him (and itself from a potential lawsuit[4]) by restraining him.

The concern was thus pragmatic: how could the team manage Alzheimer's patients on the ward? However, by depicting Mr. Weinberg as someone who needed to be restrained, they constructed a patient with little, if any, individual agency left. He became an object to be controlled and manipulated to fit into the context of the ward world. As plans were discussed to stop his efforts to walk, he lost his freedom, his independence and, in a sense, his individuality. He became another one of "the guys" strapped into a chair, passing time until he died.

Other aspects of the discourse, however, constructed Mr. Weinberg as an individual: Mr. Weinberg, who had a recent history of being able to walk independently, could still walk at that time and could potentially continue to walk in the future. Whether or not an individual with Alzheimer's disease can walk has several implications. Not only is a decline in walking a marker of the progression of the disease, it impacts on an individual's independence and sense of dignity. Thus, being able to walk independently was a crucial issue to Mr. Weinberg as an individual on the ward and in his social world. At the very least, individuals who were able to walk had the capacity to wander about the ward, to sit where they wished, to look out the window, and to engage others by walking to them. In other words, if Mr. Weinberg were perceived of as someone who could not walk, he would be construed as an Alzheimer's patient – that is, an inevitable, passive recipient of care, confined to a chair. On the other hand, if Mr. Weinberg were framed as a walking patient, he would maintain some level of independence, and he would be more active in his own care.

One important question emerged from the discourse: could Mr. Weinberg walk or not? The team vacillated between talking about him as being able to get up and walk (although his safety would be in question), being unable to walk at all, being able to walk again, and having been able to walk in the past. One might think that the team was confused and contradicting itself, or that the separate members simply viewed the situation differently. I will argue, however, that the shifts in the discourse on opinion regarding Mr. Weinberg's ability to walk were linked more with how team members constructed the problem and Mr. Weinberg. That is, if one viewed Mr. Weinberg as an Alzheimer's patient whose ability to walk would decline inevitably over the course of the disease, the goal would be simply to keep him safe, and subsequent discussion would focus how to restrain him. If, however, one viewed Mr. Weinberg as an individual who had walked quite frequently and well until his recent admission to the hospital, the goal would be to get him walking again.

## *4.1. Walking and restraint in the second review*

Let us turn now to the specific discourse about walking in the second review of Mr. Weinberg. As the meeting progresses it becomes clear that the question of his walking engenders two lines of discussion: 1) how well, if at all, is he able to walk and 2) if it is necessary to restrain him in his chair.

### 4.1.1. Does he have an unsteady gait?

The discussion about Mr. Weinberg's walking begins in line 204, when the nurse practitioner introduced the problem, as listed on the ITP.

(1)

| | | |
|---|---|---|
| 204 | NP: | unsteady gait/ |
| 205 | ?: | hmhm// |
| 206 | | (..) |
| 207 | OT: | That's really declined I think// |
| 208 | | um even since last– |
| 209 | | he's no longer ambulation ad lib, |
| 210 | | um, he's not steady enough for that// |
| 211 | | he is participating under interventions in the Merry Walker study/ |
| 212 | | um, |
| 213 | NP: | okay/ |
| 214 | | (..) |
| 215 | OT: | and we are (..) [all working] |
| 216 | KTA: | [yeah], |
| 217 | OT: | to get him stronger and increase his endurance// |

The nurse practitioner introduced the issue of Mr. Weinberg's walking through the use of jargon, "unsteady gait," and the without the use of a sentential subject. Her rising intonation functioned as an invitation for someone else to address the problem. The occupational therapist (lines 207–216) responded by presenting a picture of Mr. Weinberg as getting worse. He began by referring to the problem ("*That's* really declined") and only introducing the patient ("he") later in l. 209. When he did introduce the patient, he used stative verbs ("he's"), thereby diagnosing the patient in terms of categories that are sanctioned by the Discourse, such as "ambulation ad lib." Mr. Weinberg's act of walking was thereby codified into generic categories that could be applied to any patient on the unit. The occupational therapist ended by stating that the intervention would be for team members to work "to get him stronger and increase his endurance." Note the placement of Mr. Weinberg in the passive position, with the team as the active agents. In l. 216, the kinesiotherapist echoed this concern and supported the intervention.

Mr. Weinberg was presented as a set of problems and interventions and was diagnosed as no longer ambulating "ad lib". At the same time, however, the occupational therapist *raised* an issue that was important to Mr. Weinberg as an individual: his ability to walk. The OT shifted from speaking of the problem of unsteady gait to speaking of Mr. Weinberg as "participating under interventions in the Merry Walker study,"[5] thereby ascribing some agency to him. Thus Mr. Weinberg was portrayed as someone who was capable of walking with assistance at that time and who, with help, would be able to walk independently again.

The issue of his walking was not taken up again until the physician refocused the discussion on the question of using a posey to restrain Mr. Weinberg.

(2)

| | | |
|---|---|---|
| 218 | MD: | and what are we going to do about the posey// |
| 219 | ?LPN: | does he do? |
| 220 | OT: | He doesn't wear it at all [times], |
| 221 | ?: | [no]// |
| 222 | LPN: | PRN [that's crossed off um/] |
| 223 | MD: | [Does he need it at all/ |
| 224 | | no we cannot do that//] |
| 225 | LPN: | [what's it gonna be/] |
| 226 | NP: | [yeah we can't do now] posey that's PRN// |
| 227 | | (..) |
| 228 | | um/ |
| 229 | OT: | [what behavior does he do that he requires], |
| 230 | MD: | [{ }]// |
| 231 | LPN: | that would be at night// |
| 232 | | um |
| 233 | ?: | to prevent [falls/] |
| 234 | OT: | [so should] we [put that under]– |
| 235 | LPN: | [well {why don't we} just check it off] |
| 236 | | and monitor him for a [couple of weeks] // |
| 237 | NP: | [right] // |
| 238 | LPN: | see if [it's really necessary]// |
| 239 | ?: | [{ }]/ |
| 240 | ?: | oh I'm just/ |

When the physician asked, "what are we going to do about the posey," the nurse responded by asking for it to be used "PRN" or as needed. The physician replied, "No we cannot do that," and was subsequently supported by the nurse practitioner. In a follow-up interview, it was discovered that when the physician states that they "cannot do that," he is referring to external guidelines established by JCAHO (JCAHO 1996). These guidelines require specific reasons for restraint to be identified in the treatment plan, in order that a team may not use restraint whenever they deem it practical.[6] Thus the discussion truly revolved around the team's accountability to the institutional and governmental regulations regarding the use of restraint with patients, a practice that was common for those with

Alzheimer's. The concern only shifted away from the diagnosed patient back to Mr. Weinberg's role as an actor when the occupational therapist asked what "behavior does *he do*" to require the posey. Here, the evidence being requested was based upon how Mr. Weinberg acted as an individual: the issue at hand was refocused on the person (rather than the institutional object) to be restrained. The nurse and another team member responded that the posey would be used at night "to prevent falls." Thus the team members responded by providing an institutionally sanctioned rationale for using a posey; a rationale that could be used for any patient.

The OT further deflected his attempts to understand Mr. Weinberg as an active agent when he shifted to the task of writing the treatment plan in line 234. There was no discussion about why Mr. Weinberg might fall at night or if there was an alternative way to manage the problem. Rather, the discussion continued about how to codify the problem and its solution for the ITP:

(3)

| | | |
|---|---|---|
| 241 | LPN: | make sure we have a monitor for a couple of weeks/ |
| 242 | NP: | oh RN monitor? |
| 243 | MD: | RN monitor? |
| 244 | LPN: | not an RN mon- |
| 245 | | well, yeah we could do that or just visual, you know/ |
| 246 | | He's in the dorm he's right, |
| 247 | | He does try and- you know he does, |
| 248 | NP: | he does try to get, yeah// |
| 249 | NP: | so maybe [we should put { }]/ |
| 250 | OT: | [so we should put unaware] of-- |
| 251 | | not only unsteady gait but unaware of you know [ gait impairment//] |
| 252 | MD: | [unable to walk/] |
| 253 | LPN: | yeah// |
| 254 | | cause he likes the table down also// |
| 255 | | he really thinks he can get up and go but he can't// |
| 256 | MD: | so he needs to be in a geri-chair with table top up/ |
| 257 | LPN: | yes// |
| 258 | MD: | at all times/ |
| 259 | LPN: | yes// |
| 260 | | (5) |

The nurse described Mr. Weinberg's efforts to get out of bed (246–248) and then went on to personalize his concerns by addressing what he "liked" and "thought" (254–255). Although she appeared to be ascribing some level of mindfulness to Mr. Weinberg, in line 255 the nurse went on to discount his cognitive abilities by stating that he "really" thought he could "get up and go" when, according to her, he could not walk. She thus repositioned him as an individual for whom the team needed to think. She positioned the team as the experts on the diagnosis of Mr. Weinberg's abilities as a generic Alzheimer's patient. Because the team was more cognizant of Mr. Weinberg's limitations than he was, it was responsible for taking control of the situation by restraining him in a geri-chair. Mr. Weinberg's capacity to understand his own ability to walk, however, was not taken up as a topic of discussion. Instead, the team returned to its deliberations regarding the correct way to write the ITP, the assigned institutional task. In this manner, the patient was completely removed from the discourse, and, as one social worker commented, the team meeting became "all about the paper."

### 4.1.2. What does Mr. Weinberg 'need'?

The construction of Mr. Weinberg as a passive object was reinforced when the physician stated "he needs to be in a geri-chair with the table top up" (line 256). The verb "need" has an interesting status in this case, functioning more as a modal verb than an active verb. Although at first glance it appears that "need" is acting as a main verb with the subject being "he" (i.e., Mr. Weinberg), it is in some senses functioning as a modal. That is, the sentence effectively means "*It needs to be the case that* Mr. Weinberg sits in the chair with the table top up." In this case, Mr. Weinberg is no longer the subject; rather, he is the object and the active agent is linguistically absent. Who exactly is establishing that he should be in the chair is not indicated. In fact, here "need" may be understood not in the epistemic sense, in that it is necessary for Mr. Weinberg to sit in the chair with the tray table up, but rather in the deontic sense, in that the physician has ordered it to be the case. Thus, although the team appeared to be addressing what Mr. Weinberg really needed, they continued to treat him as a passive Alzheimer's patient, whose actions were controlled through the discourse.

Determining if and how to restrain patients was clearly within the purview of the team's authority. Hence, the discussion took on an institutional life of its own, furthering the interests of the team as the authoritative decision-maker in determining Mr. Weinberg's fate. The OT's shift to writing the report re-established the task as an institutional one. Further, his request for the physician to write the order highlighted the importance of the physician in the institutional decision-making process.

### 4.1.3. And the discussion goes on

The issue of Mr. Weinberg's ability to walk could easily have been dropped at this point. Instead, in line 269, the social worker reintroduced the topic and brought his wife into the discussion:

(4)

| | | |
|---|---|---|
| 269 | SW: | you know, I don't know/ |
| 270 | | has she talked to [you about that/] |
| 272 | LPN: | [well you know/] |
| 273 | SW: | she's identified all his problems as [related to that// |
| 274 | | is there something we can do/?] |
| 275 | LPN: | [okay well/ |
| 276 | | I don't know if there's a place where they can get a] personal chair or have |
| 277 | | [somebody { }] |
| 278 | OT: | [she's um] She's she's currently thrilled with the-- |
| 279 | | she [was up yesterday with the uh, merry walker] |
| 280 | LPN: | [uh, wonderful] |
| 281 | OT: | [study] |
| 282 | SW: | [oh, I know that] |
| 283 | | But I mean his normal life is in that chair that she feels is causing him to be |
| 284 | | unable to walk and his feet to swell and// |
| 285 | | his feet don't touch the floor/ |
| 286 | | she's very upset// |
| 287 | | and I was just wondering if there [was anything that could be done]/ |

The social worker introduced Mrs. Weinberg as a relevant actor in the discussion by requesting that action be taken on a problem that had been identified by her rather than by team members. That is, it was Mrs. Weinberg who identified the issue of the swelling in Mr. Weinberg's feet and attributed it to the kind of chair he sat in. The social worker allowed Mrs. Weinberg's voice to be heard in a discourse dominated by the medical professionals, thereby creating a dilemma for to the team: how to assert its authority under the guise of honoring *her* request.

The introduction of the problem of the chair by the social worker gave rise to a rather lengthy debate in which the team negotiated the nature of the problem as well as the treatment solution. In the extended interaction that followed, the team alternated between two constructions of the problem: one in which the team needed to determine what type of chair Mr. Weinberg should sit in for safety, and a second in which the team needed to find ways for Mr. Weinberg to walk independently on the ward. Each of these alternative conceptualizations of the problem constructed Mr. Weinberg as a different type of object, and each had a different status as actionable by the team.

Discussion of the first dilemma – what Mr. Weinberg should sit in – focused on the need for the chair to have some restraint on it for his own safety and to resolve the medical problem of the edema in his feet. The proposal of a safe chair with a posey or tray table continued to position Mr. Weinberg as a generic patient who must fit into the unit. Pragmatic concerns of the ward world dominated, and thus he was to be maintained safely and kept out of trouble.

The second problem was Mr. Weinberg's ability or inability to walk. These segments portrayed Mr. Weinberg as an agentive individual with a unique social history and relevant personal attributes. These two types of problems – those involving the chair and those concerning his ability to walk – were interspersed throughout the discourse. When the discussion focused on one problem, often someone on the team would redirect the discussion towards the other. In other words, the team members alternated in their discourse between a model of the patient as an institutional or medical object and a model of the patient as an individual.

In line 288, the team sought to solve one of Mr. Weinberg's problems by determining what type of chair he should sit in:

(5)

288 LPN: [{get him a different chair}],
289 NP: [should we get a PT consult]?
290 SW: a different chair/
291 LPN: we can have one fitted I I [think { }]
292 NP: [for a wheelchair/]
293 SW: It would mean a lot to her//
294 I don't know if it would really [make that much difference for him but,]
295 OT: [um]
296 SW: [but I don't know/]

The nurses and social worker attempted to solve the problem by getting a fitted wheelchair for Mr. Weinberg. Comments such as "we can have one [a chair] fitted for him" served to reinforce the notion that he was a passive recipient of actions taken by the team. Moreover, Mr. Weinberg, viewed as unable to walk, was considered to be a good candidate for a customized wheelchair in which he could spend his days comfortably. If he were comfortable in a fitted chair, the staff could simply place him in it and avoid dealing with the complications of an unhappy wife and perhaps an agitated patient. It would further allow the team to avoid the challenges of seeing Mr. Weinberg as an individual with the potential to walk.

In line 297, the discussion of a fitted chair was interrupted by the nurse practitioner's testimony that Mr. Weinberg had exhibited some ability to walk. Since wheelchairs, particularly customized ones, were typically given to patients who were unable to walk at all, evidence that Mr. Weinberg could walk would contradict the need for such an extravagance:

(6)

297 NP: [He walked] a little bit [for me yesterday]//
****

299 LPN: [he did walk//]
300 ?: [you know I]
301 LPN: yeah he walked to the bathroom with me this morning//
302 hunchbacked/
303 as long as he has something/
304 [every rail to the toilet]
305 NP: [and he held onto, yeah right]
306 LPN: he had {elimination} this morning he said he had to go/
307 [and did back] and as long as he does it, it's you know/
308 NP: [right]
309 LPN: watch him he did fine//
310 NP: [right]
311 LPN: he'so,
312 NP: yeah//
(..)
313 OT: that's because he was two hours in the merry walker that ***he
314 was able to do that [today]//
315 MD: [{I bet}]
316 OT/ OTH: [(laugh)]
317 ?: [(inaudible comments)]
318 SW: [he used to walk really well/]
319 OT: um um/
320 LPN: [he used to walk alone at home/]
321 NP: [well we took him off trasadone]
322 OT: [why don't]
323 ?: [he did walk at home//]
324 LPN: [I can't believe that he { } could walk at home]//
325 OT: [put a]–
326 SW: He used to go to day care [everyday and { }]
327 OT: [I think we should do],
328 I think we should do/
329 uh he is a candidate uh-
330 I mean I hate to– if he can walk I [hate to]
331 ?LPN: [no]
332 OT: put him in a custom wheelchair that–
333 ?LPN: that's true//
334 ?: { }
335 OT: I mean it's sort of like if we're trying to/
336 Are we– is that [the next review or]?
337 NP: [trying to get him walking]//

In this segment the discourse shifted from a generalized discussion of "the patient" on the ward, to a storied account (Antaki 1994) of Mr. Weinberg's ability to walk at home and, with physical support, on the ward. The nurse offered evidence of Mr. Weinberg as a capable individual through the description of an actual event in which Mr. Weinberg had managed to walk to the bathroom. Note that the "Mr. Weinberg" described here is assumed to have an active role: "he walked to the bathroom;" "he said he had to go;" and "he does it." Through the use of these subject-predicate combinations, Mr. Weinberg was animated as an active participant in the Discourse rather than simply as a passive object. Moreover, his actions counteract his construction solely as an immobile and declining Alzheimer's patient.

The social worker further supported these observations with the revelation that "he used to walk really well" before he was admitted to the hospital. Her comment highlighted the fact that the walking problem was a new one that had only emerged after Mr. Weinberg arrived on the ward. Once again, Mr. Weinberg was portrayed as an active agent: "he used to walk really well;" "He used to walk at home;" "He *did* walk at home;" "he used to go to day care everyday." Such an active construction of Mr. Weinberg served to remind the team that he was an individual with a unique history and unique needs.

One might point to such discussions then as counter to the earlier claim that his individuality was lost in the discourse. The team clearly had knowledge of the uniqueness of the individual patient and even seemed at times to value that information. However, such knowledge was most often peripheral in the discourse. Note that these individual life account segments lasted for only a few utterances. The team did not take them up as actionable items; there was no pursuit in the discourse about why Mr. Weinberg had declined so rapidly after residing on the unit for only four weeks or what approach could change this pattern of deterioration.

The occupational therapist moved to reopen the discussion of the chair by marking the contrast between the two ways of framing the problem. He contrasted the team's actions ("to put him in a custom wheelchair") with Mr. Weinberg's ("if he can walk"). His hesitation in the next few lines – "I mean it's sort of like if we're trying to/Are we" – indicated his uncertainty that the problem would be solved by putting Mr. Weinberg in the wheelchair. The hesitancy expressed by the occupational therapist, coupled with his apparent lack of certainty, reflected the conflict between the two constructions of Mr. Weinberg. If the team were to try to get Mr. Weinberg walking again, this would conflict with the goal of putting him in a wheelchair. If, on the other hand, decline was inevitable, the issue of walking would be essentially irrelevant and the only relevant action for the team would be the management of Mr. Weinberg as an object in the ward world. Placing him in the wheelchair was an action the team could take, while the prospect of improving his ability to walk was doubtful at best, and thus the team may have felt powerless with respect to the disease. The occupational therapist's hesitancy in this segment indexed his understanding that perhaps the team as an institutional entity did not have control over this issue; the decline of patients diagnosed with Alzheimer's is inevitable and not manageable in the medical model. Thus, within the confines of this institutional setting, there was no reasonable course of action to pursue with respect to restoring Mr. Weinberg's ability to walk. The problem of the chair, on the other hand, was clearly actionable in the eyes of the physician: the team could manage this problem by placing Mr. Weinberg in a chair and keeping him safely secured. Unlike the problem of how to support Mr. and Mrs. Weinberg's desire for him to walk despite his unsteady gait, the problem of the chair allowed for a pragmatic solution to be instituted by the team.

In line 338, the physician refocuses the discussion on the problem of the chair:

(7)

| | | |
|---|---|---|
| 338 | MD: | Or don't don't we have some some uh, { } uh, foot rest or something which can be added uh, for for short people? |
| 340 | | on the geri-chair? |
| 341 | | is there something that we can actually add, |
| 342 | OT: | we don't actually have 'em// |
| 343 | | I've asked um the carpentry to build some and they built them and they disappear as quickly as we put 'em out// |
| 345 | | um, |
| 346 | | but for him we can, I can ask them to get one as soon as possible and we can try again// |
| 348 | NP: | okay [so you wanna put footrest/] |
| 349 | SW: | [whatever we could try would help]// |
| 350 | NP: | footrest/ |
| 351 | MD: | foot rest// |
| 352 | (..) | |
| 353 | ?LPN: | let's try sitting in a wheelchair/ |
| 354 | | instead of a geri-chair/ |
| 355 | SW: | I think that would be fine too/ |
| 356 | LPN: | [There's no reason why we { }] |
| 357 | OT: | [You mean just one on the, from the unit rather than a custom one?/] |
| 358 | LPN: | Well if the wife's willing to maybe– |
| 359 | | if you said these things have to be purchased and special made maybe they, if she's |
| 360 | | willing to/ |
| 361 | | but otherwise let's try a regular wheelchair with him on a cushion and, |
| 362 | | just see a nice small wheelchair and [see how he does]// |
| 363 | SW: | [we can get him a] wheelchair from PT if he needs one// |
| 365 | | he's eligible// |
| 366 | | I mean, does he need a custom made?/ |
| 367 | LPN: | [well he's short] |
| 368 | NP: | [he probably–] |

369 LPN: I don't think [anything would fit him { }//]
370 SW: [so maybe we should try it]//
371 MD: do we do we have uh, restraint for the wheelchair
so he can [sit in there safely/]
372 LPN: [yeah, they would]
they would put a little, there's a strap on some of them//
374 MD: [okay so they]
375 DT: [isn't there a] wheelchair clinic?
376 MD: [so they/]
377 OT: [yeah there is/]
378 LPN: [yeah]
379 ?KT: [yes]

The physician raised the possibility of getting a footrest for the chair. However, he then went on to refer to this as a solution for "short people." The use of the term "people" indexes his attention to the generic patient, rather than to Mr. Weinberg as a particular person. In keeping with this, the rest of the team followed by continuously referring to Mr. Weinberg as a passive object. The team members were the only ones with active roles ("we have footrests"), who were "trying" various solutions: "let's try sitting in a wheel chair," and "let's try a regular wheel chair with him." Mr. Weinberg, by contrast, was described with stative verbs ("he [is] eligible," "he [is] short"). By designating Mr. Weinberg as short and as eligible from a bureaucratic standpoint, the team codified Mr. Weinberg into institutional categories. Thus the team control from an institutional standpoint and is able to take action on the problem at hand, thereby reaffirming its own authority. Mr. Weinberg became once again an institutional object that could be – and in fact needed to be – controlled.

Nevertheless, the occupational therapist (l. 381) interrupted again and reintroduced the issue of walking:

(8)
380 OT: { } the point that I made before though was uh, you know,
381 do we wanna do everything at once or do we wanna do this sorta systematically//
382 and if we're trying to get him up and walking does he really need–
383 MD: But he's not going to walk all the time//
384 (.) [right]/
385 OT: [But if] he can walk ad lib again (.) he can sit in a regular chair//
386 if he, if he gets his endurance back there's no reason he can't sit in a chair like this//
388 MD: a regular chair//
389 OT: right//
390 NP: But then isn't it hard for him to get up when he's sittin' low in a chai- in a [regular chair]

392 LPN: [If you hold] the chai-
393 no, this type of chair he could get up by himself//
394 the [wheelchair]
395 NP: [right, right]
396 LPN: he can't because he moved and the merry walker//
397 but he can lift himse- he can do this and get himself off the chair//
398 OT: I think he'd be safer,
399 I mean proceeding in a regular chair than
400 LPN: that's what he wanted to sit in [when we got back]//
401 OT: [than he]
would be in a wheelchair//
402 just in terms of [his judgment and his mobility]//
403 MD: [so what, do we have do we have regular chairs]?
404 NP: [maybe we should wait/]
405 LPN: yeah, there's these//
406 MD: [these]//
407 LPN: [you know with no strap]//
408 MD: can we put strap on?
409 or//
410 OT: not for right now/
411 he's [just]
412 LPN: [no]
413 OT: he doesn't have the balance and he doesn't have the endurance to be able to do that//
415 [right now]//
416 LPN: [he can't] get up and do it by himself yet//
417 (..)
418 OT: I mean I don't want to/
419 I mean I don't want to//
420 I'm not trying to say I ne- he I think he should not be
421 LPN: why don't we just use a chai- [a wheelchai-]
422 OT: [given a wheelchair] but//
424 NP: well since his[ { }]/
425 OT: [I'm just ] asking us to consider it//

At the beginning of this passage, the occupational therapist maintained a linguistic stance in which the team was the active agent ("do *we* wanna do everything at once"; "if *we're* trying to get him up"), with Mr. Weinberg as the object. By using the inclusive pronoun, "we," he attempted to align the team's perspective with his own, seeking to solicit support for Mr. Weinberg as a walking individual. The physician interrupted and disagreed with the occupational therapist by stating that Mr. Weinberg was "*not* going to walk all the time." By arguing that Mr. Weinberg would not walk like a normal person, he refocused on the chair as the issue at hand. Meanwhile, the occupational therapist continued to focus on Mr. Weinberg as an active agent who "may be able to walk again" (1.386). Thus there exists a tension here between the two models of Mr. Weinberg: one as the institutional object who sits passively in the chair and one who is an active walking and agentive individual. Furthermore, as the occupational therapist pushed for a more individualistic construction of Mr. Weinberg, his hesitation may have marked his attempts to counter the perspective of the physician who had greater authority in the team structure. This hierarchy is embedded in the Discourse, in which "who one is" is situated in a broad historical and institutional context; occupational therapists typically have little power, while physicians typically function as the highest authority in Discourses of medicine.

The occupational therapist responded to the physician's claim by connecting the issue of walking with the selection of a chair: "if he can walk ad lib again, he can sit in a regular chair." In doing this, the chair became a concern tied to Mr. Weinberg's personal circumstances. Instead of worrying about the medical and safety implications of a walking Alzheimer's patient, the team discussed the options in terms of what Mr. Weinberg would be able to do in each type of chair. If he was sitting in a "regular chair," "he could get up at walk by himself." The LPN, marking Mr. Weinberg as an active, mindful agent, supported this option by stating: "that's what he wanted to sit in when we got back." The occupational therapist followed by attributing some ability to make judgments to Mr. Weinberg in line 402. Between the comments of the LPN and the occupational therapist, this excerpt represents a rare instance when Mr. Weinberg was seen not only as an active patient, but also as a thinking, agentive individual with particular wishes and some capacity to judge his own abilities.

The LPN and the physician then raised the issue of whether or not a strap should go on the chair to ensure Mr. Weinberg's safety. The occupational therapist responded by focusing again on Mr. Weinberg as an individual with particular issues related to balance and endurance and indicated that these are problems that might improve over time. He then made a plea for the team "just to consider" giving Mr. Weinberg a regular chair. Thus the discussion continued to reflect a tension between the two constructions of Mr.Weinberg. Those interactional moments in the team discussions when he was treated as an active agent with a relevant personal history were notable because they interrupted a more dominant discourse in which he was regarded as a passive object whose own perspective did not have to be privileged.

#### 4.1.4. So what should we put down?

At this point in the team meeting, the nurse practitioner moved the discussion away from the functional problem of walking and re-instantiated the medical problem of the chair in line 426. Another nurse then repeated her opinion that "the hanging edema" was the primary problem motivating the use of a regular wheelchair capable of supporting his feet. Only then, based on this medical evidence rather than evidence regarding his ability to walk, did the team agree to put Mr. Weinberg in a regular wheelchair with legs that could support his feet.

(9)

| | | |
|---|---|---|
| 426 | NP: | so the problem now is that his feet are too short in the geri-chair// |
| 427 | LPN: | it's, the hanging edema// |
| 428 | | yes// |
| 429 | NP: | So maybe we have to adjust and use a wheelchair just for ***now and then hopefully he'll start walking, |
| 431 | | and he may not need it again// |
| 432 | | (.) what do you think// |
| 433 | | (.) |
| 434 | OT: | Just put him a regular [wheelchair]// |
| 435 | LPN: | [regular wheel] |
| 436 | OT: | [not a custom] |
| 437 | NP: | [we'll try it]// |
| 438 | OT: | wheelchair yet// |
| 439 | LPN: | no no, [just] |
| 440 | OT: | [okay//] |
| 441 | LPN: | a [regular wheelchair up on the floor] |
| 442 | NP: | [alright] |
| 443 | LPN: | we gotta make sure we got the legs that move up {and so we gotta [check}] |

The nurse practitioner followed the other nurse's concern about "hanging edema" by publicly drawing a conclusion from the current discussion: "so maybe we have to adjust and use a wheelchair just for now." Here, the "we" who would have to "adjust" was the team and not Mr. Weinberg. How Mr. Weinberg would adapt was not even addressed. In short, he was managed pragmatically according to ward world ways of categorizing patients – ways that were closely related to his medical diagnosis of Alzheimer's disease – and the needs of the staff. The occupational therapist had some impact on the institutional decision making process in that the team was not, for the present, going to order a custom wheelchair.

As the discussion continued, the focus shifted to determining how to write the problem on the ITP. Thus the team focused on the written instantiation of Mr. Weinberg, transforming him into a truly institutional object, one which must be accounted for through documentation:

(10)

| | | |
|---|---|---|
| 444 | NP: | [so we're] gonna take the gerichair out then/ |
| 445 | | [or what]// |
| 446 | MD: | [yeah]// |
| 447 | NP: | okay// |

448 MD: wheelchair/
449 wheelchair when/
450 ?: { }
451 MD: when unable//
452 OT: when out of bed/
453 LPN: [can we put–]
454 MD: [with ] a belt restraint//
455 LPN: we'll put that//
456 [belt ]
457 MD: [yeah]
458 LPN: restraint on the wheelchair//
459 (.)
460 NP: wheelchair with belt restraint//
461 (..)
462 ?: okay//
463 NP: alright//
464 so what's the status//
465 (...)
466 OT: declined//
467 NP: yeah//
468 (4)
469 alright/
470 OT: hopefully to get better for the [next review (laughing)]
471 LPN: [(laugh) next review]
472 OT: [(laughing) we can say improved]/
473 NP: [to be] improved//
474 LPN: [right]
475 OT/OTH: (still laughing)

In this segment, while the team was focused on the task of writing the ITP, Mr. Weinberg was not mentioned at all, not even pronominally. The ITP they were constructing would say "wheelchair when out of bed," and the physician raised the issue of "a belt restraint" again. When queried about the health status of the patient, the OT said "declined" and added that Mr. Weinberg would "hopefully get better for the next review." The banter and laughing that accompanied this remark and the next two utterances reflected the team's concern that Mr. Weinberg had gotten worse since admission and the lack of consensus regarding an approach to foster improvement. While such decline is inevitable in Alzheimer's patients and it is common for it to progress rather quickly after patients are admitted, it is clear that this decline is uncomfortable for the team members. The laughter also highlighted the tension between the two different constructions of Mr. Weinberg evident in the discourse. Moreover, it may have served to temper the conflict between the occupational therapist, who is lower in the hierarchy of the institution, and the physician, who ultimately has the power to make decisions on behalf of the team.

The banter may also serve to alleviate some of the tension between the two models of Mr. Weinberg present in this discussion – as one who could potentially "improve" and as one who will inevitably decline. In the first model, Mr. Weinberg continues to have the potential to change and improve as do most people who are well. In the second, he is the generic Alzheimer's patient. The tension revealed in these different perspectives raises an important question with respect to what it means to "help" patients who are dying: Is the goal of treatment to maintain and perhaps even improve their functioning, or is the objective to manage and warehouse patients with the least possible risk of injury as they inevitably decline? If the latter is the goal, the concern shifts to seating Mr. Weinberg safely, and he is more readily transformed into an institutional object.

## *4.2. So who is Mr. Weinberg?*

The discussion yielded a picture of Mr. Weinberg as someone who could not safely walk and who, therefore, needed to be confined to a wheelchair or geri-chair in order to be safe. He had also gotten worse since he had come to the hospital. Although the nurse revealed that he wanted to sit in a regular chair, and that he liked the tray table down, there was little additional information about how Mr. Weinberg acted when he was restrained in the chair. In fact, Mr. Weinberg had been yelling and pounding on his tray table at times, apparently angry at being restrained. By ignoring Mr. Weinberg's negative perspective on being restrained, the team denied him any agentive role. The final picture that emerged from the team meetings was one of a patient who could not walk independently and who needed to be seated and restrained in a wheelchair with his feet up in order to prevent edema. The team had in essence diagnosed him as a "non-walker."

In other words, Mr. Weinberg was transformed into a prototypical Alzheimer's patient on the ward. Despite the underlying tension between the two versions of Mr. Weinberg, the final construction yielded an objectified patient who fitted in well within the existing institutional structure. As the "institutional patient", his problems were to be solved by a team with the institutional authority to diagnose and treat individuals diagnosed with Alzheimer's disease.

In sum, Mr. Weinberg was constructed in two ways. First, as a patient who could improve and potentially walk again, Mr. Weinberg maintained a status as an individual who had some agency. Second, as a patient who was to be the recipient of the team's actions of placing him in a chair, he loses any potential for agency and declines into a purely institutional object. Overall Mr. Weinberg was more frequently portrayed as an individual with a social history and lifeworld relevant to his diagnosis and treatment in this second team review than anywhere else in all three meetings. However, for the most part, the discourse that served to individualize his condition and personalize his treatment was interrupted and rejected in favor of a more institutionally sanctioned perspective of Mr. Weinberg as a passive institutional object.

## 5. Walking and restraint in follow-up interviews

In follow-up interviews, seven team members were shown a videotape of this discussion about Mr. Weinberg. The author requested that the participant stop the tape at points they deemed relevant to the treatment of Mr. Weinberg or important to the treatment discussion. In general these viewers believed that the discussion about Mr. Weinberg's walking and the use of the posey was a productive, exemplary use of an interdisciplinary approach to making decisions in team meetings. However, their comments reflected tensions between the underlying models of patients – a tension between viewing patients as individuals with valued lifeworld concerns of their own and viewing patients as institutional objects in potential need of restraint.

Team members discussed some of the conflicts that arose in working with Alzheimer's patients with respect to issues of freedom and dignity versus restraint and safety. Nancy, the nurse practitioner, described this tension between restraint and freedom. On the one hand, she argued that freedom was essential, in that "you can't tie them [patients] up." On the other hand, restraint was needed to keep the patient safe. She repeatedly contrasted the problem of restricting an individual's freedom with protecting patients from the possibility of falling and injuring themselves. Her concern for patients' safety was cohesive with the goal of institutionalization of Alzheimer's patients – to keep them from harming themselves. She stated that patients who are unsteady walking "should be protected," indicating a real concern for the individual patient. This issue of patient safety, moreover, had become quite relevant because JCAHO (the regulating agency) was coming to review the program. JCAHO guidelines require long-term care facilities to refrain from using restraints unless it is clearly indicated for patient safety. In fact, it was this pending arrival of JCAHO that had sparked prior discussion among the team about the appropriateness of using a posey; prior to this, the nursing staff would use a posey whenever they deemed it was necessary. Thus, the issue of safety and restraint was, for Nancy, an issue of institutional accountability as well as an issue of concern for individual patients.

When the physician, Dr. Pressman, reviewed the taped meetings, he raised the specter that restraints were being used more for the benefit of the staff than the patients. Although he noted that JCAHO regulations sought to ensure that restraints were not used for the "convenience of the staff," he believed that restraints such as tray tables were being "overused" by the staff for their own benefit. Dr. Pressman did not raise the issue of Mr. Weinberg's individual freedom. Rather, it was the institution's adherence to guidelines that was at stake in the team's deliberations over restraints at the meetings. Earlier in the interview when Dr. Pressman had been discussing the dignity and free will of individuals diagnosed with Alzheimer's disease, he had confided that the issue of restraint created a dilemma. The safety of patients was a good reason to use restraints, but it was nonetheless difficult to strike a balance between freedom and "preventing injury." Issues of legal liability compounded this dilemma: to what extent would he, the team, and the hospital be held accountable if the patient were to fall? Irrespective of how much one wanted to grant patients individual autonomy, there would always be issues of safety that would transform individuals into objects of the institution.

Other team members also commented on the tension between allowing individual freedom and maintaining safety of patients. Although the written plan specified that Mr. Weinberg should not be restrained in a geri-chair, both the occupational therapist (Sam) and the nurse (Paula) noted that the following week Mr. Weinberg had been secured in a chair with the posey. In addition, Sam noted that the nursing staff had "convinced" a covering physician to increase his sedating medications. The occupational therapist believed that Mr. Weinberg's increased self-sufficiency was viewed as problematic by the staff. He characterized the staff as not being "tolerant," thereby highlighting the conflict between using restraint for the convenience of the staff and the removal of restraint in order to facilitate independence. The conflict between conceptualizing patients as institutional objects and agentive individuals was stressed in the occupational therapist's discussion of Mr. Weinberg.

Citing "controversy on the use of poseys," Paula noted a conflict between some professionals' goal to help maintain patients' independence and the staff's goal to keep patients safe and easy to control. After noting that restraint might be necessary for some patients, she directed her remarks toward Mr. Weinberg, arguing that since he was now "standing and starting to walk around," he should not be restrained. She further generalized her perspective to patients who could walk: they should be able to get up when they desired to do so. She thus placed higher value on Mr. Weinberg's ability to walk than on the convenience of restraining him.

In sum, the team members were not impervious to the conflict inherent in the discourse of restraint. They recognized the ongoing tension between different models of care and patients. If the goal of the team was to facilitate the independence and individual agency of patients like Mr. Weinberg, restraint was something to be avoided. If, however, the team's objective was to avoid injury and to maintain patients on the ward in a generic manner, restraint became not only possible but also preferable. Whereas in interviews the team members invoked a perspective in which patients were to be cared for in a way that encouraged independence and preserved their dignity, the discourse of the team meetings reflected an opposing value orientation: the view of the patient as an institutional object continued to take precedence.

## 6. Discussion

Throughout the discussion of Mr. Weinberg's walking, the team constructed him primarily as an institutional or medical object. Mr. Weinberg becomes, for the team, the generic Alzheiemer's patient and the diagnosis in essence comes to life in place of Mr. Weinberg himself. In this way the team's cultural practice takes the diagnosis and uses it to further assess, or diagnose, Mr. Weinberg's capabilities or inabilities. These constructions reflect cultural models dominant in the culture of institutionalized medical practice and these are reflected in the Discourse of the Alzheimer's treatment unit. Their roots may originate in a broader Discourse of medicine or from other Discourses associated with health care, but they co-exist in tension with an alternative model of patients as individuals with unique needs.

Determining what type of chair to place Mr. Weinberg in reflects the way that the "total institution" (Goffman 1961) defines the limited range of opportunities for patients. The categorization of his walking was limited, from an institutional perspective, to a determination of the type of chair in which he could be placed. He was transformed into an object to be placed into an appropriate chair by agentive others – the authoritative team. He was stripped of a valued freedom to move about, freedom taken for granted until removed by others. In Goffman's (Goffman 1961) terms, the institution degrades the individual such that he becomes an *other*, one who is different from the staff. In this instance, the "other" is the diagnosis, the Alzheimer's patient. In this way, the institution distinguishes between inmates and staff; Mr. Weinberg as the inmate is stripped of the freedom to determine where to sit; the staff would never consider this restriction to be applicable to them. It is the institution that constrains and facilitates certain ways of acting and talking, particularly in such ritualized contexts as team meetings. Moreover, the meetings serve explicit institutional requirements and are the instrumental means through which the team is held accountable for its actions. The discussions were driven by the institutional framework and consequently took on the form of objectification more often than might have been seen in other aspects of the Discourse.

The option of placing Mr. Weinberg in a "regular chair" was considered briefly, but discarded quickly in the ensuing team discussion. If the discourse had shifted towards placing Mr. Weinberg in a regular chair, it would have required the team to situate him as an active, agentive individual with critical judgment, wishes and abilities rather than an anonymous patient declining into passivity. A patient who was agentive and willful was viewed as problematic in the ward world, as he might have threatened the ongoing pragmatic management of patients on the unit, and would have further challenged the relevant categories set up in the institutional framework. When Mr. Weinberg was willful and yelled to be let out of the geri-chair, he was seen as problematic for the ward and was consequently sedated. Such action does not facilitate his personhood. If the team had considered him as an agentive individual, the institutional categories would no longer have been sufficient, and the team would have had to reach beyond the Discourse and the dominant models of patients as diagnoses in order to come up with new approaches to solving problems. Such a change would have challenged the authority of the team and the institution to manipulate patients as objects of the ward world, as diagnoses with immutable trajectories.

The assessment of an Alzheimer's patient's ability to walk depends upon the context in which such a judgment is rendered. In the context of the institution and the ward world, Alzheimer's patients need to be manipulated and restrained in various ways to keep them safe. Within the context of the lifeworld – a context in which issues of individual experience and agency are important – assessment must be altered to reflect the definition of a patient as a unique individual with personal concerns that may require distinctive particular solutions.

The discourse of the team meetings was "multivoiced" (Bakhtin 1981; Wertsch 1981), with different voices representing varying models of patients and constructing different versions of ill patients in order to diagnose and treat them. These voices manifested themselves as the tension between patients as objects of the institution and individuals as active participants in the lifeworld. Although it was the former perspective that dominated the discourse of the meetings, the team members acknowledged the potential conflict inherent in these different ways of constructing patients.

Although the dominant cultural models – and the discourse analyzed here – construct Mr. Weinberg as first a medical diagnosis and then an institutional object, these models do not exist in a vacuum. Shore (1996) argues that communicative practices emerge not out of unilateral cultural models, but out of the "problematical and always partial resolution of dilemmas proposed by the existence of competing models" (Shore 1996: 302). Thus the actions of the team members proceed from both the dominant cultural models and competing models. Through the negotiation of these alternative understandings of patients, compassionate assessment and treatment emerges.

When the health care professionals experienced patients as individuals with unique features, histories, and personalities, they employed a model of patients that lies in tension with the dominant models sanctioned by the Discourse, those sanctioned by the institutional framework and its associated practices. Certain professionals voiced a model of patient as person more often than others, raising conflicts with those who were more reliant on objectifying models. The tense exchanges between the occupational therapist and the physician highlighted yet another dimension of the Discourse, the rigid hierarchy inherent in medical settings. But these tensions also existed in the interviews – each individual practitioner found tension in their own voices between these different models of patients.

We see these tensions between conflicting ways of thinking, believing, acting, and speaking in the actions of professionals on the wards as well as in the meetings. It is out of such tensions that change becomes possible. Fairclough (1992) argues that discourse is a tool for social change. Through discussions such as the one about Mr. Weinberg's walking, individuals within the Discourse can begin to change the ways in which other members of the Discourse experience and think about the objects of their care. In other words, the language is not simply a reflection of dominant institutional procedures, but it also serves as a means by which professionals instantiate alternative models of clinical practice, providing the opportunity for dominant models to be revised. Changes in the institution and institutional structure can be motivated by the different ways in which members "push" different ways of conceptualizing and constructing patients. The discourse may yet shift from one grounded in diagnosis toward one in which individuals suffering from illness emerge as central to all decisions.

Although the dominant cultural models led to an assessment of Mr. Weinberg primarily as medical diagnosis and institutional object, alternative constructions of him in his lifeworld did emerge. Jewson (1976) observed that throughout the history of medicine the "sick man" has gradually disappeared. While aspects of the discourse surrounding the care of Mr. Weinberg did support this ironic disappearance, there is reason to believe that all is not lost. If we can look beyond the view of Mr. Weinberg the seated generic Alzheimer's patient to be manipulated for safety, we may yet locate Mr. Weinberg the dancer.

## *Acknowledgments*

This material is based upon research supported by the Office of Academic Affairs and Health Services Research and Development, the Department of Veteran's Affairs. The views expressed in this chapter are those of the author and do not necessarily represent the views of the Department of Veterans Affairs.

## Notes

1. This name and all others in this manuscript are pseudonyms.
2. The description that follows here is based upon a period of participant observation of the units during which time I was fortunate to have some interactions with Mr. Weinberg. As I write about the construction of patient in the discourse of the teams, it is important to note that my description of Mr. Weinberg is a construction in itself based on the perspective of a single researcher with a research agenda.
3. A posey is a restraint device that looks something like a harness. Typically it consists of a vest made of a fabric mesh and attached to the vest are four fabric belts that can be tied together and tied onto a chair or a bed. This prevents individuals from getting up independently.
4. The physician noted this in his follow-up interview when he said that the staff members "don't want to be blamed for a patient's injury."
5. The "Merry Walker study" is a study that the occupational therapist was conducting at the time with patients on the unit. The Merry Walker is a walking device that looks much like a typical walker with wheels, except that it also has a seat attached to it. Thus, when someone walks with the Merry Walker, he can sit down easily and safely when he gets tired. It is important to note here that Mr. Weinberg is also being constructed here as a research subject. This status again brings into question the role of the institution in caring for individual patients as opposed to being a site for research which could potentially help all Alzheimer's patients. Foucault (1975) argues in *The Birth of the Clinic* that with the shift to treating patients in the modern clinic or hospital came the ability of physicians to learn about diseases as decontextualized from bodies, as bodies who are inhabited by the disease would be gathered together in one place where they could be examined and studied. Here we have an instance where patients are now research subjects, and clinicians are able to use them as research objects to further their own knowledge.
6. JCAHO sets the following guideline as the standard for the use of restraints: "The organization uses a system to achieve a restraint-free environment." Moreover, restraint is defined as "[a]ny method (chemical or physical) of restricting a resident's freedom of movement, including seclusion, physical activity or normal access to the body." (JCAHO 1996, TX.8)

## References

Antaki, Charles
1994 *Explaining and Arguing: The Social Organization of Accounts.* Thousand Oaks, CA: Sage Publications.

Bakhtin, Mikhail
1981 *The Dialogic Imagination* (M. Holquist, ed.). Austin: University of Texas Press.
Bokhour, Barbara G.
1998 Locating patients in the discourse of health care teams: Where is Mr. Weinberg? Unpublished doctoral dissertation, Clark University.
Cassell, Eric J.
1991 *The Nature of Suffering and the Goals of Medicine.* New York: Oxford University Press.
D'Andrade, Roy and Claudia Strauss
1992 *Human Motives and Cultural Models.* New York: Cambridge University Press.
Fairclough, Norman
1992 *Discourse and Social Change.* Cambridge, MA: Basil Blackwell/Polity Press.
Foucault, Michel
1975 *The Birth of the Clinic: An Archeology of Medical Perception* (A. M. Sheridan Smith, trans.). New York: Vintage Books.
1977 *Discipline and Punish.* London: Allen Lane.
Gee, James Paul
1992 *The Social Mind: Language, Ideology and Social Practice.* New York: Bergin and Harvey.
1996 *Social Linguistics and Literacies: Ideology in Discourses* (2nd ed.). London/Bristol, PA: Taylor and Francis.
1999 *Introduction to Discourse Analysis: Theory and Method.* New York: Routledge.
Goffman, Erving
1961 *Asylums: Essays on the Social Situation of Mental Patients and Other Inmates.* New York: Anchor Books, Doubleday.
Hanks, Willliam F.
1996 *Language and Communicative Practices.* Boulder, CO: Westview Press.
Helman, Cecil
1991 *The Body of Frankenstein's Monster: Essays in Myth and Medicine.* New York: W. W. Norton Company.
Holland, Dorothy and Naomi Quinn
1987 *Cultural Models in Language and Thought.* New York: Cambridge University Press.
JCAHO
1996 *1996 Comprehensive Accreditation Manual for Long Term Care.* Joint Commission on Accreditation of Health Care Organizations.
Jewson, Norman D.
1976 The disappearance of the sick-man from medical cosmology, 1770–1870. *Sociology* 10, 225–244.
Mishler, Eliot G.
1984 *The Discourse of Medicine.* Norwood, NJ: Ablex Publishing.

Mishler, Eliot G., L. R. Amara Singham, S. T. Osherson, S. T. Hauser, N. E. Waxler, and R. Liem
1981 *Social Contexts of Health, Illness and Patient Care.* New York: Cambridge University Press.
Shore, Bradd
1996 *Culture in Mind: Cognition, Culture and the Problem of Meaning.* New York: Oxford University Press.
Wertsch, James V.
1991 *Voices of the Mind.* Cambrige, MA: Harvard University Press

# Chapter 4
# From diagnostic to aesthetic: Moving beyond diagnosis*

*Ozum Ucok*

*Ozum Ucok, like Barbara Bokhour, shows how the discursive practices of medical diagnosis can contribute to a diminished sense of self. Here the initial diagnosis and treatment of an artist with breast cancer reduce her to a physical object. Ucok goes on to trace how the artist's identity is reformulated post surgically through the development of another aesthetic sense of herself. Early discourse, immediately following the surgery, focused on what was wrong with the artist's body and the objective success of surgical treatment, while later discourse reflected the emergence of a more positive, reintegrated sense of self.*

> Diagnosis represents a linguistic moment of great import in disability: It articulates the key distinction between being abled and disabled; it labels the condition for the purposes of medical, educational, and legal institutions; and fuses identity and disability in the social experience of the individual and those in contact with him or her. (Barton 1999: 260–261)

The above quotation points to the impact of diagnosis on the positioning of individuals in terms of social capacity. Diagnosis not only serves to identify the nature of a disease or disorder and suggest potential courses of action, but transforms an ordinary adult into an ill patient (Charmaz 1989). A physician's validation of illness through diagnosis puts a person into the "sick role" (Parsons 1953). Thus, being diagnosed with a serious illness like cancer carries significant implications on issues of identity and self. From the moment of diagnosis, there is the potential for identity disintegration and transformation:

> Chronic illness can not help but separate the person of the present from the person of the past, and affect or even shatter any images of self held for the future (especially if the illness is severe or debilitating.) ... the who I was in the past and the who I hoped to be in the future, in whole or in part, are rendered discontinuous with the me of the present. New conceptions of who and what I am, past, present, and future must arise out of what remains. (Corbin and Strauss 1987: 272)

It is this potential for "identity reconstitution" when the person begins to reintegrate the self and regain a sense of wholeness (Corbin and Strauss 1987) that will be discussed. With a diagnosis of cancer and the chronic illness that often ensues, people work toward regaining a sense of balance and control over their disrupted lives. Selma R. Schimmel, a cancer survivor and the creator of a nation-wide radio talk show on cancer, wrote about the impact of diagnosis on the lifeworld of the individual:

> Before cancer or a life-threatening illness, we kind of tap dance through life ... When we get cancer, the dance changes ... And then you realize that areas of your life need reprioritizing. The diagnosis adds new stress to your personal, professional, and financial responsibilities. Issues of mortality come to mind, and, in addition to your emotions, you must also deal with everyone else's. And somehow in the midst of this emotional upheaval, you still have to keep a clear head in order to make decisions about your medical care. As your health takes center stage, your days may be a series of doctor's appointments, consultations, and continued medical evaluation. You've become a cancer patient. (Schimmel 1999: 3–4)

In a similar vein, one artist explained changes in her life from the moment of diagnosis onward: "When I was diagnosed with my breast cancer in 1992, I was forced to stop and reconsider my life. The first change I made was to drop out of the fashion business and paint full time. I began to paint with obsessive urgency as if making up for lost time" (Ades 2000: Artist's Statement, para. 1).

The personal reflections of Schimmel (1999) and Ades (2000) emphasize the impact of diagnosis and chronic illness on everyday life. This chapter focuses on the transformation and reconstitution of self after a diagnosis of breast cancer. As opposed to viewing the self as a constant set of attributes that are internally circumscribed within a biological organism, the position taken here is that questions of identity can be studied fruitfully as they arise in social interaction (Carbaugh 1996). From the work George Herbert Mead (1934), Kenneth Gergen (1991), and others (Blumer 1969; Burkitt 1991; Harre and Gillet 1994), the notion of a socially situated, mutable self that is subject to change through interactions with others and the vicissitudes of human experience has emerged (Winkler 1999).

Similar to Charmaz (1987), consideration is given to the notion of self in chronic illness as "an emergent structure or organization" that "may shift or change as the person reflexively interprets the identifications and images that self and others confer upon him or her" (p. 284). Although a number of authors have examined the transformation of self in the experience of illness (Charmaz 1985, 1991, 1994a, 1994b, 1995; Corbin and Strauss 1987; Denzin 1987a, 1987b; Fallowfield and Clark 1991; Frank 1991; Orona 1990; Radley and Green 1985; Yoshida 1993), the construction of an aesthetic self in response to a chronic illness has not yet been addressed. This chapter describes the emergence of an aesthetic self through aesthetic discourse as a means of reunifying body and self, and facilitating integration and wholeness of being in illness.

The remainder of this chapter is organized as follows. First, there is a discussion of people's responses to diagnosis. Next, excerpts from the Stephanie Project – a visual and verbal documentary of a woman's experience with breast cancer – are analyzed with an eye toward the transformation of self. It will be argued that the construction of an aesthetic self served as a turning point for moving beyond initial diagnosis and identity disintegration. Contrary to diagnostic discourse that focused on what was wrong with the body, aesthetic discourse helped transform one individual's way of seeing her own body as beautiful.

## 1. Responses to diagnosis

Diagnosis doesn't come alone. It is accompanied by a broad spectrum of emotions including fear, anger, disbelief, and loneliness (Varricchio 1997). Each of these reactions is discussed briefly.

### *1.1. Fear and anger*

Among the most immediate reactions to the diagnosis of cancer is fear: Fear of dying, fear of the unknown, fear of pain, and fear of losing control (Charmaz 1991; Kahane 1990; Schimmel 1999).

> I'm afraid of everything. I am fifty-seven and newly diagnosed with prostate cancer – I'm having surgery in a few days. I'm afraid I'm going to die before the surgery, I'm afraid I'm going to die during surgery, I'm afraid they won't get all the cancer, I'm afraid I'll be impotent and incontinent forever, I'm afraid I'll be "cured," then get it again. I'm even afraid that it won't come back, but I'll live the next twenty years afraid that it *will* come back. (Schimmel 1999: 93)

Sometimes, anger precedes fear as indicated by this cancer patient:

> I'm too angry to be afraid. I've been mad at everyone and everything since my diagnosis. I'm only in my early thirties. I eat perfectly, I work out everyday, and gear my life toward staying healthy, but I still got "ball" cancer! That pisses me off. (Schimmel 1999: 94)

### *1.2. Disbelief*

Despite the intensity of the emotions experienced upon diagnosis, the "meaning" of diagnosis might not be clear initially. Rather, the unexpected news and an improbable present might throw people in a separate reality where events seem unreal (Charmaz 1991). This is well illustrated by the following lines from a cancer survivor: "... The diagnosis changes your life in a split second. When you hear those words 'You have cancer,' everything stops. Nothing feels real" (Schimmel 1999: 4). Similarly, Murphy (1987: 24) recounted his own experience of being diagnosed with a benign spinal cord tumor:

> ... Many are unable to assimilate the full meaning all at once and may sit dazed for hours until the heavy weight of truth finally sinks in. It took time for me to realize the significance of what I have heard, enough time for my psychic defense system to become mobilized and throw up a wall between me and an unpalatable reality.

In response to these initial disorienting experiences, physicians may let their patients discover the meaning of the diagnosis over time:

> I said, "Well, what is this problem?" And they put me in a hospital and took a lot of tests, and they said, "Everything is fine Ron, but- so we've come up with multiple sclerosis, a possible multiple sclerosis." I said, "What is that?" And they said, "You'll learn about it." And I did. (Charmaz 1991: 18)

### *1.3. Loneliness*

Feelings of loneliness and isolation also accompany the diagnosis of a life-threatening illness. One cancer survivor recollected that her first feeling upon diagnosis "was total isolation. I didn't feel like anybody knew what I was going through, how I was feeling" (Schimmel 1999: 14). Another individual revealed that feelings of separation continue as one goes through treatment:

> You can't just call up somebody and say "Gee, I am feeling rotten because I had chemo today." They have no idea what you're talking about. I went to a concert when I still had the drainage under my arm from lumpectomy. I thought I was the only person in the world that had cancer. I felt absolutely alone. (in Schimmel 1999: 130)

In response to reported experiences of loneliness that accompany the diagnosis of a life threatening illness, some patients take a more active role against isolation. As Stephanie Byram, a breast cancer survivor explained: "When told they have a life threatening illness, some people withdraw into themselves. I on the other hand seek connections outside of myself both physically and spiritually" (Byram and Brodsky 1996a: photo.10.html).

Sandstrom (1990) discussed how the diagnosis of AIDS resulted in especially painful and extreme feelings of isolation. Upon revealing their diagnoses, many people with AIDS were ostracized by parents, siblings, or colleagues. Furthermore, several of them were asked not to return home for visits. For people with AIDS, support group relationships became the central source for emotional support and the formation of social ties (Sandstrom 1990). Sandstrom argued that people diagnosed with AIDS were able to construct identities linked to their lived experience and to sustain a sense of self-worth by taking an active role in developing social relationships with others. On the other hand, those patients who adopted defensive identity management strategies by disguising or restricting their interactional involvements with others were less successful in building a positive self-image. Thus, seeking and creating social connections allowed people to affirm and embrace their new identities and preserve a sense of dignity.

## 2. Diagnosis and transformations of self: The Stephanie Project

As discussed previously, the diagnosis and subsequent treatment of a serious medical condition has a transforming effect on the self. The moment of diagnosis may signal the transition to a "disabled" (Barton 1999), "marginal" (Sandstrom 1990) self through which the individual gets socially re-positioned as a medical body. In keeping with this, the term "diagnostic self" will be used to refer to the transforming state of an individual post diagnosis; a "medical" self that may be "disabled," "diseased," "differentiated," and even "lost."

Stephanie Byram chronicled her personal experiences with breast cancer over time through photographs and a series of interviews (Byram and Brodsky 1996a, 1996b, 1997). The image of a diagnostic self revealed itself in her early photographs of her chest after surgery. She characterized the photograph in Figure 1 as one of her "least favorite" and most "clinical" (see Figure 1):

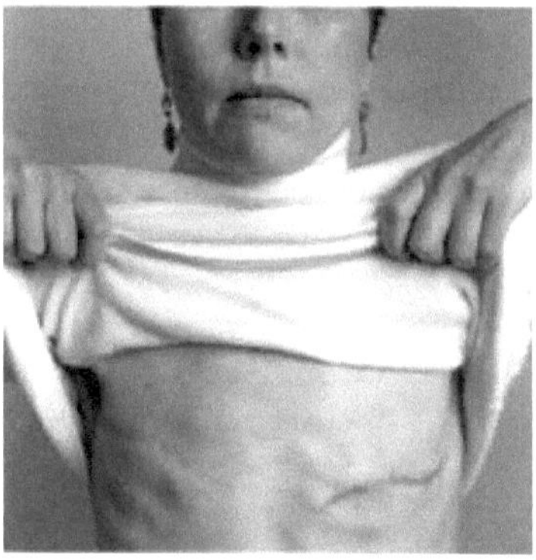

*Figure 1.* Shock
Source: http://www.cmu.edu/cfa/design/people/sford/stephanie/high/shock.html

This is one of my least favorite photographs. It's a very sterile photograph you can't see my eyes. The audience is not allowed to see any emotion from me, instead the reason for doing that is that it forces or allows perhaps the audience to

> be voyeuristic in looking at my chest, in looking at something that might be very uncomfortable to look at had my eyes been there. This photograph is very sterile and clinical this is perhaps something you might expect to see in a medical textbook. It's not a passionate photograph at all. (public speech, January 16, 2001)

In exposing her chest after surgery, Stephanie emphasized the absence of her eyes and related that to the sterility of the photograph. By cutting off the eyes and depersonalizing the image, Charlee Brodsky, the visual artist of the Stephanie Project, literally and figuratively framed Stephanie as a "medical body," a specimen to be analyzed. In short, the whole person is reduced to a medical sample, a diagnostic body. In reporting that she posed like this for women who had never seen a mastectomy (Byram and Brodsky 1996: interview.1.html), this "clinical" portrayal of self was intended to invite others to examine the body-as-object and was represented by Stephanie as a "diagnostic self" that had experienced both physical and emotional loss.

The construction of a diagnostic self, created by viewing the body in terms of what is wrong with it (or what is missing), reveals itself in two themes in the talk of cancer survivors: "divergence of self and body" and "loss."

## 3. The divergence of body and self

Being diagnosed with a chronic illness shakes previous assumptions about the relation between body and self (Charmaz 1995; Kelly and Field 1996); the sense of wholeness of body and self is disturbed (Bury 1982; Brody 1987; Charmaz 1991, 1994a, 1994b, 1995; Gadow 1982; Murphy 1987), the integrity of self is threatened (Kestenbaum 1982), and the ordinary features of everyday life are disrupted (Anderson and Bury 1988; Charmaz 1991; Davis 1972; Davis and Horobin 1977; Finlayson and McEwen 1977; Kelly and Field 1996; Lawrence 1958; Radley 1993).

In the verbal and visual documentary of her breast cancer experience, Stephanie Byram (in Byram and Brodsky 1997) wrote:

1 Cancer Destroys.
2 It ravaged my sense of Self.
3 My body betrayed me: it could no longer be trusted,
4 especially since I had treated it so well.
5 Suddenly, every body part was suspect.
6 I was no longer a whole.

These comments revealed the devastating effects of cancer on Stephanie's self-concept and her body. In lines two and three, she stated that cancer damaged her sense of self by betraying her expectations and her trust. In doing this, Stephanie created a distinction between her body ("my body") and her self ("betrayed *me*"): the self and the body were no longer a single unit. The body was construed as an object ("it"), rather than the subject of her being. And this objectified body was not responsive to how it was cared for (line 4).

The divergence of the body and the self resulted in uncertainty and doubt; the body was no longer reliable and the status of each body part was questionable (line 5). Not only was the body objectified; it was also under suspicion. The body was framed as a willful being that had betrayed her trust. In short, the body was personified as a conscious object acting against Stephanie.

Consequently, in the final line, Stephanie explicitly stated that her sense of self had been fragmented: "I was no longer whole." Stephanie's sense of being as an integrated self had changed to the point where she no longer trusted her body: "bodies change in chronic illness" and so do "self-conceptions which are reciprocal to bodily experiences, feelings and actions ... self conceptions undergo considerable transformation" (Kelly and Field 1996: 247).

Such identity changes have been noted by others. Charmaz (1995), for example, cited the experiences of a woman with asthma: "... I felt like my body had betrayed me ... like my body was sort of foreign territory – it was not the body that I knew" (p. 662). The taken-for-granted idea of a body that serves the needs of the self is altered dramatically. This conflicted separation of body and self continues as people seek to distance their feelings about themselves from their bodies. Rather than living with their bodies, they experience fragmented selves where the body and self are separated. The diagnostic self of Stephanie described here was not only fragmented, there was also a sense of loss on a variety of personal fronts.

## 4. Loss

After being diagnosed with a highly malignant and aggressive form of breast cancer, and having surgery to remove both breasts, Stephanie experienced loss. Even though the following photograph was taken seven years prior to a talk she delivered to a local church group in Pittsburgh, she confided that it was still a very difficult picture for her to see:

> I look at my eyes and what I see is all of the- all of the feelings of loss that I was going through at the time and in particular I was ruminating I guess on lost womanhood, lost sexuality and lost motherhood. The most obvious markers of my womanhood were gone. I'd never be able to breast-feed a kid and my sex life would be unalterably changed for the rest of my life. And this photograph captures for me all of that. (public speech, January 16, 2001)

In recounting feelings that surfaced soon after her diagnosis of breast cancer and the immediate surgery that followed, Stephanie revealed how physical changes diminished her sense of self: she lost her womanhood, her motherhood, and her sexual life.

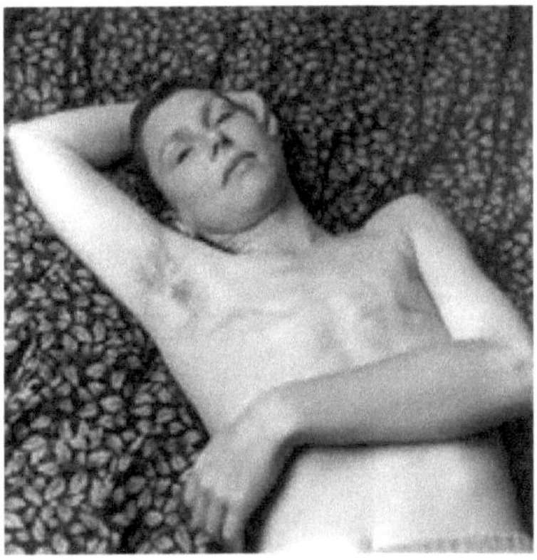

*Figure 2.* Why am I so sad?
Source: http://www.cmu.edu/cfa/design/people/sford/ stephanie/ high/shock.html

The feelings of loss expressed by Stephanie were similar to those observed personally at a meeting of the "Look Good Feel Better" project of the American Cancer Society. At this gathering licensed cosmetologists helped cancer survivors address problems with respect to hair loss, skin, and a variety of other image-related issues. The theme of a lost self emerged repeatedly through comments such as "I don't feel like myself" or "I feel like I am losing myself."

With these experienced feelings of loss, some women refrain from looking at their altered bodies after mastectomy, and avoid being seen by their intimate others: "I tend not to look at myself," "it upsets me that I don't look like a woman anymore," "Oh, I don't let him see me, oh no. I couldn't. He'd be horrified. I always undress in the bathroom now" (Fallowfield and Clark 1991: 66). In hiding their appearance from themselves and intimate partners, ill people may seek to reduce the effects of surgery on themselves and their social identities (Charmaz 1995: 667).

By way of contrast, a physician's post-surgery perspective may be viewed as radically different from that of the patient: different in ways that only serve to heighten the dissonance experienced after a mastectomy:

> When I did wake up from surgery I thought the scars I would have from removing three tiny little growths would be minimal, that my breast would look pretty much the same as it did before surgery .... Not so! I wasn't prepared for the ugliness of my breast or the dramatic change in its configuration. The nipple was in the wrong place. I felt misshapen, mutilated. When Dr, Sachs told me after surgery that the breast looked beautiful – from a surgeon's point of view, I guess – I decided from a woman's point of view that the man was crazy. He found it hard to understand my reaction. (Blumberg 1991: 27)

In sum, the divergence between the objective body and the subjective self, coupled with the experienced sense of loss and dissonance, are all part of the transformation to a diagnostic self. However, the emergence of this diagnostic self does not necessarily mark the end of an individual's identity transformation. In what follows, the manner in which Stephanie's diagnostic self changed over time to reveal a more positive sense of identity will be described.

## 5. Moving beyond the "diagnostic self"

The following image represented a significant turning point in Stephanie's self-perception. Through conversations with the photographer who took this picture, she began to develop a new way of "seeing" her body: the image of a disfigured body was transformed into an aesthetic body. In short, a positive aesthetic meaning and sensibility was constructed through interaction:

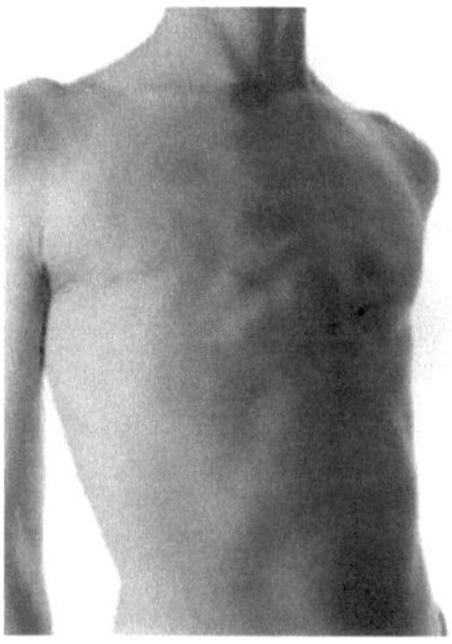

*Figure 3.* Venus
Source: http://www.cmu.edu/cfa/design/people/sford/stephanie/high/venus.html

> After learning my story, many people glance at my chest almost despite themselves, making me feel embarrassed and ashamed. Then we did the "Venus" photo. Like a Michelangelo sculpture with the arms knocked off and the head missing, I now see my torso as a work of art. Although I'm missing some pieces, I no longer feel disfigured. This image was a turning point for me.

By pointing to a similarity between the representation of her body and Michelangelo's famous sculpture "Venus," Stephanie forged a link between the two: both were missing pieces and both were works of art. By viewing her body as artwork, she was now able to see it as beautiful sculpture.

Although art served as a catalyst for Stephanie's transformation to a more aesthetic self, this change did not happen in isolation. Rather, it was an interactional achievement built, in part, through her conversations with the photographer of the project:

> I remember when Charlee (the photographer) and I did this photograph u:h we had done a whole series of me turning around in a circle with this backlighting. A:nd I remember her saying "*Ste*phanie these are so beautiful these are just *so beautiful*" and I was thinking yeah yeah yeah. Uhm you know because it's my disfigured chest. A:nd when we got the photographs back and started looking at them she started pointing out the *shadows* and the *softness* and the *grace* and the *curves* and all of the things that she as a photographer was seeing and I began to internalize that (.) message so that rather than seeing my body as mutilated I began to see it as uhm a beautiful body. (public speech, January 16, 2001)

Stephanie's body was situated as a beautiful object through the interactive sharing of its aesthetic qualities; its shadows, softness, grace, and curves. In contrast to the traditional discourse of diagnosis with its focus on what is wrong with the body, aesthetic discourse, through its emphasis on the pleasing, gracious and artistic qualities of the body, framed a new way for Stephanie to see her body as beautiful. "Through the discursive activity of aesthetic sensemaking ... the viewer[s] [are] fashioning a *self* vis-à-vis the artwork-as-other" in which "they position themselves in the face of the artwork they interpret" (Bruder and Ucok 2000: 355). The interactive nature of jointly viewing and reacting to artwork permits the viewers to construct a mutual self-sense through their talk about art. The interactive quality of the aesthetic experience permits "viewers [to] cooperate in the mutual formation of their self-sense through art talk" (Bruder and Ucok 2000: 356). By viewing the photograph of Stephanie's body together and constructing an image of her body as beautiful, the interactants facilitated the transformation of Stephanie's sense of self.

This transformation of self manifested itself in interaction with others in different contexts:

> Self-acceptance happened suddenly. Sitting in a hot tub, I revealed my new body hesitantly to a group of women; none had seen anyone with a mastectomy. To my amazement, no one fainted or looked shocked, no one pitied me. It was a simple meeting of women comfortable with nudity, accepting their bodies and mine. I began to realize how little I had lost. (Byram and Brodsky 1997: Breasts Equal Sexuality, para. 2)

The perceived reactions of others in this intimate and public setting was a watershed experience for Stephanie. Doubts about her own body and the potential negative reactions of others disappeared. This acceptance by other women foreshadowed other positive experiences:

> Later I discovered that I still lusted after the same men who were attractive to me before my diagnosis. Unexpectedly acting on those feelings, I experienced an awakening that liberated me from the stereotypes and fears of owning a "mutilated" body. My flat torso simply didn't matter; the chemistry and intense passion were the same. (Byram and Brodsky 1997: Breasts Equal Sexuality, para. 3)

During my interview with her, Stephanie revealed that incidents like those mentioned above gave her the external validation she needed and allowed her to believe that not having breasts was irrelevant to who she was and what she wanted to do. Moreover, she wrote in her journal that her sexuality and self-esteem had become more secure (Byram and Brodsky 1997). The nature of this reconstructed self became more apparent in the final text of the Stephanie Project (1997):

1 Cancer Builds
2 My body, soul, and mind do not function as separate parts.
3 Struggling for a sense of balance,
4 I pieced together a new Self, unified and wonderfully alive.
5 Reflection has been my salvation.

In this excerpt, Stephanie explicitly mentioned construction of a new self that was no longer disintegrated. Through reflection, her body, mind, and soul had been unified and balanced. In the final line, Stephanie states "reflection" as the source of her recovery. By keeping a journal, creating visual representations of the processes she went through with her photographer friend, and reflecting upon the nature of her disease, Stephanie was able to move beyond a diagnostic self victimized by cancer to an aesthetic self that was reintegrated and capable of positively experiencing social life.

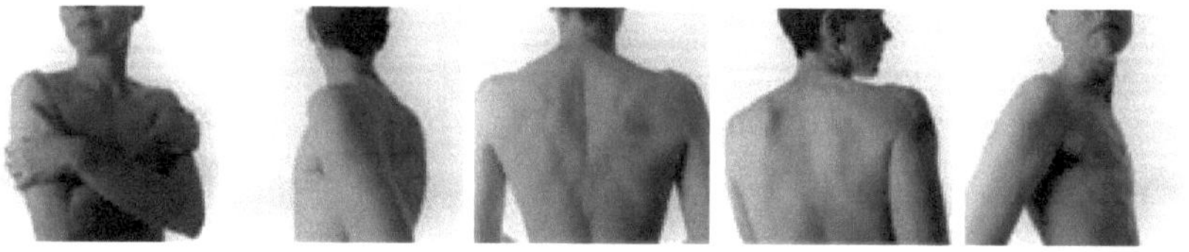

## 6. Conclusion

Being diagnosed with a serious illness carries significant implications for the construction of identity and self. Changes in the relation between the body and the self can result in the emergence of a diagnostic self dominated by a sense of loss, fragmentation, and a perceived lack of grounding in social reality. Yet there exists a potential for the constitution of a renewed and transformed self through discursive practices.

One way of moving beyond the debilitating impact of a catastrophic diagnosis was found in the construction of aesthetic discourse; through the interactive creation of beauty in reaction to Stephanie's physical appearance in a photograph, a reintegrated and positive sense of self began to emerge. As Stephanie became more able to view her altered body in a new and positive way, she gained enough confidence to participate in other positive social activities. In contrast to a diagnostic discourse that focused on what was wrong with her body, aesthetic discourse, through its emphasis on the pleasing, gracious, and artistic qualities of the body allowed Stephanie to construct a new and positive way of viewing her changed appearance. Thus, her "disfigured" body was transformed into an aesthetic body, and the "diagnostic self" into an "aesthetic self."

This chapter serves to document that social interaction and relationships – from medical, to aesthetic, to everyday conversations in a hot tub – are central to the constitution and transformation of identity. Through discursive practices that reinforce the creation of an integrated identity, even devastating experiences such as being diagnosed with a life-threatening illness might result in the realization of new meanings about one's self and life.

## *Note*

*This study is dedicated to Stephanie Byram, a loving soul.

## *References*

Anderson, Robert and Michael Bury (eds.)
1988 *Living with Chronic Illness: The Experience of Patients and Their Families.* London: Unwin Hyman.

Ades, Melissa
2000 Homepage. Retrieved April 2001 from www.keig.com.au/melissa/artist.htm.

Barton, Ellen L.
1999 The social work of diagnosis: Evidence for judgments of competence and incompetence. In Kovarsky, D., J. Duchan, and M. Maxwell (eds.), *Constructing (In)Competence: Disabling Evaluations in Clinical and Social Interaction.* Mahwah, NJ: Lawrence Erlbaum, 257–288.

Blumberg, Rena
1991 *Headstrong: A Story of Conquests and Celebrations – Living Through Chemotherapy.* Shaker Heights, OH: HB Press.

Blumer, Herbert
1969 *Symbolic Interactionism.* Englewood Cliffs, NJ: Prentice-Hall.

Brody, Howard

1987 *Stories of Sickness*. New Haven: Yale University Press.

Bruder, Kurt A. and Ozum Ucok

2000 Interactive art interpretation: How viewers make sense of paintings in conversation. *Symbolic Interaction* 23(4), 337–358.

Burkitt, Ian

1991 *Social Selves: Theories of the Social Formation of Personality*. Newbury Park, CA: Sage.

Bury, Michael.

1982 Chronic illness as biographical disruption. *Sociology of Health and Illness* 4, 167–182.

Byram, Stephanie and Charlee Brodsky

1996a Cancer destroys, cancer builds. *Cultronix* 4. Retrieved July 10, 2001 from http://eserver.org/cultronix/stephanie/PhotoEssay/

1996b Cancer destroys, cancer builds. *Cultronix* 4. Retrieved July 10, 2001 from http://eserver.org/cultronix/stephanie/interview/

1997 *Stephanie*. Retrieved January 2001 from http://www. thestephanieproject.org.

Carbaugh, Donal

1996 *Situating Selves: The Communication of Social Identities in American Scenes*. Albany, NY: State University of New York Press.

Charmaz, Kathy

1985 The body, identity, and self: Adapting to impairment. *The Sociological Quarterly* 36(4), 657–680.

1987 Struggling for a self: Identity levels of the chronically ill. *Research in the Sociology of Health Care* 6, 283–321.

1989 The self in time. In Denzin, N. K. (ed.), *Studies in Symbolic Interaction*. Greenwich, CT: JAI Press, 127–141.

1991 *Good Days, Bad Days: The Self in Chronic Illness and Time*. New Brunswick, NJ: Rutgers University Press.

1994a Discoveries of self in chronic illness. In Dietz, M. L., R. Prus, and W. Shaffir (eds.), *Doing Everyday Life: Ethnography as Human Lived Experience*. Mississauga, Ontario: Copp Clark Longman, 226–242.

1994b Identity dilemmas in chronologically ill men. *The Sociological Quarterly* 35, 269–288.

1995 The body, identity, and self: Adapting to impairment. *The Sociological Quarterly* 36(4), 657–680.

Corbin, Juliet and Anselm Strauss

1987 Accompaniments of chronic illness: Changes in body, self, biography, and biographical time. *Research in the Sociology of Health Care* 6, 249–281.

Davis, Alan and Gordon Horobin

1977 *Medical Encounters: The Experience of Illness and Treatment*. London: Croom Helm.

Davis, Fred

1972 *Illness, Interaction, and the Self*. Belmont, CA: Wadsworth.

Denzin, Norman K.

1987a *The Alcoholic Self*. Newbury Park, CA: Sage.

1987b *The Recovering Alcoholic*. Newbury Park, CA: Sage.

Fallowfield, Lesley and Andrew Clark
1991 *Breast Cancer.* London: Tavistock.
Finlayson, Angela and James McEwen
1977 *Coronary Heart Disease and Patterns of Living.* London: Croom Helm.
Frank, Arthur W.
1991 *At the Will of the Body.* Boston: Houghton Mifflin.
Gadow, Sally.
1982 Body and self: A dialectic. In Kestenbaum, Victor (ed.), *The Humanity of the Ill: Phenomenological Perspectives.* Knoxville: University of Tennessee Press, 86–100.
Gergen, Kenneth
1991 *The Saturated Self: Dilemmas of Identity in Contemporary Life.* New York: Basic Books.
Harré, Rom and G. Gillett
1994 *The Discursive Mind.* Thousand Oaks, CA: Sage.
Kahane, Deborah H.
1990 *No Less a Woman: Ten Women Shatter the Myths about Breast Cancer.* New York: Prentice Hall Press.
Kelly, Michael P. and David Field
1996 Medical sociology, chronic illness and the body. *Sociology of Health and Illness* 18(2), 241–257.
Kestenbaum, Victor
1982 The experience of illness. In Kestenbaum, V. (ed.), *The Humanity of the Ill: Phenomenological Perspectives.* Knoxville: University of Tennessee Press, 3–38.
Lawrence, P. S.
1958 Chronic illness and socio-economic status. In Jaco, E. G. (ed.), *Patients, Physicians and Illness: Sourcebook in Behavioral Science and Medicine.* New York: Free Press, 37–54.
Mead, George Herbert
1934 *Mind, Self and Society: From the Standpoint of a Social Behaviorist.* Chicago: Chicago University Press.
Murphy, Robert
1987 *The Body Silent.* New York, NY: Henry Holt.
Orona, Celia J.
1990 Temporality and identity loss due to Alzheimer's disease. *Social Science and Medicine* 30, 1247–1256.
Parsons, Talcott
1953 *The Social System.* Glencoe, Ill: Free Press.
Radley, Alan (ed.)
1993 *Worlds of Illness: Biographical and Cultural Perspectives on Health and Illness.* London: Routledge.
Radley, Alan and R. Green
1985 Styles of adjustment to coronary graft surgery. *Social Science and Medicine* 20, 461–472.

Sandstrom, Kent L.
1990 Confronting deadly disease: The drama of identity construction among gay men with AIDS. *Journal of Contemporary Ethnography* 19(3), 271–294.
Schimmel, Selma R.
1999 *Cancer Talk*. New York: NY: Broadway Books.
Varricchio, Claudette G. (ed.)
1997 *A Cancer Sourcebook for Nurses*. Sudbury, MA: Jones and Bartlett Publishers.
Winkler, C. J.
1999 How opposing perceptions of communication competence were constructed by Taiwanese graduate students. In Kovarsky, D., J. Duchan, and M. Maxwell (eds.), *Constructing (In)competence: Disabling Evaluations in Clinical and Social Interaction*. Mahwah, NJ: Erlbaum, 83–110.
Yoshida, Karen K.
1993 Reshaping of self: A pendular reconstruction of self and identity among adults with traumatic spinal cord injury. *Sociology of Health and Illness* 15, 217–245.

# Section 2. Doing diagnoses

# Chapter 5
# Revisiting authority in physician–patient interaction

*John Heritage*

*In this chapter, John Heritage studies the interactions between doctors and patients in medical interviews. In particular, he examines the contextual factors that affect the degree of authority expressed in physician-centered discourse. Heritage concludes that the doctors frame their discourse differently depending upon the transparency of the relationship between the tests and the diagnosis. In contexts where doctors can point to test results that allow them to infer the diagnoses, they use authoritarian language (by baldly stating the diagnosis, e.g. "you have a broken bone"). In contexts where the test results are less obviously related to the diagnosis, the doctor uses less authoritarian language (by explaining a diagnosis or using evidential verbs, e.g., "it appears that..."). Heritage finds a delicate balance between authority and accountability; the degree to which doctors assume an authoritarian stance in delivering the diagnostic news will depend upon the degree to which they need to account for how they arrived at their diagnostic conclusion.*

As both physicians and social scientists have noted, the physician–patient relationship is marbled through with the exercise of authority. An orientation to authority begins when the patient, who has experienced some potential medical symptoms and perhaps formed some theory of their nature and etiology, makes an appointment and visits the doctor. At the moment when they present a medical problem, patients face the problem of justifying the medical visit and, in particular, of showing that their concerns are neither irrational nor motivated by external, instrumental considerations (Heritage and Robinson, forthcoming). During the history-taking phase of the visit, patients' reported symptoms are validated (or not) as medical 'signs' relevant to a diagnosis. And at the point of diagnosis, the patient's 'illness' ("the innately human experience of symptoms and suffering" (Kleinman 1988: 3)) becomes a medically validated 'disease' ("an alteration in biological structure or functioning" (Kleinmen 1988: 5)). All these activities are impregnated with the exercise of authority, but its exercise arguably becomes most explicit during the physician's rendering of a diagnosis and subsequent recommendations for treatment.

In his book *The Social Transformation of American Medicine* (1982), Paul Starr argues that medical authority involves each patient in what he calls "the surrender of private judgment" (p. 10). By that he means that when patients get a recommendation from their doctor, they end up abandoning whatever private beliefs, uncertainties, fears, and misgivings they may have about their medical condition, and accept the physician's diagnosis and treatment recommendation. This medical authority, Starr observes, has two main sources. First, there is the dependency of patients who are sick, demoralized, and fearful, and who are not capable of understanding or solving their health problems without expert assistance. The second derives from the cultural authority of science. Cultural authority, says Starr, involves the rights of certain individuals, groups or professions to describe the world: that is, to make definitive pronouncements about the nature of the world, or about specific objects or qualities to be found in the world. Physicians have been trained as scientists in regimes of seeing and recognizing complexes of signs (cf. Barnes 1982; Kuhn 1970, 1977) and have been so certified. Starr argues that medical authority doesn't simply derive from the fact that certain medical techniques work, but rather from the more general scientific basis of medical knowledge which empowers doctors to describe and define the nature of health and illness and the causes of both.

Doctors have not always possessed the kind of authority they wield today. As Edward Shorter (1985) observes, before the rise of scientific medicine in America starting around 1880, patients avoided doctors as far as possible and only went to see them under very severe circumstances. By the turn of the century, the improvement of medical technique resulted in improvements in diagnosis and prognosis and, some time before the development of significant drugs like antibiotics and the development of surgical techniques, the status of the profession rested primarily in its ability to diagnose rather than to treat disease (Shorter 1986). In the opinion of many commentators (Friedson 1986; Shorter 1985; Starr 1982), medical authority and status, powered by the emergence of new drugs, surgical techniques and other treatments, reached its zenith around 1960 – the 'golden age of doctoring' (McKinlay 1999) – and subsequently entered a long process of decline. While many factors have contributed to this process, two stand out. First is the rise in 'consumerist' attitudes among patients who are prepared to 'shop around' for doctors, and to evaluate and disagree with their medical conclusions by looking at the internet or in medical textbooks (cf. Roter and Hall 1992: Ch. 2). The second is the rise of managed care, which allows corporations to subject medical judgments to bureaucratic and financial evaluation, and involves sanctioning doctors for the use of inappropriate treatments (Light 2000).

In this chapter I will examine medical authority in relation to the process of diagnosis and treatment recommendation. There is broad agreement among medical sociologists and practitioners that diagnostic reasoning in medical settings is an activity based on special knowledge possessed and controlled by the profession of medicine. A number of authors also argue that the knowledge gap between the physician and the patient is so wide that diagnostic reasoning is inherently opaque to the layperson. As Parsons (1951) put it, "The physician is a technically competent person whose competence and specific measures cannot be competently judged by the layman. The latter must therefore take these judgments and measures 'on authority'." So then it is this point in the visit – where the physician counsels the patient and proposes treatment – that we arguably reach the point where the patients truly "surrender their private judgment," as Starr puts it. By the same token, it is this point where physicians most completely deploy their cultural authority to define the nature of the patient's problem. Most medical sociologists therefore suggest that the patient is at best a marginal participant in the diagnostic process, and that physicians are not obligated to present, to explain or justify their medical reasoning to patients or to persuade them of the rightness of their decisions. It is sufficient for them simply to pronounce a diagnostic judgment.

Our questions in this chapter are: How do physicians wield their cultural authority at this point? What sort of information do they give patients? On what sort of a basis do patients surrender their private judgment at this point in the interaction? And what are the dynamics of the physician's assertion of cultural authority in the interaction? To answer these questions, discussion will focus on primary care. Here, we are dealing only with moderate illnesses that are not normally life-threatening. The story is likely to be significantly different with more serious illnesses.

With respect to these moderate, primary care illnesses, preliminary evidence from studies of recordings of medical encounters suggests that patients do indeed abrogate their own judgments and more or less surrender with a blindfold on. Roter and Hall (1992) cite a number of studies showing that patients are badly informed about their medical conditions, that physicians tend to use too much medical jargon that patients do not understand, and that physicians underestimate the amount of information patients want about their diagnoses. Most of these studies are based on survey data, but they have been confirmed by studies that rely on recordings of physician–patient interaction which, given the deficiencies of memory, should be regarded as the 'gold standard' in these matters. One of these (Waitzkin 1985) based on 330 recordings, found that physicians spent about 9 percent of their time (on average 1 minute 20 seconds) giving information or explanations to patients about their condition. Notwithstanding the relatively little time they spent in these activities, the physicians believed that they had spent a good deal of their time in giving information. When asked to estimate it, the average estimate was just under 9 minutes (an overestimate of nearly seven times!). Initially, then, it seems apparent that physicians imagine that they do a great deal of explaining, while patients are reluctant to initiate explanations by asking questions. This study also found that physicians significantly underestimated the patient's desire for information. Thus, in addition to their erroneous perception of the amounts of information they have given to patients, physicians also generally do not recognize the amount of information which patients actively desire.

What factors impacted this situation? There were two main sorts of factors focused on (i) patient characteristics and (ii) situational characteristics. With regard to patient characteristics, older patients tended to get more information than younger ones, women received more information than men, and middle class patients received more information than working class patients. In terms of situational characteristics, length of acquaintance with the physician was strongly associated with information giving and busy case loads were strongly associated with less information giving (Waitzkin 1985).

In what follows, I will explore the process of diagnosis and treatment recommendation as an interactional negotiation. I will do so, first, with the aid of three significant studies of the 'diagnostic moment' in the medical visit which give strong, though qualified, support for the idea that patients show strong recognition of medical authority during the process of diagnosis. Second, I will qualify these observations by reference to studies of diagnosis and treatment recommendations in patients with upper respiratory tract infections (URTIs), which are common medical conditions in which many patients may claim some expertise.

## 1. Three studies of the interactional management of diagnosis

### *1.1. Patrick Byrne and Barrie Long: Doctors talking to patients (1976)*

I want to begin by considering a British study conducted about twenty-five years ago by Patrick Byrne and Barrie Long (1976). Byrne and Long's study was large scale (over 2000 medical visits were examined) and pioneering in that it focused on the need for patient-centered medicine (see Mead and Bower 2000 for a review of contemporary literature on this topic). The study focused on a range of physician behaviors across the medical visit, but in relation to the diagnostic phase Byrne and Long asked two questions:

(1) Did the physician identify and explain the diagnosis and treatment?
(2) Did the physician design these descriptions so as to invite the patient to ask questions or participate in a discussion or negotiation of the treatment?

Using these criteria, Byrne and Long formulated seven diagnostic styles, which they arrayed in terms of whether they were physician-centered (focusing on the physicians' knowledge and expertise) or patient-centered (attending more to the patients' interests and concerns).

*Table 1.* Diagnostic styles (Byrne and Long (1976)

| | |
|---|---|
| 1. The physician makes a decision about the patient and his treatment and then instructs the patient to see some service. | 31% |
| 2. The physician makes a decision and announces it. | 36% |
| 3. The physician sells his decision to the patient. | 4% |
| 4. The physician presents a tentative decision subject to change. | 14% |
| 5. The physician presents the problem, seeks suggestions, and makes decisions. | 8% |
| 6. The physician defines the limits and requests the patient to make a decision. | 4% |
| 7. The physician permits the patient to make his own decision. | 1% |

As Table 1 indicates, most of the cases fall into styles 1 and 2, which are the most doctor-centered styles. Below are some examples of these:

*Style 1: [Diagnosis is not named, treatment is not explained]*

Doc: Well now, take this along to the chemist. Take them three times daily after meals. Bye bye.

Doc: I'll make an appointment for you to have an X-ray. Now don't worry. We'll be in touch.

*Style 2: [Diagnosis is named, but not explained. Treatment is not explained, discussed, or negotiated]*

Doc: Well now you seem to have nothing more than a bout of flu. Take this to the chemist on your way home. Go to bed for a few days and I'll look in from time to time.

Doc: This is an infection of the lung. I want you to go upstairs and have an X-ray now. When you've had that, come back here and I will detail some more treatment.

*Style 4: [Diagnosis is presented and explained: treatment options are given in a more exploratory, tentative fashion]*

Doc: Now then, you appear to be having some more trouble with that leg of yours. This is, I think, a consequence of the fact that you're still trying to work as you did ten years ago. Now you are fifty-five and you ought really to start taking things a little easier. I think you ought to have a long rest. Now then, how do you think you can cope with that?

As will be clear from these examples, physician-centered styles of diagnosis are those that involve little or no explanation to patients, and that invite little or no participation from them. Patient-centered styles involve more of both. The two most physician-centered styles are by far the most common, amounting to a total of two thirds of all the diagnoses in Byrne and Long's 2000+ recordings. And, as Table 1 shows, in nearly a third of these, no diagnosis was given at all. This study strongly reinforces the general claim from within medical sociology that physicians tend to be highly authoritarian in their delivery of diagnoses and that they, in effect, compel patients to surrender their private judgment to the physician because they leave the patient little other choice.

## *1.2. Christian Heath: Diagnosis in the general practice consultation (1992)*

This idea that diagnosis involves the exercise of authority is also addressed by the second study, Heath's investigation of how patients respond to medical diagnoses (Heath 1992). His central observation concerns the remarkable passivity of patients in the face of diagnoses by physicians. Most obviously, Heath notes that in a significant proportion of the videotapes he looked at, patients remained completely silent in the face of a diagnosis. Note the arrowed silence at line 2 in (1) below, which is a point at which the patient could have responded.

(1) [Heath 1992: 239]

| | | |
|---|---|---|
| 1 | Doc:→ | Er::::::: Yeas:: (0.3) this one's blocked (.) the other one's not. |
| 2 | → | (1.2) |
| 3 | Doc: | Well when would you like to have them done |
| 4 | | (.) |
| 6 | Doc: | Next week sometime:? |
| 7 | Pat: | Yers (.) yes please. |

Patients also responded to diagnoses with a minimal form of acknowledgement token, a downward intoned "er", "uh", or "yeh' ".

(2) [Heath 1992: 240]

| | | |
|---|---|---|
| 1 | Doc: | hhhh You've got erm: (0.8) bronchitis::. |
| 2 | Pat: → | °er:.° |
| 3 | → | (4.5) ((Dr begins to write prescription)) |
| 4 | Doc: | .hhh (0.3) I'll give you antibiotics: to take for a week. hhh |
| 5 | | (0.8) |
| 7 | Doc: | How long are you here for? |

Heath notes that there are several other response types that are completely absent. Patients could, for example, respond with "oh," a form of acknowledgement that treats what they have just heard as new information (Heritage 1984). Another response could be with a 'newsmark' (Heath 1992), for example, "it is?" or "oh really," which show interest in the diagnosis and invite some expansion of its details by the physician. And, of course, there are explicit questions patients might ask in response to a newsworthy item: "What's that?", "What causes it?", "Is it contagious?", "Is it serious?", "How long will it last?" All of these response types are largely absent. These patients have just been given a diagnosis, but they don't even acknowledge it as information.

Why is this the case? Heath considers the bodily and other nonverbal behavior of the physician. For example, the physician could be writing notes or a prescription, and appear unavailable. This, however, was not the case. Physicians were normally gazing directly at the patient – something which ordinarily solicits response. Heath argues that patient passivity is directly related to the design of the diagnostic utterance – the feature stressed in the Byrne and Long study. For example, in (1) and (2) the diagnoses are simply delivered as authoritative assertions of fact. As expert opinions, authoritatively delivered, they do not offer a context that is ripe for subsequent enquiries. If we had to classify these designs in Byrne and Long's terms, we would probably suggest that they are 'style 2' diagnoses.

Heath confirmed this observation by looking at cases in which the diagnosis is offered in a less authoritative way as in (3):

(3) [Heath 1992: 247]

| | | |
|---|---|---|
| 1 | Doc:→ | .hhh It's not a totally typical story of a |
| 2 | → | wear and tear arthritis, but I think that's: |
| 3 | → | what it's going to turn ou[t to be::::. |
| 4 | Pat: | [(Well that (.) but that en right wouldn') wife and nurse |
| 5 | | says hhh[h |
| 6 | Doc: | [Oh well [I think we ought to get an X-ray as a check. |
| 7 | Pat: | [.hh heh Yers |
| 8 | Doc: | You've not had this done on that ankle before? |
| 9 | Pat: | No:. |

Here the physician offers a tentative diagnosis that will require confirmation by X-ray, and the patient responds quite actively.

Heath also shows that similarly active responses also emerge when the physician's diagnosis is different from the patient's lay understanding of the problem. In (4), the patient has an eye problem that he thought was due to a vein: the physician determines that it's a muscle problem, and this engenders some discussion between physician and patient.

(4) [Heath 1992: 250]

| | | |
|---|---|---|
| 1 | Doc:→ | It's not a vein: (.) it's a muscle in spas:[m. |
| 2 | Pat: → | [Is it? |
| 3 | Doc: | Yeah. |
| 4 | Pat: → | Oh: |
| 5 | Doc: | And I think what's cau[sing it to be in spasm |
| 6 | Pat: → | [I've had it for about |
| 7 | → | three or fou[r weeks, and n[ow (or something like that.) |
| 8 | Doc: | [Yeah [Yeah |
| 9 | Doc: | You've got a low grade inflammation of the eye:::: |
| 10 | | (0.3) the front of the eye and this is probably making the spasm come. |

A third environment in which patients offer elaborate responses to physician's evaluations emerges when these evaluations undermine the legitimacy of the patient's reasons for visiting the doctor. In (5) the patient who is in effect told he's well, counters with a report that his symptoms arise at night.

(5) [Heath 1992: 255]

| | | |
|---|---|---|
| 1 | Doc: | Well yer ches:t is:: (.) absolutely cle:ar: today::, |
| 2 | | (1.0) |
| 3 | Doc: | which is helpful: (0.4) and your pulse is: (0.7) only eighty .thhhh (.) which is er:: (1.2) not so bad. |
| 5 | | (1.2) |
| 6 | Pat: | (Right it's::) there:: night time (uh) (.) it's:: 'ts not clear there, I've got er::: ( ) (1.4) ( ) (0.3) I've more |
| 7 | | or less gone to bed when it starts: on us:? |
| 8 | | (2.5) |
| 9 | Pat: | I wake all the way through the night without getting any sleep (un open)) |
| 10 | | (0.5) |
| 11 | Doc: | Mm |
| 12 | Pat: | (I don't know what's fetchin it up) during the nights (.) but it comes in at the nights. |

Even here the patient avoids an overt challenge to the status of the evaluation, but instead vigorously asserts that his, currently undetectable, symptoms emerge at night. Similar responses emerge when physicians offer diagnoses that appear to "question the severity of their symptoms and suffering" (Heath 1992: 255), though these rarely eventuate on overt disagreement or challenge.

To summarize, both the Byrne and Long and the Heath studies suggest that diagnosis is a prime site for the expression of medical authority. Byrne and Long show that the majority of diagnoses are delivered in a highly authoritarian fashion, offering little explanation and seemingly designed to occlude patient participation. Heath shows that patients respond to these diagnoses very passively. Patients rarely ask questions about the diagnosis and almost never question it or challenge it. So they tend to remain outside of and uninvolved in diagnostic reasoning. Heath finds only two types of exceptions to this: (1) if physicians are more patient-centered, patients become more involved; (2) if the diagnostic process threatens the legitimacy of the patient's complaint.

### *1.3. Anssi Peräkylä: Authority and accountability (1998)*

More recently a further perspective on medical authority and diagnosis has been offered by Anssi Peräkylä, a Finnish sociologist studying the physician–patient relationship. Peräkylä starts by establishing clearly that the simple unelaborated diagnostic statement is the basic or default kind of diagnostic statement that physicians most commonly make. Peräkylä calls these kinds of diagnoses "straight assertions." They are the most common kind of diagnosis in primary care and they are illustrated in (6):

(6) [Peräkylä 1998] "Straight factual assertion"

| | | |
|---|---|---|
| 1 | Doc: | Here's (.) luckily the bone quite intact, |

However, Peräkylä also notes two other ways in which physicians can frame their diagnoses. One involves reference to the experience of the physician in coming to a decision. This type involves the use of what linguists term 'evidentials' (Chafe and Nichols 1986). These are expressions where people make reference to what they are seeing, feeling, hearing, smelling or sensing. In this format, Peräkylä writes that evidential verbs "operate in a border area, as it were, between the speaker's inner world on the one hand, and the external, objective world on the other. Thus, they are verbs capable of expressing how the external world is revealed to the inner world of the speaker-observer." This type of diagnosis is illustrated by (7).

(7) [Peräkylä 1998] "Evidential formulation"

| | | |
|---|---|---|
| 1 | Doc: | Now there *appears to be* an (1.0) infection at the contact point of the joint below it in the sac |
| 2 | | of mucus there in the hip |

A third type of diagnostic format involves laying out some of the reasoning that stands behind the physician's judgment. Peräkylä calls this the "evidence formulating pattern," as illustrated by (8).

(8) [Peräkylä 1998] "Evidence formulating pattern"

| | | |
|---|---|---|
| 1 | Doc: | As tapping on the vertebrae didn't cause any .pain |
| 2 | | and there aren't any actual reflection symptoms |
| 3 | | in your legs it corresponds with a muscle h (.hhhh) |
| 4 | | complication so hhh it's only whether hhh (0.4) you |
| 5 | | have been exposed to a draught or has it otherwise= |
| 6 | Pat: | =Oh yes, |
| 7 | Doc: | .hh got irritated, |

Although the straight factual assertion format is the most common, the other two formats are also quite common. The relative frequencies of these formats is found by Peräkylä is given in Table 2:

*Table 2.* Frequency of types of diagnostic turns (Peräkylä 1998)

| Turn design | Frequency | Percentage |
|---|---|---|
| 1. Plain assertion | 31 | 44 |
| 2. Evidential | 12 | 17 |
| 3. Evidence formulating | 28 | 39 |
| Total | 71 | 100 |

How are we to explain this general pattern? Peräkylä argues that we have to start from a different place than the traditional discussions of medical authority that I have discussed so far. He argues that physicians' authority is not unbounded, but is balanced by their accountability. By accountability, Peräkylä means that physicians have some obligation to index the grounds on which their conclusions are formed. In practice, he suggests physicians' diagnoses incorporate a balance between the authority of their conclusions, and the social accountability of their judgments. This accountability of medical judgments is limited, Peräkylä argues, because laypersons cannot fully recognize the symptoms the physician is seeing, or make fully valid inferences about the causes of those symptoms: these things belong to the realm of expert knowledge. Nonetheless, Peräkylä finds that physicians are accountable to patients in the more limited sense of indicating to them the general basis of the judgements they are making.

Peräkylä argues that even the diagnoses that are formatted as straight factual assertions and look really quite authoritarian, can embody this balance between authority and accountability. He shows that when there is a close and relatively transparent relationship between the examination and the diagnosis that results from it, the diagnosis will be presented as straight factual assertion. For example, in (6) the physician's assertion "Here's (.) luckily the bone quite intact," is made while he is holding up an X-ray picture between himself and the patient. The patient can clearly see the evidence on which the diagnosis is based, though in keeping with his limited capacity to 'read' X-ray plates he only briefly glances at it.

In this case, there is close a relationship between the evidence and the diagnostic conclusion without any great leap of inference. Peräkylä calls this relationship between evidence and conclusion the 'inferential distance' between the two, and in the X-ray example case it is extremely short. In this case the authority of the physician's diagnosis is expressed in the *verbal design* of his diagnostic turn. The accountability of the diagnosis is managed through the *context* of his utterance, which conveys without stating so in so many words that the diagnosis is based in evidence that both parties have in front of them, though they have differential abilities to make use of it.

Let me repeat here that Peräkylä is not claiming that the patient has an exact understanding of the physician's diagnosis. Quite the contrary, the patient mainly does not understand them, but the patient does know what the physician looked at in arriving at the diagnosis: the patient knows that the diagnosis is based on something specific, even though he may not know exactly what its relevance is. In Peräkylä's words, the patient knows from what direction the evidence comes.

Peräkylä shows that in the vast majority of cases where the inferential distance between examination and diagnosis is short – for example, the physician looks in the patient's ear and then announces she has an infection – physicians tend to use the simple factual assertion format. And his argument is, as I have suggested, that this does not embody flat-out authoritarianism, but rather a particular balance between authority and accountability.

What are the contexts then in which physicians move away from the simple factual assertion to the more elaborated formats, using evidentials or evidence formulating? Let's start with the evidentials. Peräkylä argues that physicians use evidentials when the inferential distance between the examination and the diagnosis is greater. This greater distance can be the result of two factors, either separately or together. The first involves what Peräkylä calls temporal separation between the exam and the diagnosis. For example in (9), the physician conducted a physical examination of the patient, then he spent a while working on the computer preparing a referral for an X-ray, and at line 14, quite a while after the examination, he describes his diagnosis using an 'evidential formulation' – "there *appears to be* an infection ..."

(9) [Peräkylä 1998: Expansion of (7)]
((Before this extract, the physician conducted the physical examination, after which he worked on his computer, telling the patient that he was preparing a referral to the X-ray lab))

| | | |
|---|---|---|
| 1 | Doc: | Has your hip ever been X-rayed before. |
| 2 | | (0.5) (Dr picks up some papers)) |
| 3 | Pat: | hhhh erm::hhh (1,0) I don't really rememb- |

4 I don't think it has.
5 (0.8)
6 Pat: I don't think it has.=.hh My knee has been X-rayed
7 as it #erm# yea:rs (0.2) .hh years
8 ago as riding a bicycle was so painful
9 that it couldn't put up (.) with it, .h but
10 then nothing was found there.=As far as I remember there has never been an
11 X-ray of my hip hh.
12 (1.2)
13 ?Pat: .mth
14 Doc: Now there appears to be an (1.0) infection at the contact
15 point of the joint below it in the sac of mucus
16 there [in the hip.
17 Pat: [Oh right .hh that's what I thought myself
18 too that <it probably must be an infection>.
19 [.hhhhh
20 Doc: [And, because you have had trouble this [long we will
21 Pat: [hhhhh
22 Doc: make sure and take an X-[ray.
23 Pat: [Yes:.

Peräkylä argues that through this evidentialized turn design the physician verbally retrieves the earlier examination of the patient as a context for his diagnosis. In other words, the construction *there appears to be* reinvokes the examination where the physician got his evidence, and indicates that this event can be understood as the context for the diagnostic conclusion. The same is true for evidence formulating. Here evidence is explicitly retrieved. So when the diagnosis is temporally distant from the exam, physicians use the more expanded 'evidential' or 'evidence formulating' diagnostic designs.

The second aspect of greater inferential distance between exam and diagnosis involves what Peräkylä calls the 'opacity' of diagnostic reasoning. By the term 'opacity,' Peräkylä means to refer to cases where the patient knows what was examined, but does not know what it was being examined for. This is what happens in (10). Here the patient complained about a pain in her foot and physician has been looking at it.

(10) [Peräkylä 1998]
((The physician has just examined the patient's foot))
1 Doc: Okay:. .h fine do put on your,
2 (.)
3 Doc: the pulse [can be felt there in your foot so,
4 Pat: [Thank you.
5 Doc: .h there's no, in any case (.) no real circulation
6 proble[m

Pat: [Yes I don't understand then
[really .hh I was wondering whether (.) I should
Doc: [is <involved>.

Peräkylä reports that the patient's foot looks quite normal and it's not clear what the examination was aimed at. At the end of it, the physician describes a result of the examination, stating that he can feel a pulse in her foot, and then concludes with a diagnostic evaluation, telling the patient that she doesn't have a circulation problem. In this way, he connects his diagnostic conclusion to the physical exam, whose point is now revealed. Once again, Peräkylä finds that this is a quite general pattern where the purpose of physical examinations is opaque to patients.

Another kind of relationship between evidence formulating diagnoses and their circumstances will be more predictable in light of Heath's findings. It occurs when the diagnosis is uncertain, or when the diagnosis is controversial. By controversial Peräkylä means the diagnosis runs against the patients' beliefs about what is wrong with them, most often when the patient believes that the diagnosis is more serious than the physician seems to think, or the diagnostic evaluation may seem to undermine the legitimacy of the patient's medical visit.

Peräkylä's study does two things. It revises our mind-set about the nature of authority. If we do not look at interactional data, it is all too easy to see authority as an all-or-nothing phenomenon. Peräkylä reminds us that accountability goes with authority – in the medical office just as much as the Oval Office. And he also shows us how subtle that accountability can be. It can simply be a matter of the context in which a diagnosis is offered. And that kind of subtle accountability may be just enough when the problem isn't that serious and does not (or should not) require a vast amount of discussion or joint decision-making.

Peräkylä also shows how physicians expand the verbal accountability of their diagnoses when the context cannot or will not do the job. He points out that physicians treat themselves as more accountable when their diagnoses are problematic, uncertain or disputed. Some researchers believe that physicians restrict the flow of information to patients as a means of bolstering their authority. But research by Howard Waitzkin (1985) suggested that when their diagnoses are tentative or under attack, physicians actually give more information to their patients. This finding is underlined by Peräkylä's study. Peräkylä shows that in these situations, physicians don't give orders or simply "assert their authority," rather they engage in persuasion: they treat their judgments as founded in an authority that is, after all, accountable.

## 2. How authoritative are physicians? A case study

All the papers described so far have deployed interactional data to give at least qualified support to the traditional sociological understanding of the relationship between diagnosis and medical authority. But more recent studies of medical visits involving relatively mild conditions, e.g., upper respiratory tract infections (URTIs) suggests some further adjustments to this picture.

A large body of research suggests that patients find ways to convey a demand for certain medications, particularly antibiotics, and that as a result the medical visit can take on the character of a tacit negotiation. The starting point for this research is that antibiotics are more commonly prescribed when patients want them and/or convey that they want them to the physician (Britten and Ukoumunne 1997; Cockburn and Pit 1997; Hamm, Hicks, and Bemben 1996; Himmel, Lippert-Urbanke, and Kochen 1997; Macfarlane, Holmes, Macfarlane, and Britten 1997; Schwartz, Freij, Ziai, and Sheridan 1997; Virji and Britten 1991). As Stivers and colleagues have shown, this desire is not always conveyed explicitly (Stivers 2002a, 2002b; Stivers, Mangione-Smith, Elliott, McDonald, and Heritage 2003). But, as Table 3 shows, when physicians perceive such a desire, they commonly adjust their diagnoses in the direction of bacterial illness and prescribe accordingly.

*Table 3.* Impact of perceived parental expectations on diagnosis and treatment of pediatric upper respiratory infections (Mangione-Smith, McGlynn, Elliott, Krogstad, and Brook 1999)

| | Physician believes parent expects ABX (%) | Physician believes parent does not expect ABX (%) |
|---|---|---|
| Otitis media Dx (all cases) | 49 | 13 ($p<.001$) |
| Sinusitis Dx (all cases) | 38 | 5 ($p<.001$) |
| ABX prescribed (viral cases) | 62 | 7 ($p<.001$) |

Recent research by Stivers (forthcoming a, b) confirms Heath's earlier findings that patients rarely question physicians' diagnoses. However, she also shows that they more frequently contest treatment recommendations, and that this is one of the factors involved in inappropriate antibiotics prescribing. In one of her examples, (11) below, it is clear from the way in which the physician formulates his diagnosis (lines 1–8) that he perceives that the patient would like an antibiotic for her child. And, shortly after he has stated that the condition is viral "so we can't make it go *away* any faster," the mother makes a guarded request for antibiotics at lines 14–15:

(11) [Stivers 2000]

1 DOC:→ *Well* you know it's sort of one of those *good* news
2 → *bad* news scenarios. On one han:d thuh *good* news is
3 → that she [doesn't have any serious in*fec*tion. I=
4 GIR: [( ).
5 DOC: =mean her ears are fi:ne, so she can *fly*: an' .hh=
6 MOM: =(an-)=
7 DOC:→ =everything *el*se looks okay. Thuh *bad* news is that
8 → it's probably *vi*ral so we can't make it go a*way* any faster,
9 (.)
10 MOM: Mkay.
11 (0.4)
12 MOM: .hh -.h Now-
13 GIR: ( [ )
14 MOM:→ [should I- (0.4) just as uh preventative *thi:ng*,
15 → should I give them some- antibi*o*tics?, or: [(does that-)
16 DOC: [It wouldn't
17 do *a*nything for thi[s.
18 MOM: [No?=
19 DOC: =An' if [*a*nything it'd make: her diarrhea [worse=
20 MOM: [Okay. [#huh huh#

While the physician succeeds in resisting the mother's pressure for antibiotics in this case, in others physicians reverse their diagnoses and/or prescribe inappropriately (Stivers 2002b, forthcoming a). In such cases, patients have exerted pressure for prescriptions and coerced physicians into prescribing against their better judgment. This is the reverse of the 'surrender of private judgment' with which we began, and represents, in effect, an abrogation of medical authority.

In recent work, Heritage and Stivers (1999) have suggested the use of 'online commentary' as a means of resisting patient pressure to prescribe. Because a good deal of patient pressure is exerted through the problem presentation stage of the visit (Stivers, Mangione-Smith, Elliott, McDonald, and Heritage 2003), physicians often perceive patient pressure early on. In such cases, online commentary, in which the physician describes the physical examination as it is happening 'online' can be a means of defeating patient expectations. In the following case, the physician describes what he is seeing, in the process indicating that the patient's signs are mild. While this may reassure the mother that her child is not very sick, it also builds a case against antibiotics prescribing and 'forecasts' (Maynard 1996) an eventual 'no antibiotics' treatment recommendation:

(12) [Heritage and Stivers 1999]

1 Doc: Can you op'n your mouth for me agai:n,
2 (0.3)
3 Doc: °'ats i:t°

| | | |
|---|---|---|
| 4 | | (0.7) |
| 5 | Doc:→ | °*Lit*tle bit re:d (.) hm° |
| 6 | | (1.6) ((moving sounds)) |
| 7 | Doc: | °°Alri::ght(h)°° |
| 8 | | (2.8) ((more moving sounds)) |
| | | ((32 lines omitted)) |
| 9 | Doc: | Ari:ght Michael. Can I loo:k >in your< *ears* |
| 10 | | (0.3) |
| 11 | Mom: | °This o:n[e:° |
| 12 | Doc: | ['ank you |
| 13 | | (0.9) |
| 14 | Doc:→ | 'ats fi:ne the other one? |
| 15 | | (4.5) |
| 16 | Doc: | ktch °okha::yh° |
| 17 | | (0.5) |
| 18 | Doc:→ | They're alri::ght(h). I mean there's a *just* a *li:(*tt)le |
| 19 | → | redness in his *throa:t* an:d and just a little pinkness ther:e |
| 20 | → | which (.) means he's got one of tho:se *co:lds* that make them |
| 21 | → | cou:gh a lot .hh Because his chest is pe:rfectly all ri:ght |
| 22 | → | he *ce:r*tainly doesn't need (.) peni*cil*lin |
| 23 | Mom: | N:o[: |
| 24 | Doc: | [°'r anything like tha:t° .hhhh hh I think the *cough*ing ... |
| | | ((talk continues)) |

Here the online comments (lines 5 and 17) 'forecast' the diagnostic outcome, which explicitly retrieves them as part of the case against prescribing (lines 21–24). Here, we might say, Peräkylä's 'evidence formulating' starts earlier in the medical visit and is used ancillary to a 'no treatment' recommendation. Preliminary findings suggest that this kind of online evidence formulating can reduce inappropriate prescribing (Mangione-Smith, Stivers, Elliott, McDonald, and Heritage 2003).

## 3. Conclusion

What conclusions are to be drawn from this array of conversation analytic studies of medical practice? First, it is clear that the act of diagnosis remains a fulcrum in the exercise of medical authority. None of the studies reviewed here shows a significant incidence of explicit disagreement with medical diagnoses. This is so even though the medical conditions being addressed are the relatively minor staples of primary care medicine in which patients may have some experience and 'expertise,' and it may be surmised that in more serious, unusual or life-threatening conditions the conclusion holds with still greater force. The older Byrne and Long study shows physicians exercising this authority in a fashion which is quite authoritarian, though this observation and those of Heath's later study need to be seasoned with Peräkylä's observations, which suggest more of a balance with social accountability than is traditionally observed in the sociological literature.

The studies of antibiotics prescribing qualify these observations significantly. They suggest that in cases of mild illness which patients have frequently experienced in the past, medical authority is compromised by a tacit bargaining process, in which the perception that patients may become dissatisfied with their medical care may outweigh the exercise of clinical judgment. Paradoxically, if the results of the 'online commentary' study are borne out by further research, physicians can redress the balance by a more fundamental exercise of the cultural authority of medicine: the capacity to 'name the world' which in this case takes the form of unchallengeable observations about patient signs and symptoms. Yet this too involves a revision of physician authority. 'Online commentary' is 'evidence formulating' and reveals a process of diagnostic reasoning to the patient, thus further redrawing the balance between authority and accountability a little further in the direction of accountability.

## *References*


Barnes, Barry
1982 *T. S. Kuhn and Social Science.* London: Macmillan.

Britten, N. and O. Ukoumunne
1997 The influence of patients' hopes of receiving a prescription on doctors' perceptions and the decision to prescribe: A questionnaire study. *British Medical Journal* 315, 1506–1510.

Byrne, Patrick and Barrie Long
1976 *Doctors Talking to Patients.* London: Her Majesty's Stationary Office.

Chafe, Wallace and Johanna Nichols (eds.)
1986 *Evidentiality: The Linguistic Coding of Epistemology.* Norwood, NJ: Ablex.

Cockburn, J. and S. Pit
1997 Prescribing behavior in clinical practice: Patients' expectations and doctors' perceptions of patients' expectations – a questionnaire study. *British Medical Journal* 315, 520–523.

Friedson, Eliot
1986 *Professional Powers: A Study of the Institutionalization of Formal Knowledge.* Chicago: University of Chicago Press.

Hamm, R., R. Hicks, and D. Bemben
1996 Antibiotics and respiratory infections: are patients more satisfied when expectations are met? *Journal of Family Practice* 43, 56–62.

Heath, Christian
1992 The delivery and reception of diagnosis in the general practice consultation. In Drew, P. and J. Heritage (eds.), *Talk at Work.* New York: Cambridge University Press, 235–268.

Heritage, John
1984 A change-of-state token and aspects of its sequential placement. In Atkinson, J. M. and J. Heritage (eds.), *Structures of Social Action*. Cambridge: Cambridge University Press, 299–345.

Heritage, John and Jeffrey Robinson
forthcoming Accounting for the visit: Patients' reasons for seeking medical care. In Heritage, J. and D. Maynard (eds.), *Practicing Medicine: Structure and Process in Primary Care Consultations*. Cambridge: Cambridge University Press.

Heritage, John and Tanya Stivers
1999 Online commentary in acute medical visits: A method of shaping patient expectations. *Social Science and Medicine* 49(11), 1501–1517.

Himmel, W., E. Lippert-Urbanke, and M. M. Kochen
1997 Are patients more satisfied when they receive a prescription? The effect of patient expectations in general practice. *Scandinavian Journal of Primary Health Care* 15, 118–122.

Kleinman, Arthur
1988 *The Illness Narratives: Suffering, Healing and the Human Condition*. New York: Basic Books.

Kuhn, Thomas
1970 *The Structure of Scientific Revolutions*. Chicago: University of Chicago Press.
1977 Second thoughts on paradigms. In Kuhn, T., *The Essential Tension*. Chicago: University of Chicago Press, 293–319.

Light, Donald W.
2000 The medical profession and organizational change: From professional dominance to countervailing power. In Bird, C. E., P. Conrad, and A. M. Fremont (eds.), *Handbook of Medical Sociology*. Upper Saddle River, NJ: Prentice Hall, 201–216.

Macfarlane, J., W. Holmes, R. Macfarlane, and N. Britten
1997 Influence of patients' expectations in antibiotic management of acute lower respiratory tract illness in general practice: Questionnaire study. *British Medical Journal* 315, 1211–1214.

Mangione-Smith, Rita, Elizabeth McGlynn, Marc Elliott, Paul Krogstad, and Robert H. Brook
1999 The relationship between perceived parental expectations and pediatrician antimicrobial prescribing behavior. *Pediatrics* 103(4), 711–718.

Mangione-Smith, Rita, Elizabeth McGlynn, Marc Elliott, and Laurie McDonald
2002 An observational study of antibiotic prescribing behavior and the Hawthorne effect. *Health Services Research* 37(6), 1603–1623.

Mangione-Smith, Rita, Tanya Stivers, Marc Elliott, Laurie McDonald, and John Heritage
2003 Online commentary on physical exam findings: a communication tool for avoiding inappropriate antibiotic prescribing? *Social Science and Medicine* 56(2), 313–320.

Maynard, Douglas
1996 On 'realization' in everyday life. *American Sociological Review* 60(1), 109–132.
McKinlay, John B.
1999 The end of the Golden Age of medicine. *New England Research Institutes Network* Summer, 1, 3.
Mead, Nicola and Peter Bower
2000 Patient centredness: A conceptual framework and review of the empirical literature. *Social Science and Medicine* 51, 1087–1110.
Parsons, Talcott
1951 *The Social System*. New York: Free Press.
Peräkylä, Anssi
1998 Authority and accountability: The delivery of diagnosis in primary health care. *Social Psychology Quarterly* 61(4), 301–320.
Roter, Debra and Judith Hall
1992 *Doctors Talking with Patients/Patients Talking with Doctors: Improving Communication in Medical Visits*. Westport, Conn: Auburn House.
Schwartz, R. H., B. J. Freij, M. Ziai, and M. J. Sheridan
1997 Antimicrobial prescribing for acute purulent rhinitis in children: A survey of pediatricians and family practitioners. *Pediatric Infectious Disease Journal* 16, 185–190.
Shorter, E.
1985 *Bedside Manners: The Troubled History of Doctors and Patients*. New York: Simon and Schuster.
Starr, Paul
1982 *The Social Transformation of American Medicine*. New York: Basic Books.
Stivers, Tanya
2000 Negotiating antibiotic treatment in pediatric care: The communication of preferences in physician–parent interaction. Unpublished PhD dissertation, Department of Applied Linguistics, University of California, Los Angeles.
2002a 'Symptoms only' and 'Candidate diagnoses': Presenting the problem in pediatric encounters. *Health Communication* 14(3), 299–338.
2002b Participating in decisions about treatment: Overt parent pressure for antibiotic medication in pediatric encounters. *Social Science and Medicine* 54, 1111–1130.
forthcoming a Parent resistance to physicians' treatment recommendations: One resource for initiating a negotiation of the treatment decision. *Health Communication*.
forthcoming b Treatment decisions: The interactional process of reaching a treatment decision in acute medical encounters. In Heritage, J. and D. Maynard (eds.), *Practicing Medicine: Structure and Process in Primary Care Consultations*. Cambridge: Cambridge University Press.
Stivers, Tanya, Rita Mangione Smith, Marc Elliott, Laurie McDonald, and John Heritage
2003 What leads physicians to believe that parents expect antibiotics? A study of parent communication behaviors and physicians' perceptions. *Journal of Family Practice* 52(2), 140–148.

Virji, A. and N. Britten
1991 A study of the relationship between patients' attitudes and doctors' prescribing. *Family Practice* 8, 314–319.
Waitzkin, Howard
1985 Information giving in medical care. *Journal of Health and Social Behavior* 26, 81–101.

# Chapter 6
# "I just wanna know *why*": Patients' attempts and physicians' responses to premature solicitation of diagnostic information

*Charlotte M. Jones and Wayne A. Beach*

*Picking up on the issue of authoritarianism raised by Heritage in the previous chapter, Jones and Beach examine how authoritarianism gets enacted throughout physician–patient encounters. A collection of instances are analyzed where patients solicit diagnostic information during initial moments and phases of medical interviews. In response, doctors treat such actions as premature and generally avoid addressing patients' concerns. The authors then examine instances where patients take the initiative, despite discouragement, to pursue diagnostically relevant responses. For the most part physicians continued to not respond willingly to patients' pursuits, revealing their dispreference for ongoing patient-initiated questions (and related actions). But the authors also describe interactional environments wherein patients shape their initiations in ways that doctors treat as acceptable. After exploring specific features of interactions resulting in more positive responses by physicians, it becomes clear that mutual involvement and decision-making can be enhanced through collaborative approaches to medical care.*

During medical interviews patients seek assurance, solicit diagnostic information from physicians, and even proffer their own diagnosis of an illness. We examine a range of soliciting techniques employed by patients as they pursue understandings about their medical condition, and in response, how physicians treat such contributions with hesitation and indirectness. At times, physicians are also shown to disattend patient-initiated topics by moving back to biomedical agendas. Acting as though patients' contributions are untimely and/or altogether inappropriate, physicians appear to treat patients as resisting adherence to a biomedical model in which *physicians* address diagnoses, and only subsequent to data-gathering and physical examination. The result is a marked contrast in orientations to communication in medical interviews, where patients' lay concerns and diagnoses get raised but only minimally acknowledged by clinicians (Beach 1995, 2006; Beach and Mandelbaum 2005; Jones 2001; Lutfey and Maynard 1998; Peräkylä 1991).

Moments where patients solicit, and physicians withhold providing "premature" diagnostic information, are deserving of close analytic inspection. We begin by overviewing five central issues underlying the need to examine these interactional involvements.

First, while clinicians are traditionally understood to be the "officially" designated participants responsible for regulating emergent phases of a biomedical encounter (Byrne and Long 1976; Drew and Heritage 1992; McWhinney 1989; ten Have 1989) – (a) opening, (b) data-gathering or question-answer, (c) physical examination, (d) diagnosis and treatment, and (e) closing – such phases are interactionally produced and thus not necessarily linear nor constrained by role (see Heath 1992; Modaff 1996a; 1996b; Peräkylä 1997; Robinson 1998; ten Have 1991a). Just as medical professionals predominantly ask more questions, offer "formal" diagnoses, and prescribe treatment regimens, so too has it become increasingly clear that patients should be treated as active collaborators throughout interviews (Beach 2001a; Drew 2001; ten Have 2001). At times patients extend and may even abandon physicians' attempts to constrain answers focusing on lifeworld experiences (Beach and Dixson 2001; Heritage and Stivers 1999). More commonly, however, patients avoid intruding on the prescriptive judgment of a physician (Robinson 2001), hint at rather than directly state their requests (Gill et al. 2001), and limit their questions to provided opportunities such as "Is there anything else today?" (Frankel and Beckman 1988). Nevertheless, it is undeniable that patients influence the course an interview might take by somehow initiating talk about their background, present concerns, and future anxieties (Beach and Dixson 2001; Beach and LeBaron 2002).

Second, researchers from diverse disciplines have investigated what has for some time been characterized as patient desires and expectations when seeking medical care.[1] Patients report that receiving medical explanations from physicians about what is wrong with them is one of, if not *the* top priority in medical visits (Beisecker and Beisecker 1990; Eisenthal et al. 1990; Good and Good 1982; Good et al. 1983; Like and Zyzanski 1987; McKinley and Middleton 1999; Mockapetris and Craigie 1986). A large survey revealed that sixty-nine percent of seven hundred and fifty-six general practice patients wanted an explanation for their problem (McKinley and Middleton 1999). In a study of four primary care clinics, patients cited the need for "explanation twice as frequently as medical tests and half again as frequently as medication" (Good and Good 1982: 293). Furthermore, a majority of patients from two primary care practices reported wanting information regarding their conditions (e.g., "I'd like to be told what's causing this rash") (Eisenthal et al. 1990).

Third, since reduction of uncertainty about a medical condition is a natural inclination (Babrow 2001; Babrow et al. 1998), it should not be surprising that many patients may require assurance, diagnostic information, and/or clarification during care. Hurting bodies are constant sources of uncertainty and anxiety (Frank 1991; 1997). Outside of the clinic, considerable time and effort may have been invested in reflecting upon and talking with others about what might potentially be wrong (Beach 2001b). Of course, receiving an explanation may itself be not just an anticipated but a "dreaded" experience, in hopes that a particular diagnosis such as AIDS or cancer is *not* delivered (see Peräkylä 1995). However, in other cases patients may (more or less proactively) enact their own agendas by soliciting assurance or information, during moments when clinicians are orienting to tasks such as opening an encounter and gathering data about a medical condition. It will be shown that these moments contribute to disjunctures between "business as usual" and "business at hand" within the clinic (see Beach 1996; Button and Casey 1989; Pomerantz 1984a; Stivers and Heritage 2001).

Fourth, although many patients report wanting explanations and diagnostic information, research has shown that patients do not often ask questions (Beisecker and Beisecker 1990; Frankel 1990; ten Have 1991a; Todd 1983; West 1983, 1984). For example, Beisecker and Beisecker (1990) found that patients rarely asked direct questions or initiated a topic to gain information, or asked the physician for clarification (an average of three questions per interaction). In fact, almost one third of their sample made no attempts to seek information. In a study of family practice interviews, West (1984) discovered that only nine percent of all questions asked were initiated by patients, just as Frankel (1990) observed that patients initiated questions only one percent of the time. For numerous reasons (e.g., intimidation of the physician's expertise or social standing, fear of looking ignorant, fear of "bothering" or wasting the physician's time), patients seem to ask few, if any, direct questions. Two central questions thus arise: Might patients be seeking information in ways other than direct questioning? Or, alternatively, are patients the passive recipients they have been construed to be in medical encounters (Parsons 1951)?

Fifth, it seems reasonable to assume that patients seek assurance and information in ways other than by asking direct questions to medical experts. Several studies have observed that patients who make requests do so indirectly (Cegala 1997; Cegala et al. 2000; Gill et al. 2001; Robinson 2001), but little research has examined *how* patients might go about soliciting assurance and information, in specific, diagnostic data. An exception is the work of Gill and colleagues (Gill 1998; Gill et al. 2001; Gill and Maynard in press). For example, in a single case analysis Gill et al. (2001) found that a patient's request for medical action involving diagnostic testing was delicately oriented to. Instead of directly asking for a diagnostic test, the patient mentioned the concern of a third party (i.e., her children) as a reason for taking such action. In addition, Gill (1998) identified three types of explanation strategies employed by patients to solicit diagnostic information: speculative (common), unmitigated (less usual), and explanations embedded in overt questions (rare). The first two turn designs, not involving straightforward questions, only tentatively establish "conditional relevance" (Schegloff 1972) for a physician's evaluation. Moreover, explanations embedded in overt questions were not found in the data-gathering portion of the interviews. Yet all types of explanations were tailored to exhibit caution and to avoid disaffiliative responses (e.g., being ignored, being disagreed with). In essence, patients "cautiously downplayed their knowledge about the causes of their problems" (Schegloff 1972: 344) by exhibiting claims of uncertainty ("I don't know if ...", "whether"), attributions to third parties, and/or positioning the explanation as an aside (see also Haakana 2001).

It has also been observed that patients "frequently formulate their 'ignorance' or 'doubts' in various medical matters" by using "covert questioning" approaches that "do not have a question form and do not create a conditional relevance for an answer in the next slot. But they do display what the patient would like to know ..." (ten Have 1991a: 146). As ten Have examined one instance of a patient offering two lay diagnoses, it thus remains to be more fully explicated how patients' diagnoses or lay explanations get employed as practices designed to solicit assurance and/or diagnostic information from physicians (e.g., in contrast to asking direct questions).

We address alternative interactional strategies employed by patients as they seek assurance, and solicit diagnostic information, during openings and data-gathering activities within medical interviews. The moments we analyze reveal that patients do not necessarily "play by the book," at least in traditional and biomedical terms. For example, they may seek assurance even before being examined, and/or during other interview phases, prior to normal "slots" when medical professionals deliver diagnoses and formulate treatment strategies. And as noted above, physicians' responses to such "premature" solicitations confirm their problematic nature. Considering ongoing attempts to foster physician–patient partnership building that stresses shared participation and decision-making (see Emanual and Emanual 1992; Hall et al. 1988; McWhinney 1989), it seems warranted to further investigate how patients solicit physicians' responses for care and diagnosis.

Below we briefly describe the data and methods employed for this investigation, analyze a series of moments wherein patients solicit physicians' responses, and conclude by raising study limitations and implications for clinical application.

## 1. Data and methods

This study is based on videorecordings of naturally occurring medical visits between physicians and patients.[2] Transcriptions from these recordings follow Jefferson's notation system (Sacks et al. 1974).

Conversation analytic methods are employed (e.g., see Drew and Heritage 1992; Heritage and Atkinson 1984; Sacks 1992), and priority is given to locating and substantiating participants' methods for organizing and thus accomplishing social actions. This mode of analytic induction is anchored in repeated listenings of recordings, in unison with systematic inspections of carefully produced transcriptions. It is an explicit and working feature of this research method that participants continually and instrinsically achieve, through an array of interactional practices, displayed understandings of emergent interactional circumstances. The overriding goal is to identify patterned orientations to moment-by-moment contingencies of interaction comprising everyday life events.

The data set includes 25 videotaped patient–general practitioner interviews (preceded with an S in the heading of reported data instances), supplemented by six medical student/actor videotaped interviews (preceded with an F). Medical staff are relatively young (thirty-six years or less), and include eight males and three females. Patients include males and females of a wide age range, experiencing a variety of health concerns (e.g., allergic reactions, back problems, high blood pressure, suspected pregnancy, growths, pregnancy check-up, heart palpitations, constant coughing, chest tightness). No grave or imminently life-threatening cases were present in the data set (cases that were perhaps referred to outside specialists). Instances of patient solicitations during opening, and data-gathering or question-answer phases (i.e., approximately the first ten minutes) of the visits were identified and collected for analysis.

## 2. Soliciting assurance about "hope" and acknowledgment of "pain"

We begin our analysis with two instances drawn from different medical interviews – the first from the opening moments, and the second from the data-gathering portion of a clinical encounter.

In Excerpt (1), consider how the patient (P) expresses his "hope" that the physician (Dr) "can find out what's wrong with me" (1 →):

(1) S14:1

|  |  |  |
|---|---|---|
|  | Dr: | H'lo Mister Steen.= |
|  | P: | =Good morning. |
|  |  | (2.0) |
|  | Dr: | I'm Doctor Krone. |
|  |  | (0.2) |
|  | P: | Pleased to meet sir. |
|  | Dr: | Nice to meet you.= |
| 1→ | P: | =Well I hope you can find out what's wrong with me. |

2→ Dr: We(h)ll I hadn't even seen you yet.
3→ P: (Ats whuh) I say I still say I hope you can find
out what's wrong with me.
[
4→ Dr: O:h, okay. (0.4) Well we will.
5→ P: Whatever you think whatever yo:- (0.5) u:h (0.3)
whatever it is tell me: so I can- (0.7) eh- (0.7)
(keepn gih-) get somethin done about it. Cause (.)
ma:n (0.4) it's worrying me.

That the patient takes the initiative to raise his concerns, immediately following greetings and thus as a first item of business, suggests the importance of securing diagnostic information about what is assumed to be "wrong with me". With surprise marked by laughter and "We(h)ll" (2→), the physician does not treat the patient's prior utterance as an expression of anxiety and request for assurance. Rather, with "I hadn't even seen you yet.", the physician states the obvious with a factual statement in lieu of addressing the patient's unease. Next (3→), however, the patient does not abandon but pursues the consolation that the physician has withheld. By prefacing with "I still say," the patient proceeds to reiterate (1→) word-for-word.

Only then (4→) does the physician offer reassurance, apparently in recognition of the patient's steadfastness, though not without some hesitation. With "well we will" notice also that the physician depersonalizes his acknowledgment of the patient's expressed need for "hope," employing the lexical "we" to signify institutional affiliation (see Drew and Heritage 1992), rather than a personal commitment to provide care for a patient who has twice requested that "I hope you can find out." As the patient continues (5→), however, he retains "you" and shifts from what the physician might "think" to an explicit request to "tell me." In response to the apparent ambiguity between the physician's impersonal acknowledgment, and the patient's personalization with "you," the patient also produces numerous pauses and dysfluencies, amounting to what the patient eventually specifies: "ma:n (0.4) it's worrying me."

Of interest here, particularly in the context of expressed "hope," are the lexical affiliates "we," "you," and "me." The enactment of these usages display delicate, and potentially troubling connections, as these speakers manage what appear to be contrasting orientations to just what constitutes the physician–patient *relationship*: In what ways is the physician acting as a bureaucratic representative unwilling (and/or unable) to treat this patient with "personal" care?

In Excerpt (2), from the data-gathering portion of another medical interview, a patient responds to a physician's question by describing the location of the pain, and how hurting his back in an accident has resulted in a limited range of movement:

(2) S6:3

| | | |
|---|---|---|
| | P: | From here down. (0.4) pt And I can't *turn* from side to s*i*de like I *u*sually do because it, it gets re:al (0.3) painful you know. I can turn so *far* and then I just can't go that way anymore. |
| 1→ | | (0.5) |
| 2→ | P: | I'm just *won*dering because I never had any ↑back problems before (0.2) what the *prob*lem is. |
| 3→ | | (0.5) |
| 4→ | Dr: | Okay .h you noticed that immediately. |

As the physician does not verbally respond to the patient's "painful" description (1→), the patient continues (2→) with "I'm just *won*dering because I never had any ↑back problems before." This explanation accomplishes two key actions: (a) the patient provides an account, essentially a justification for the prior description, that is an upshot of the physician's failure to respond in (1→); and (b) the patient expresses a desire for an explanation and thus diagnosis from the physician. Akin to "fishing devices," which seek yet fall short of directly requesting information (Pomerantz 1980), the patient has solicited but not received from the physician either an acknowledgment or diagnosis for his pain (see Heath 1988).

As the interview continues, the physician further withholds a response in (3→). With an "Okay"-prefaced question, the physician then shifts attention away from what the patient has solicited and toward a data-gathering agenda. The physician, however, does not treat the request as a matter of business at hand for her. She minimally acknowledges the patient's solicitation ("Okay") before continuing with what is treated as business as usual for her, that is, the diagnostic inquiry. Prior research on institutional interactions has demonstrated that "okay"-prefaced questions function to ensure completion of a previous answer as sufficient, while also initiating next-positioned and agenda-relevant matters (Beach 1992, 1995; Hopper et al. 1993; Jones 1994b; Sorjonen and Heritage 1991).

To summarize thus far, it is clear that patients may proactively (Excerpt 1) or more indirectly (Excerpt 2) solicit a variety of responses – assurance about hopes and anxieties, personal care, acknowledgment and information about "pain" – that are responded to by physicians in ways that neither assuage patients' unease nor provide diagnostic information prior to the "officially" designated time near the end of the medical visit. Both during opening and data-gathering phases of interviews, patients' solicitations create a dilemma for physicians. As physicians display an unwillingness and/or inability to temporarily place their agendas aside to address patients' stated concerns, contrasts in "agendas" are readily apparent. These instances are aligned with extant findings that patient-initiated questions are in general dispreferred by physicians (i.e., do not always elicit a direct answer) (Frankel 1990; West 1983, 1984; West and Frankel 1991), particularly in the data-gathering phase when "covert" questioning utterances are most often ignored by physicians yet sometimes addressed later in the interview (ten Have 1991a). Similarly, Gill (1998) observed that physicians rarely responded immediately to speculative explanations – though again, sometimes did attend to them much later in the visit – or to unmitigated explanations, but did respond to rarely used explanations embedded in overt questions.

## 3. Patients' solicitations and physicians' withholdings of diagnostic information

Our data suggest that when patients solicit "early" diagnostic information but not by asking overt questions, physicians recognize that requests are being made yet withhold providing a diagnosis. Five distinct yet overlapping interactional environments are identified where patients pursue diagnostic information: (a) expressing an interest in and/or need for an "early" diagnosis; (b) offering a self-diagnosis; (c) attempting to assist with the inquiry; (d) adding evidence and observations; and (e) stating uncertainty and a lack of medical knowledge. Patients' attempts to solicit diagnostic data vary in displayed tentativeness. Throughout, patients treat their diagnostic solicitations as delicate interactional business, just as physicians display differing types of resistance to indirectly formulated diagnostic requests during interviews.

### *3.1. Expressing an interest in and/or need for diagnostic information*

In pursuit of diagnostic information, it has been noted that patients overwhelmingly do not use overt questions directed specifically to the physician. For example, requests for diagnosis do not typically appear as "Doctor Baker, do I have meningitis?" or "What is the reason for this problem, Doctor Gonzalez?" Rather, patients enact indirect requests during elaborations often involving the personal pronoun "I": my-world depictions of what patients have been feeling, thinking, and noticing about their condition. One routine usage includes the word "just" (e.g., "I just"), which may function to minimize and (literally) *justify* a request for information.

Consider Excerpt (3), which begins with a patient stating "I'm hoping that it's nothing."

(3) F2:5
→ P: pt .hhhhh- Well- uhhh .hh I'm hoping that
→ it's nothing. But it's just sorta been
bothering me and I thought I maybe should

| | | |
|---|---|---|
| | | (0.2) .hhhhhhh check into what's going on.= |
| | | The last um (1.2) bout three months .hhh I've |
| | | noticed that I have b*ee*n: br*ui*sing a lo:t |
| | | more easily than I ever did before in my life. |
| | | (1.2) |
| → | P: | .hhhhhh A:nd it's: not a- major problem. But I |
| | | just wonder if:: there's n a *rea*son for this. |
| | | [ |
| | Dr: | Um hm. |
| | | (1.0) |
| | Dr: | O:kay where have you been br*ui*sing. |

The patient continues by reporting that because her bruising has been bothering her, "I thought I maybe should (0.2) .hhhhhhh check into what's going on." This depiction reflects some uncertainty but also, as evident in her extended inbreath (".hhhhhhh"), a resolve to seek assistance with what may be a medical condition requiring treatment. The patient also utilizes an extreme qualifier to characterize her bruising ("more easily than I ever did before in my life") that solicits but does not receive uptake (e.g., in the form of an assessment or commentary) from the physician (see Jones 2001).

In response to more than a full second pause, the patient continues by minimizing her problem (almost apologetically). She then indirectly pursues diagnostic information by stating "But I just wonder if:: there's n a *rea*son for this." By not requesting from the physician an immediate and direct explanation for bruising, but instead articulating that she is "wondering" what might be the problem, the patient accomplishes two key actions: she hedges by assuming responsibility for her inquiry, and actively avoids putting the physician "on the spot" to offer diagnostic insights.

Through an extended pause, once again the physician withholds response to the patient's obvious request for diagnostic-relevant information. And with an "okay-prefaced" next question, she seeks instead data about the location of the patient's bruising.

It has been observed that patients' utterances such as "But I just wonder if:: there's n a *rea*son for this," as summarized in Excerpt (3), and "I'm just *won*dering because I never had any ↑back problems before (0.2) what the *prob*lem is" (Excerpt 2), are recruited to achieve a number of social actions: displaying my-world concerns (i.e., cognitive concerns via "wonder/*won*dering" in these two instances), explicitly avoiding direct requests, and imposing less conditional relevance or responsibility on the physician to generate diagnostic insights in response to these indirect ruminations. Even when it was clear that patients were making requests (via expressions of an interest/need for diagnosis), physicians tended not to provide diagnostic "answers."

In the following Excerpt (4) (an extension of Excerpt 2, above), it becomes further clarified that even when a patient repeatedly pursues information about a diagnosis relevant to back injury, such information is not forthcoming from this physician. Additional attempts to become informed about their case, i.e., an extension of "pursuit of response" (see Beach 1996; Pomerantz 1984a), don't compel physicians to revise a protocol in which "diagnosis" is slotted to occur *only* following data-gathering and physical examination:

(4) S6:3,4
P: From here down. (0.4) pt And I can't *turn* from<br>
*si*de to *si*de like I usually do because it, it<br>
gets re:al (0.3) *p*ainful you know. I can turn<br>
*so far* and then I just can't go that way anymore.<br>
(0.5)<br>
P: I'm just *won*dering because I never had any ↑back<br>
problems before (0.2) what the *prob*lem is.<br>
(0.5)<br>
1→ Dr: Okay .h you noticed that immediately.<br>
(0.4)<br>
P: Yes ma'am.<br>
[<br>
1→ Dr: Following? Or later: (0.2) that night.<br>
2→ P: We:ll it got *wor*se as ti:me (0.2) you know, went<br>
*on* (0.2) but I've *no*ticed *it* (0.2) at the time<br>
it *hap*pened. But- you know- (0.2) I just didn't pay<br>
any attention because you know (.) usually (0.2)<br>
stuff like that just go a*way*.<br>
3→ Dr: Mm hm.<br>
3→ (0.8)<br>
4→ P: But it hadn't went away yet (0.2) and I just<br>
want to know *why*.<br>
5→ Dr: .hh The reason why: you waited til Monday to<br>
come into the emergency room?

It was earlier noted that in (1→) the physician does not offer an assessment nor commentary, but shifts back to data-gathering by focusing on *when* the patient noticed back-related problems. The patient responds (2→) that it got worse with time, and noticed when it happened, but didn't attend to the discomfort "because you know (.) usually (0.2) stuff like that just go a*way*." In (3→) the physician minimally acknowledges the patient's description, withholds further commentary, and in these ways facilitates continuation by the patient.

Here the patient constructs a more direct and even command-like request, but carefully so. With "I just want to know *why*," the patient's "I" assumes responsibility and in this environment, "just" minimizes his request. This bolder statement may very well be the upshot of the patient not having received, in a prior and first attempt to solicit diagnostic information ("I'm just *won*dering"), an adequate response from the physician. Yet the patient is no more successful at securing such an explanation. Indeed, the patient's utterance is responded to with an almost accusing question from the physician (5→). It is curious that the physician responds with a "why" of her own, as though she is positioning herself as an expert for whom it is appropriate to ask "why" questions. In this sense, the physician displays resistance by treating the patient's second, and more direct attempt to solicit diagnostic information, as a "breach" of order and protocol.[3]

### *3.2. Offering a self-diagnosis*

In a study of general practice patients surveyed before they went into their visits, almost forty percent offered opinions about what they believed to be wrong with them (McKinley and Middleton 1999). Hence, many patients have conceptions of what is wrong with their health prior to medical consultation, and may make their opinions or self-diagnoses available for the physician's consideration (e.g., agreement or disagreement).

Similar to the request strategy of expressing an interest/need for diagnostic information, self-diagnoses also display patients' reflections or my-world summaries of their conditions. Likewise, it is clear from the instances above, and other available data, that patients' self-diagnoses are often built tentatively and with marked uncertainty. These utterances are commonly constructed as speculative self-diagnoses and self-proclaiming diagnostic assertions ("I think it's x") (Gill 1998). They routinely include features such as self-referent qualifiers ("I think"), modals ("may," "maybe"), verbal hesitations or dysfluencies ("uh"), pauses, and attempts to acknowledge limitations of their explanations as being only "part of it" (i.e., the medical problem). With the exception of overt questions – a rarity in the data set employed for this analysis, as only two overt questions were identified that were designed by patients to address a possible diagnosis – these solicitations do not directly request an evaluation. Thus, less pressure is imposed on physicians to confirm or disconfirm the lay diagnoses. In short, physicians' responses to patients' self-diagnoses, including both non-responses (i.e., questions shifting topic) and cautious evaluations, display some degree of resistance to patients' diagnostic solicitations.

In the following segment, a patient's self-diagnosis gets no immediate response from the physician.

(5) S18:5

P: <I don't know it's probably because this: (0.2)
I don't know why but (0.2) my left nostril *blee*ds.

| | | |
|---|---|---|
| | | (0.4) |
| | P: | Pretty of*t*en. |
| | | (0.4) |
| → | P: | ((sniff)) And that may be the reason I dunno. |
| | | (0.2) |
| | Dr: | You been taking anything, (0.2) any medicine?= |

Here the physician has asked the patient about a second health problem, a sore throat. After a sufficient and newsworthy answer concerning the problem and a possible cause, we see a gap as the patient withholds speaking and the physician does not provide an assessment or commentary. The patient then pursues a response by noting the frequency of the bleeding, and again after no uptake from the physician states that the bloody nostril may be the reason for the bloody phlegm (→). In other words, he offers a "candidate" diagnosis of the problem (see Pomerantz 1988). Notice that the patient mitigates his utterance by adding "And that may be the reason I dunno," discounting actions confirming the adage that while patients may not be assumed capable of understanding medical causation, physicians are and may thus be expected to share their knowledge.

Instead of immediately addressing the patient's concern, however, we see the physician disattending the patient's explanation and, by asking a question concerning his taking of medication, resisting any elaborated response to it. The result is that a patient's self-diagnosis receives no adjacent uptake or evaluation from the physician.

Physicians' responses may vary, of course, but in general terms they display resistance to directly address patients' self-diagnoses. However, in approximately forty percent of self-diagnostic instances in this category, physicians did display an orientation to the relevance of an answer. These responses included cautious evaluation of patients' self-diagnoses, confirming or disconfirming the possibility fashioned with a noncommittal quality. The confirming, affiliative remarks tended to involve short responses followed by the physician quickly getting back to business as usual (i.e., asking a question). The disconfirming, disaffiliative comments, on the other hand, seemed to require a bit more interactional work. They were longer, usually including some type of medical evidence or rationale for the disagreement or disconfirmation, and often were prefaced with delay devices (e.g., "well," "you know"). Despite the lack of commitment or conviction, these responses may nevertheless indicate physician interest in and attention to patients' ideas and opinions.

In the next three instances, for example, patients' diagnostic attempts elicit a brief confirmation (Excerpt 6), but also recurring evidence of disconfirmation in Excerpts (7) and (8). Beginning with Excerpt (6), a woman visits the clinic for a pregnancy checkup. She has noted some "spells" where she sweats "like crazy" and feels like she's going to faint:

(6) S10:2
Dr: Wai- when do you usually notice that.
(0.8)
P: Well usually I get it- (0.3) when I go to class.
It's- this *one* buildin I don't know if it's-
→ it may just be because I go from the cold
into that. (That's part of it)
[ ]
Dr: A::h that's a possi bility.
(0.3)
P: (That's so stupid.) Huh hah.
[
Dr: S- so it's usually the same place every time?

After being asked by the physician "when do you usually notice that," the patient offers a diagnosis that her spells may result from going into a presumably hot building from the cold outside (→). Her "I don't know"-prefaced description (see Beach and Metzger 1997) is uncertain and tentative (i.e., marked with a halting and repaired "it's- it," a limiting phrase, and qualifier).

This solicitation for diagnostic information is somewhat successful. The physician offers a short confirmation ("that's a possibility"), albeit lacking in conviction. He attends to and treats the patient's diagnostic idea as potentially relevant. After a (0.3) pause, he continues by asking a question to specify the location.

Excerpt (7) involves a patient with a swollen foot:

(7) S2:5
Dr: >>It's n^ot<< (0.3) a *rea*l: common place
for- (1.0) One of two things that we (0.6)
have to kind of distinguish (.) between is
uh (0.2) problems like this is whether or
not this is a *ca*llus?
(1.0)
Dr: From- (from way- here or down.)
[
→ P: Or a cancer.
Dr: Bahhh hah (h) are you(h) afraid it's cancer?
huh huh uhh Doesn't look like cancer,
alright?
(0.2)
Dr: Bu what we call a pl*a*nter's *wart*
(0.2)
P: That's no-
[
Dr: Are you familiar with that?

After the physician states one of the two diagnostic possibilities she will "distinguish (.) between" (callus), the patient offers a lay diagnostic possibility ("cancer") (→), in anticipation of the physician's second option.

The physician does respond to the patient's candidate possible diagnosis by disagreeing with it. She initially addresses the patient's probable fear by asking him if he is "afraid it's cancer?" However, she treats it as an irrational, or perhaps even "silly" suggestion, by displaying laugh tokens before, during, and after her question. Subsequently, the physician does address the issue with some seriousness as she tells him that it "doesn't look like cancer," even including an "alright" (displaying emphasis and reassurance, with a mild response-elicitation quality). She next explicates her second diagnostic option, a planter's wart, by implying it is a more likely diagnosis.

Interestingly in this instance, the physician explicitly addresses the patient's potential fear, quickly offers an "early" diagnosis, and continues to discuss it with the patient. She displays some sensitivity (albeit oddly designed) to the patient's candidate explanation, perhaps in response to the serious and extreme nature of it.

Next, in a follow-up visit, a patient experiencing tightness in his chest and stomach area has been told, at the beginning of the encounter, that his heart test came back negative. The patient showed initial resistance to this evaluation by noting the continuing nature of the problem:

```
(8)      S4:11
  1→     P:       Well I think it's just that (0.6) flare
                  up from that (0.5) gout a little bit
                  maybe (   ).
                        [
         Dr:            We:ll hh you know r: you really expect your
                  uric acid to be a lot higher though on that.
                                                     [
         P:                                          Yeah.
                  (0.6)
         Dr:      .hh So I really can't hang it off on that.(0.2)
                  The: uric acid's just not high enough. (0.2)
                  .hh It may be that- (0.2) that- you know either you
                  did something that you're not used to doin,
  2→     P:       What about ulcers.
                            [
         Dr:                .hh (And it has    )
                                            [
         P:                                 Is ulcer (.) wull it
                  wouldn't fit (          ).
                            [
         Dr:                Wull it doesn't really sound like an
                  ulcer though.
```

In this later segment, the patient offers two candidate diagnostic possibilities (1→, 2→), gout or ulcers. After delaying ("Well"), he takes responsibility for the first suggestion by saying "I think," pauses, diminishes the self-diagnosis ("a little bit"), and finally qualifies it with "maybe" (1→).

Although the physician responds by disconfirming the patient's explanation, he does orient to the relevance of an evaluation by quickly addressing it. He begins his utterance with delay, and offers a medical rationale for his disagreement in a cautious manner. The disconfirmation is repeated with reference to the test findings, and by offering a candidate causation.

In (2→) the patient does not respond to the physician's possible explanation, and instead offers another one of his own. Notice that this solicitation is designed as a direct request, not proffered in a tentative manner. Perhaps this is an expression not only of the patient's frustration from a "failed" first self-diagnosis, but also an upshot of simply attempting to deal with the inevitable *uncertainty* of continued discomfort following an informing of negative test results. The patient's assertiveness may thus be a consequence of both the "difficult" nature of the visit with the "no problem" initial finding, but also the inevitable *indeterminancy* that Maynard and Frankel (in press) have described as being associated with "symptom residue":

> ... potential irrationality is evoked when physicians *don't know* or are *uncertain* about the answers to medical questions... Despite the good news that some disease is not present, patients still have pains and symptoms, and doctors cannot yet assert anything definitive to account for them. (Maynard and Frankel in press: 27, 31)

Notice also that the patient eventually backs down from his second candidate diagnosis, which the physician next and immediately responds to with a more assured position – that the problem "doesn't really *sou*nd like an ulcer though." This response by the physician may itself be one way of asserting some certainty in the face of hanging doubts and thus "symptom residue" (see also Excerpt 14, below).

Researchers have identified other and related practices that physicians employ in situations of anticipated patient resistance to diagnosis (Heritage and Stivers 1999; Peräklyä 1998). Of particular interest here is that while the physician may not be able to eliminate the indeterminacy which negative test results have created about the patient's tightness in his chest and stomach, a lack of diagnostic capability may itself promote collaborative involvement in the medical encounter. In Excerpt (8), we observed that the patient twice offers a self-diagnosis and the physician responds with disconfirmation. Although they are disagreeing responses, they do reveal that the physician is treating the patient's participation in the visit as potentially relevant and useful – a source of information that, in essence, allows the physician to act (albeit through disconfirmation and disagreement) with *some* authority in the midst of unresolved diagnostic problems and resulting indeterminacy.

### *3.3. Attempting to assist with the inquiry*

Patients attempt to assist physicians with diagnostic inquiries in ways other than by offering self-diagnoses. For example, they may ask about medical test results, suggest factors that may be aggravating their current medical problems, and inquire about physical examination findings. In these ways, patients actively elicit diagnostic information by raising and inquiring about potential factors that may facilitate physicians' diagnoses.

These solicitations are enacted through direct questions, and speculative assertions, regarding specific medical findings. As with the data examined previously, these actions are also initiated with tentativeness and uncertainty. Tag questions, restarts, verbal hesitancies, and remarks deferring to the physician's expertise ("that you could tell") are apparent.

For example, Excerpt (9) involves the same patient with chest and stomach tightness that was examined in Excerpt (8):

```
(9)      S4:3
  →      P:       =What is- what is the uric acid on this.
         Dr:      pt This one's six point fo:ur. hh
         P:       Yeah so that about-
                                  [
         Dr:                      Which is bout where that last
                  one was also.
```

As noted above, the physician has stated earlier that an EKG test came back negative (i.e., no cardiac or heart problem). After discussing this and continuing symptoms, the patient asks about the results of another test (uric acid), mitigated with a restart displaying some hesitation (Jones 2003). The physician provides a specific response with "Pt this one's six point fo:ur. hh," displaying not resistance but alignment with the patient's solicitation for diagnostically relevant information. Of course, such information is not only readily available and retrievable by the physician, but is a small portion of data that needs to be considered to construct an overall diagnosis of the problem.

In another patient's follow-up visit in Excerpt (10), the patient has been told that his heart palpitations are "normal" and "happen to a lot of people." Similar to the patient in Excerpt (8) (above), he initially resisted the "no problem" diagnostic report by noting the extreme nature of his continuing symptoms, but received no explanation from the physician:

(10) S31:3

→ P: But the- the blood pressure uh a- appears
to be good doe sn't it.
[
Dr: Uh huh exactly. .hh You
don't seem to- be having any symptoms of
like congestive heart failure. .hhh Don't
have a history
[
→ P: I never had nothing like that other than this.
[
Dr: Yeah (0.2) exactly.

In this later segment, by asking a question regarding the results of his blood pressure reading, the patient raises another possibility for consideration. Again, the query is tentatively constructed with restarts, a verbal hesitation, and a tag question (see Winefield et al. 1989). The physician treats the assertion and tag question as a request and responds to it. He agrees with the patient and continues by noting that the patient is "exactly" correct, and offers his medical opinion regarding the lack of symptoms and history. The patient next confirms by declaring his lack of history, yet qualifies with "other than this" that is quickly affirmed in overlap by the physician. Interestingly, after some initial hesitancy on the part of the patient, this brief segment illustrates a trajectory of agreement and support.

In short, unlike the previously described patient methods of attempting to solicit diagnostic information, physicians in Excerpts (9) and (10) were responsive to patients' efforts to assist with diagnostic inquiry. Both physicians offered immediate, direct, and somewhat expanded answers rather than display resistance to patients' attempts to seek diagnostic information. Several explanatory influences seem plausible. First, it should be noted that these brief instances involve "difficult" or "hard" follow-up medical visits, ones involving "no problem" diagnoses. As alluded to earlier, it is possible that physicians were displaying sensitivity to patients' frustration about indeterminate health predicaments, evident in part by overtly phrased patient questions imposing more "pressure" on physicians to respond more directly. Second, being focused on particular and specific medical findings (e.g., test or exam results as opposed to an overall diagnosis), the questions and speculative assertions might be more straightforward and therefore easier for physicians to address.

### *3.4. Adding evidence and observations*

An alternative way to seek diagnostic information from a physician is to offer additional evidence and observations that a patient considers potentially relevant to the inquiry. These self-initiated observations seem to occur in two environments: (a) in "nonproblematic" moments during data-gathering, with patients appearing to be "helpful," and (b) in "problematic" instances, displaying a disagreeing quality or resistance to the physician's stance. In both environments patients exhibited only mild levels of tentativeness or discomfort, actions standing in contrast to other and previously examined solicitation strategies. Although possibilities for physicians' disagreements and disconfirmations remain, patients appear to be more assured when presenting evidence derived from knowledge of and experiences with their own bodies (Gill 1998). In the following examples, patients self-initiate by volunteering different kinds of personal experiences and observations.

In Excerpt (11) a patient is reporting, to her regular physician, about an emergency room visit the day before:

```
(11)      S3:4
          P:        Yeah (.) they gave me shot.
          Dr:       They gave ya a shot.
                                [
          P:                     For the headache and the (0.4) vomiting.
                    But it didn't help any.
          Dr:       It didn't help the headache either?
                    (0.3)
          P:         No:.
                    [
          Dr:        Or the vomiting.
   →      P:        N- I had chills all night so I think I'ms (0.4)
                    probly got the flu.
          Dr:       .hhhhh Did you: (1.0) take your insulin today?
```

After confirming for the physician that the shot she received in the ER did not relieve her symptoms of headache and vomiting, the patient volunteers an additional symptom (chills) and concludes with a candidate explanation (flu) (→). Notice that the first part of her utterance, where she expresses her physical experience is stated with no hesitations. However, her subsequent self-diagnosis (flu) is offered with mitigation and hesitancy. When comparing the two, then, it is evident that while the patient displays entitlement and expertise about her body, she is more tentative when offering her diagnosis for the physician's consideration.

In response, the physician does not offer any diagnostic commentary on the patient's reported evidence (chills) and lay diagnosis (flu). Instead, she continues with the next question about "*in*sulin" and thereby resists the patient's bid for evaluation as an indirect request for diagnositic confirmation or disconfirmation.

Next, a patient is visiting a physician for the first time for a previously diagnosed problem of high blood pressure:

(12) S25:12

Dr: And the top figure below a hundred an three.
[
→ P: But see ↑I had it ch^ecked yesterday (0.7) and it was a hundred and three over eighty: eight.
(1.0)
Dr: Yeah.
(0.6)
Dr: Aga:in (0.4) it's hardta (0.3) ta make the diagn*o*sis of (0.3) high blood pressure with one (0.3) reading.
P: Mmkay.
(1.2)
Dr: U::h may:be (0.3) we have another one h^ere when you were h^ere back in May.

After the physician comments that her blood pressure is "n^ot too bad," the patient quickly offers (in overlap with the physician's turn) self-initiated information emphasizing the volatility of her problem (→). With the exception of her (0.7) pause, the patient displays no signs of being tentative, hesitant, or reluctant to state her experience.

With an extended (1.0) pause, followed by "Yeah," the physician's minimal response declines to immediately confirm or deny the evidence the patient has articulated. Following another (0.6) pause, the physician reemphasizes a position that a single reading does not constitute a diagnosis, essentially discounting the patient's earlier offering. Yet with "Mmkay," the patient nevertheless acquiesces to the physician's unwillingness to take seriously her single reporting of yesterday's results. Notice, though, that during another long pause the physician does inspect the medical chart, and locates a possible blood pressure reading from a previous visit.

The following encounter involves a patient who has just received a negative test result for chest pain (see also Excerpts 8 and 9). Similar to earlier observations, the patient appears to be resisting the negative result by offering further information, including a self-diagnosis about "h*ea*rt palpitation" (1→):

(13) S31:1,2

P: Yeah but I- I don't tuh seem to (1.0) um
1→ (0.7) (feel it's- it's it's like a (0.3) extraordinarily (0.3) uh (1.0) h*ea*rt
[
Dr: Uh huh
1→ P: palpit*a*tion of the heart. 's It's- (0.2) it's more of a (1.0) (          )

[
2→ Dr: Like a little fibrillation.=
1→ P: =Fibrillation (.) for a period of time.
(.) And then I also have a- (.) a- (0.4)
very prominent tuh (0.4) *sur*ge there.
[
Dr: Uh huh.
1→ P: Or a h*ea*rt (0.6) *beat.*
[ [
Dr: Uh huh. Exa-
Dr: Exactly.=
P: =But I noticed that tuh (0.4) very
[
Dr: Uh hmm.
P: predominant.
3→ Dr: Yeah.
(0.2)
P: You see u h
[
3→ Dr: Uh (1.4) I really can't tell you
why (.) those things happen.

The physician offers an alternative description, "fibrillation" (2→), one form of a delayed and collaborative completion (Lerner 1989), as he displays attentiveness to the patient's description by attempting to complete his thought. The patient next adopts "fabrillation" en route to offering additional details, which the physician monitors and first minimally acknowledges with "Uh huh." before more fully displaying recognition with "Exactly." But as the patient moves to summarize his reporting, the physician's "Uh hmm" and "Yeah" (3→) give rise to "Uh (1.4) I really can't tell you why (.) those things happen." Thus, even though the physician treats the patient's overview as a reporting deserving close monitoring, it is noticeably more: an indirect request for a diagnosis (i.e., a direct question has not been asked) that is not granted by the physician. Indeed, such a diagnosis is explicitly declined because of the physician's disclosed lack of knowledge. So doing leaves as indeterminate, of course, not only why test results failed to confirm the patient's experiences, but also other plausible explanations for his "prominent surges."

In Excerpt (14), the patient begins with "Wh- one ques:-" (1→), but does not fully articulate the "question" because it overlaps with the physician's utterance:

(14) S4:2
1→ P: Wh- one ques:-
[
Dr: You know there's:

|  |  |  |
|---|---|---|
|  |  | (0.8) |
|  | P: | When it went- ↑*I felt like-* (0.2) last night-<br>(0.7) right around my (0.2) my belly<br>right here it was. |
|  |  | [ |
|  | Dr: | Mm hm. |
|  | P: | When I when I went *ho*me a:nd a:h pt h:h<br>(1.0) u:h that seems strange it just like ah °hh<br>I got a little so- I got a s:- certain little<br>soreness. And it- kinna comes an goes. I'll have |
|  |  | [ |
|  | Dr: | Right. |
|  | P: | it here and then I'll have it in the back. |
|  | Dr: | Uh huh. |
|  | P: | .hh And then I might ha- have it right across here. |
| 2→ |  | I dunno that may be because I'm: (.) getting<br>(.) towards dinnertime. I dunno that might be<br>part of it guh huh. |
| 3→ | Dr: | Yeah. |
|  | ?: | hh |
| 3→ | Dr: | Well let me think. |

Though the question never gets asked, the patient elaborates about "soreness" (location, duration), which is closely monitored by the physician. The patient ends his self-initiated symptomatic observations with his own diagnosis (2→) that his discomfort may be occasioned by "dinner time" that is then followed with laughter ("guh huh"). Of interest here is that the patient is not inviting the physician to share in the laughter (Haakana 2001), and such shared laughter is not forthcoming. Rather, the patient treats the offering of additional observations and a self-diagnosis as delicate interactional business. It cannot be unequivocally determined whether the delicacy is an upshot of such matters as an atypical disclosure about eating, and/or hesitancy about volunteering a diagnostic possibility for the physician's consideration. What can be observed, and with some certainty, is that the patient's symptomatic descriptions and own explanation is in pursuit of a diagnosis that the physician – at this juncture of the interview – minimally acknowledges ("Yeah") but is unable and/or unwilling to provide ("Well let me think") (3→).

To summarize excerpts (11–14), it has been observed that physicians responded in two ways to patients' further evidence and observations. First, physicians did not respond to the additional data and instead asked other questions (as in Excerpt 11), commented on another part of the patient's utterance, or moved onto a physical test or examination. Second, physicians at times verbally declined to provide a diagnostic evaluation, as with excerpts (12) ("Aga:in (0.4) it's hardta (0.3) ta make the diagnosis of (0.3) high blood pressure with one (0.3) reading"), (13) ("I really can't tell you why (.) those things happen"), and (14) ("Let me think"). With these latter responses, physicians displayed explicit resistance to attempted solicitations for whatever reasons (e.g., lack of an explanation, not being ready yet, and/or lack of sufficient medical data). It should be noted that all the instances in the second response type are from "difficult" clinical visits involving a "no-problem" test result or further testing.

### *3.5. Stating uncertainty and a lack of knowledge*

In several previously examined excerpts (5, 6, and 14), patients have been shown to express a lack of knowledge en route to soliciting diagnostic explanations from physicians. These claims of insufficient knowledge (Beach and Metzger 1997; Metzger and Beach 1996), achieved in part through "I don't know" or "I dunno," occur in an array of interactional environments, but particularly are positioned at the end of some volunteered observations or at the end of an answer to a physician's question. Thus, patients qualify the positions they are forwarding for physicians' consideration and invite them to share their medical expertise. First, patients display an ability to describe certain bodily symptoms, and at times associated feelings about irregularities and/or discomforts. Yet in so doing they may also display recognition that their "medical" knowledge, and consequently their lay diagnoses about and explanations for health conditions, are not only limited but potentially wrong. Second, by claiming insufficient knowledge, patients orient to physicians as medical experts possessing two key attributes: comparatively more technical knowledge, and as bureaucratic representatives, authority to manage treatment and care.

Consider Excerpt (15), for example, as a physician inquires about previous testing on one of the patient's presenting complaints, blurry vision:

```
(15)    S34:10,11
        Dr:     Have you ever had your eyes checked.
                (0.6)
        Dr:     By: Doctor ((name)).
        P:      U:::m no no never ((name)) no.
                (0.2)
        Dr:     ↑Al right.
                   [
        P:         It's just when I come over to his
                office and he just (look at me). When I come
        Dr:     Uh huh.
        P:      they check my my my eyes over here an everything
                my ears an everything.
```

| | | |
|---|---|---|
| | | (.) |
| | Dr: | Okay. |
| → | P: | But I don't know what's goin on. |
| → | Dr: | °Kay.° Do you have any problems with uh-<br>your thyroid gland. (.) ((continues)) |

After answering negatively, the patient revises his answer by offering that during a past medical visit "they" had checked his eyes and ears. Receipted by the physician with "Okay," the patient qualifies "But I don't know what's goin on." This utterance distinguishes between the patient's ability to *report* on an examination, and actually *knowing* what the exams revealed. As a result of not being personally capable of rendering a diagnosis, in unison with his apparently not being informed of the diagnostic outcome by examiners, the patient facilitates the interview moving forward by making it obvious that it is the physician's medical and expert opinion that is required.

Notice, however, that no such opinion is offered in the physician's next response, a quiet "°Kay.°" preceding a shift to "thyroid gland" and thus away from rendering a diagnosis at this moment.

Again, in Excerpt (16), following a physician's query about symptom location, a patient's statements of uncertainty receive only minimal uptake:

| | | |
|---|---|---|
| (16) | S4:8-9 | |
| → | P: | (I'o'know) as I said it doesn't it's not there all<br>the time. |
| | Dr: | Mm hm. |
| | | [ |
| | P: | It'll be there for an hour or so and it'll seem<br>like it'll go away. But .hhhh then I have this (.)<br>cross around mah-. °hh But that was fine when I went<br>home, that was: yesterday was just (0.4) just *right.*<br>Like there was a kinna *fire* around there.= |
| | Dr: | =Mm hm. |
| → | P: | I don't know what that was. |
| | | (0.5) |
| | Dr: | Have you *no*ticed it at all when you eat your meals. |

Following the physician's first "Mm hm," the patient elaborates by describing location, duration, and severity of his pain. After a second withholding with "=Mm hm," however, the patient states "I don't know what that was." which not only disclaims his own knowledge, but creates an opportunity for the physician to offer an informed explanation. Rather than doing so, however, the physician exhibits resistance to pursue any diagnostic commentary in favor of seeking additional information about "meals."

When compared with earlier examined soliciting actions (i.e., expressing an interest in/need for diagnostic information, adding evidence and observations), it has become clear that when patients provide follow-up statements of insufficient knowledge (as in Excerpts 15 and 16), they too are unsuccessful. Physicians do not treat these qualifications as indirect solicitations deserving of immediate diagnostic remarks. Rather, they continue to pursue further information that may eventually be relevant for a diagnosis to be offered only when the physician determines that sufficient topics and concerns have been addressed.

## 4. Discussion

Patients have been shown to pursue what physicians treat as "premature" diagnostic explanations. In various ways, patients demonstrate subtle yet proactive capabilities transcending stereotypic notions of "passive involvement." By displaying interactional resistance to distinct and mandated phases of clinical interviews, traditional and biomedical procedures are repeatedly challenged. In turn, physicians routinely resist opportunities to expand upon actions soliciting early requests for diagnostic information. Therein lies a communicative disjuncture between patients and physicians, creating what is perhaps a universal set of interactional problems across daily medical encounters. Such appears to be the case even though we have identified moments wherein patients who enact a more active and participatory role are accommodated by physicians displaying flexibility when organizing interview structures. Instances were analyzed (about one third of the cases) where physicians answered overt questions with direct answers (albeit all in "difficult" visits), and cautiously dis/confirmed patients' lay diagnoses.

Patients have a variety of methods at their disposal to express their informational needs to physicians. By seeking diagnostic information at the outset and during data-gathering phases of interviews, an unwillingness is displayed to wait for physicians' "official" diagnoses to be revealed near the interview's conclusion. As patients are overwhelmingly tentative in their various solicitations, they reveal distinct orientations to their actions as delicate maneuvers while also legitimating physicians' authority and expert knowledge. Our analysis revealed that requests were rarely expressed as overt questions, and if so, were during "difficult" and repeat visitations exemplifying patients' frustration and/or determination to simply find out what is wrong.

More commonly, patients' soliciting actions were variably disguised as speculative assertions, statements of potentially medically-related observations, and/or expressions of the patient's my-world concerns and insufficient knowledge. These enacted devices are commonly associated with such notions as discomfort (Pomerantz 1984b), deference and powerlessness (O'Barr and Atkins 1980), politeness (Brown and Levinson 1989), delicateness and hesitancy (Jones 2003; Peräkylä 1995; 1998; Schegloff 1980). The majority of examined instances included an array of tentative markers: restarts, minimizing tokens ("just"), self-referent qualifiers ("I think"), modals, verbal hesitations, pauses, qualifying phrases ("part of it"), justifications, tag questions, and remarks deferring to physician expertise ("that you could tell"). Just as previous research has suggested that patients appear to have trouble "spitting out" their questions (West 1983), and that patients express their lack of entitlement to knowledge about causation (Gill 1998), so too have we evidenced that and how patients orient to soliciting diagnostic information as inherently delicate in the face of physicians' resistance.

These diverse forms of patient solicitations have different sequential implications for subsequent interaction. Solicitations phrased as various indirect requests, such as those found in the categories of offering a self-diagnosis and attempting to assist with the inquiry, are produced as though physicians are capable of hearing and responding with diagnostically relevant explanations. In these less frequent cases, physicians expressed cautious confirmation or disconfirmation of lay solicitations, offered direct answers (in "difficult" visits), or explicitly declined to provide requested information. In contrast, solicitations designed as assertions regarding additional evidence and patient concerns (i.e., expressing a lack of knowledge) seem to impose less constraint on physicians' next turns, evident in how physicians routinely shift away from patients' concerns and next ask questions forwarding their agenda. Patients' solicitations were generally unsuccessful, in such cases, apparent in the way they were treated by physicians as irrelevant, problematic, and/or inappropriate. The majority of physician responses were thus produced in such a manner as to display some level of resistance to patients' early solicitations of diagnostic information. As ten Have (1991b) suggested, physicians commonly "lay off" or do not comment on patients' complaints or solicitations, but instead passively tolerate such contributions before shifting to other aspects, topics, or activities. It is possible and perhaps likely that physicians would simply prefer that patients wait for an invited opportunity to add their observations and experiences. Similarly, physicians are not compelled to address patients' expressions of their my-world conditions, since psychosocial considerations are too infrequently treated as related to biomedical symptoms (Beach and Dixson 2001).

In most general terms, therefore, it appears warranted to conclude that physicians' actions do not yet reveal a proclivity toward "partnership building" emphasizing joint participation and decision-making during medical interviews. This is not a novel observation. Nor is it surprising to suggest that our study contributes to ongoing investigations delineating the intricately woven asymmetry evidenced in physician–patient interaction (ten Have 1991a; Maynard 1991; Modaff 1996b; Roberts 2000; Robinson 2001; Stivers and Heritage 2001; Treichler et al. 1984).

Such inquiries into clinical encounters share common concerns with findings uncovered in this chapter: repeated evidence that and how patients tentatively design diagnostic solicitations (indirectly and directly), and physicians' lack of, cautious, and/or topic-shifting responses. Our results describe one more way in which "asymmetries are produced *in and through the details* of the physicians' and patients' situated interactions" (ten Have 199la: 138). Through the examination of such details, we can observe "power relations as negotiated within the context of face-to-face interaction," rather than "established a priori by the differential position of individuals or groups within the social structure (e.g., patients and physicians)" (Treichler et al. 1984: 63).

We acknowledge several limitations of this project, and the opportunities available for future research endeavors. One limitation involves the examination of only traditional general practice interviews. It would be interesting to investigate patient diagnostic solicitations in other styles of medical encounters, such as Health Appraisal visitations in a Health Maintenance Organization (HMO) (see Beach and Dixson 2001; Beach and LeBaron 2002). Several questions arise: Would we find early solicitations of diagnostic information across alternative interview formats (e.g., health appraisal, surgical, pediatric, holistic, alternative, oncological, ophthalmological, osteopathic)? If so, how would these differently trained medical professionals respond (see Stivers 2002)? A related limitation of our study is that data did not include medical visitations involving severely ill patients. Severity of illness may impact patients' behavior in relation to their desire for diagnostic information, as with "difficult" problems requiring return visitations examined herein. As Good and Good (1982) concluded twenty years ago, "[p]roviding help in answering troubling questions and making sense of threatening life conditions is a very fundamental characteristic of medical care" (Good and Good 1982: 293).

Descriptive analyses such as the current study – providing findings illustrating momentary "breaches" in the conduct of the traditional biomedical interview (e.g., see Stivers and Heritage 2001), and how patients' methods of diagnostic information-seeking occasion alternative responses physicians exhibit to them (e.g., resistance) – could have important applications to diverse forms of clinical interaction in light of "new" partnership models, innovative patient education programs, medical resources available on the Internet, and drug advertisements on television:

- In what ways and in what situations do physicians' routinely respond by not attending to patients' early diagnostic solicitations, thus failing to show alignment with patients' actions?
- How might such disattending actions by physicians contribute to low patient satisfaction, return visitations (and thus expensive, "high volume" patients), and malpractice litigations? For example, Hickson et al.

(1994) discovered that patients' complaints about physicians with prior malpractice claims included receiving inadequate explanations or advice.

- Are resistant attempts to offer "early" diagnostic explanations associated with patients' perceptions that physicians are unsupportive and/or "unfriendly"?
- How might physicians' resistant actions be related to patients' unwillingness to follow treatment regimes, dissatisfaction, diminished health outcomes, healing, and "physician shopping"? Years ago, for example, Like and Zyzanski (1987) described how physicians' fulfillment of patients' requests was strongly related to patient satisfaction.

Recent research has also provided evidence that not all patients are concerned primarily with diagnostic explanations. Some are more interested in treatment of their conditions. Eisenthal et al. (1990) suggested that patient satisfaction and treatment adherence may be related to physicians' ability to distinguish between patients who are focused on medical explanations, versus patients who are focused on treatment. Specifically, "[a] patient focused on the problem only may feel misunderstood if treatment options are explained in detail while the problem is barely touched" (Eisenthal et al. 1990: 404). Being able to recognize various patient solicitations could help physicians identify patients' particular informational needs.[4]

Once it is evident to a physician that patient is seeking early diagnostic information, based on the interactional and inquiry needs of the moment, the physician can more clearly choose among response options at these junctures. For example, the physician may decide to put his/her line of questioning on hold to address the patient's request and/or alter an ongoing line of questioning. The research findings of Levinson et al. (1997), addressing remarks involving "orientation about the flow of the visit," point to an additional and potentially helpful option for physicians. Processual comments like "I'll have to ask you some more questions before I can comment on that," or "I'll need to take a look at it before I can tell," may function to assure the patient that the physician has "heard" the request but isn't able to address it immediately. In addition to addressing patient needs these utterances could also be time efficient for the physician, only momentarily sidetracking the diagnostic line of questioning. Levinson et al. (1997) noted that such orienting statements may "help the patient develop appropriate expectations about a medical visit. They may also inform the patient about when during the interview to raise concerns ..." (1997: 558). Moreover, processual or orientation utterances were linked with fewer malpractice claims (Levinson et al. 1997).

Finally, in addition to allowing medical professionals to observe and examine in detail these interactional moments, our findings may be of interest to patients. The physician responses we have identified illustrate the impact of various patient solicitation strategies, and may assist in patients' participative decisions. Patients who may desire to express their concerns early in the visit might somehow alter their behaviors in light of the phasic and processual nature of the medical history-taking. How might patients better negotiate with physicians about their "premature" concerns? In what ways might patients alter their expectations toward receiving early answers about diagnostic evaluation, and perhaps be less disappointed with physicians' responses? These queries only begin to address the need to take seriously a basic notion: Just as medical encounters are collaborative endeavors, so should educational opportunities be provided for patients to learn how to efficiently and successfully achieve their communicative needs regarding health and illness.

## *Notes*

1. See Uhlmann et al. (1984) for a discussion of the differences between the terms "patient expectations" and "patient desires."
2. Acknowledgement is extended to Richard Street and Richard Frankel for contributing materials employed in this analysis.
3. This moment is similar to how judges "regulate court traffic," at times "sanctioning" what they treat as inappropriate interactional conduct (e.g., speaking at the same time as the judge), and in this way instantiating their role, status, and power (see Beach 1995).
4. Although not a focus of the current project, instances involving patients requesting treatment information in the data-gathering phase were found.

## *References*

Babrow, A. S.

2001 Uncertainty, value, communication, and problematic integration. *Journal of Communication* 51, 553–573.

Babrow, A. S., C. R. Kasch, and L. A. Ford

1998 The many meanings of uncertainty in illness: Toward a systematic accounting. *Health Communication* 10, 1–23.

Beach, W. A.

1992 Agenda-based "institutional" relevancies of "okay-prefaced" queries. Paper presented at the annual meeting of the Speech Communication Association, Chicago.

1995 Judges' sanctions: Interactional techniques for regulating court traffic. Unpublished manuscript.

1996 *Conversations about Illness: Family Preoccupations with Bulimia*. Hillsdale, NJ: Lawrence Erlbaum.
2001a Introduction: Diagnosing "lay diagnosis". *Text* 21, 3–12.
2001b Stability and ambiguity: Managing uncertain moments when updating news about mom's cancer. *Text* 21, 221–250.
2006 (ed.). *Handbook of Patient–Provider Interactions: Raising and Responding to Concerns about Life and Illness*. Cresshill, NJ: Hampton Press.

Beach, W. A. and C. N. Dixson
2001 Revealing moments: Formulating understandings of adverse experiences in a health appraisal interview. *Social Science and Medicine* 52, 25–44.

Beach, W. A. and C. LeBaron
2002 Body disclosures: Attending to personal problems and reported sexual abuse during a medical encounter. *Journal of Communication* 52, 617–639.

Beach, W. A. and J. Mandelbaum
2005 (*in press*). "My mom had a stroke": Understanding how patients raise and providers respond to psychosocial concerns. In Harter, L. H., P. M. Japp, and C. M. Beck (eds.), *Constructing our Health: The Implications of Narrative for Enacting Illness and Wellness*. Mahwah, NJ: Lawrence Erlbaum Associates.

Beach, W. A. and T. R. Metzger
1997 Claiming insufficient knowledge. *Human Communication Research* 23, 562–588.

Beisecker, A. E. and T. D. Beisecker
1990 Patient information-seeking behaviors when communicating with physicians. *Medical Care* 28, 19–28.

Brown, P. and S. C. Levinson
1989 *Politeness: Some Universals in Language Usage*. New York: Cambridge University Press.

Button, G. and N. Casey
1989 Topic initiation: Business-at-hand. *Research on Language and Social Interaction* 22, 61–92.

Byrne, P. S. and B. E. L. Long
1976 *Physicians Talking to Patients: A Study of the Verbal Behaviors of Physicians in the Consultation*. London: HMSO.

Cegala, D. J.
1997 A study of physicians and patients communication during a primary care consultation: Implications for communication training. *Journal of Health Communication* 2, 169–194.

Cegala, D. J., L. McClure, T.M. Marinelli, and D. M. Post
2000 The effects of communication skills training on patients participation during medical interviews. *Patient Education and Counseling* 41, 209–222.

Drew, P.
2001 Spotlight on the patient. *Text* 21 (1/2), 261–268.

Drew, P. and J. Heritage
1992 Analyzing talk at work: An introduction. In Drew, P. and J. Heritage (eds.), *Talk at Work: Interaction in Institutional Settings*. Cambridge: Cambridge University Press, 3–65.

Eisenthal, S., C. Koopman, and J. D. Stoeckle
1990 The nature of patients requests for physicians help. *Academic Medicine* 65, 401–405.
Emanual, E. J. and L. L. Emanual
1992 Four models of the physician–patient relationship. *Journal of the American Medical Association* 267, 2221–2226.
Frank, A.
1991 *At the Will of the Body: Reflections on Illness.* Boston: Houghton Mifflin.
1997 *The Wounded Storyteller: Body, Illness, and Ethics.* Chicago: University of Chicago Press.
Frankel, R. M.
1990 Talking interviews: A dispreference for patient-initiated questions in physician–patient encounters. In Psathas, G. (ed.), *Interaction Competence: Studies in Ethnomethodology and Conversation Analysis.* Lanham, MD: University Press of America, 231–262.
Frankel, R. M. and H. B. Beckman
1988 The pause that refreshes. *Hospital Practice* 71, 62–67.
Gill, V. T.
1998 Doing attributions in medical interaction: Patients explanations for illness and physicians' responses. *Social Psychology Quarterly* 61, 342–360.
Gill, V. T., T. Halkowski, and F. Roberts
2001 Accomplishing a request with making one: A single case analysis of a primary care visit. *Text* 21(1/2), 55–81.
Gill, V. T. and D. W. Maynard
i. p. Patients' explanations for health problems and physicians' responsiveness in the medical interview. In Heritage, J. and D. W. Maynard (eds.), *Practicing Medicine: Structure and Process in Primary Care Consultations.* Cambridge: Cambridge University Press.
Good, M. D. and B. J. Good
1982 Patient requests in primary care clinics. In Chrisman, N. J. and T. W. Maretzki (eds.), *Clinically Applied Anthropology.* London: D. Reidel, 275–295.
Good, M. D., B. J. Good, and A. J. Nassi
1983 Patient requests in primary health care settings: Development and validation of a research instrument. *Journal of Behavioral Medicine* 6, 151–168.
Haakana, M.
2001 Laughter as a patient's resource: Dealing with delicate aspects of medical interaction. *Text* 21(1/2), 187–219.
Hall, J. A., D. L. Roter, and N. R. Katz
1988 Meta-analysis of correlates of provider behavior in medical encounters. *Medical Care* 26, 657–675.
Heath, C.
1988 Embarrassment and interactional organization. In Drew, P. and A. Wootton (eds.), *Erving Goffman: Exploring the Interaction Order.* Boston: Northeastern University Press, 136–160.
1992 The delivery and reception of diagnosis in the general-practice consultation. In Drew, P. and J. Heritage (eds.), *Talk at Work: Interaction in Institutional Settings.* Cambridge: Cambridge University Press, 235–267.

Heritage, J. and J. M. Atkinson
1984 Introduction. In Atkinson, J. M. and J. Heritage (eds.), *Structures of Social Action: Studies in Conversation Analysis.* Cambridge: Cambridge University Press, 1–15.
Heritage, J. and T. Stivers
1999 Online commentary in acute medical visits: A method of shaping patient expectations. *Social Science and Medicine* 49, 1501–1517.
Hickson, G. B., E. W. Clayton, and S. S. Entman
1994 Obstetricians' prior malpractice experience and patients' satisfaction with care. *Journal of the American Medical Association* 272, 1583–1587.
Hopper, R., W. R. Thomason, and J. A. Ward
1993 Demographic questions in telephone calls to a Cancer Information Service. *Southern Communication Journal* 58, 115–127.
Jones, C. M.
1994a Assessments in everyday talk: Initiating supportive trajectories. Paper presented at the annual meeting of the Western States Communication Association, San Jose, CA.
1994b Supportive communication in physician–patient interviews: The case of the missing assessments. Doctoral dissertation, University of Texas at Austin. Dissertation Abstracts International 55, 1420A.
2001 Missing assessments: Lay and professional orientations in medical interviews. *Text* 21(1/2), 113–150.
2003 Utterance restarts in telephone conversation: Marking topic initiation and reluctance. In Glenn, P., J. Mandelbaum, and C. LeBaron (eds.), *Excavating the Taken-for-Granted: Essays in Language and Social Interaction. A Festschrift for Robert Hopper.* London: Erlbaum, 137–149.
Lerner, G.H.
1989 Notes on overlap management in conversation: The case of delayed completion. *Western Journal of Speech Communication* 53, 167–177.
Levinson, W., D. L. Roter, J. P. Mullooly, V. T. Dull, and R. M. Frankel
1997 The relationship with malpractice claims among primary care physicians and surgeons. *Journal of American Medical Association* 277, 553–559.
Like, R. and S. J. Zyzanski
1987 Patient satisfaction with the clinical encounter: Social psychological determinants. *Social Science and Medicine* 24, 351–357.
Lutfey, K. and D. W. Maynard
1998 Bad news in oncology: How physician and patient talk about death and dying without using those words. *Social Psychology Quarterly* 61, 321–341.
Maynard, D. W.
1991 Interaction and asymmetry in clinical discourse. *American Journal of Sociology* 97, 448–495.
Maynard, D. W. and R. M. Frankel.
i. p. On the edge of rationality: Bad news, good news and uncertainty in primary care encounters. In Heritage, J. and D. W. Maynard (eds.), *Practicing Medicine: Talk and Action in Primary Care Encounters.* Cambridge: Cambridge University Press.

McWhinney, I.
1989 The need for a transformed clinical method. In Stewart, M. and D. Roter (eds.), *Communicating with Medical Patients.* Newbury Park: Sage, 25–40.

McKinley, R. K. and J. F. Middleton
1999 What do patients want from physicians: Content analysis of written patient agendas for the consultation. *British Journal of General Practice* 49, 796–800.

Metzger, T. R. and W. A. Beach
1996 Preserving alternate versions: Interactional techniques for organizing courtroom cross-examination. *Communication Research* 23, 749–765.

Mockapetris, A. M. and F. C. Craigie
1986 Patient requests in a family practice setting. *Family Practice Research Journal* 5, 216–225.

Modaff, D. P.
1996a The slots in a canonical physician–patient interview opening. Paper presented at the annual meeting of the Western States Communication Association, Pasadena, CA.
1996b Some systematically-asymmetrical activities in the physician–patient interview opening. Paper presented at the annual meeting of the Speech Communication Association, San Diego, CA.

O'Barr, W. M. and B. K. Atkins
1980 "Women's language" or "powerless language"? In McConnell-Ginet, S., R. Borker, and N. Furman (eds.), *Women and Language in Literature and Society.* New York: Praeger, 93–110.

Parsons, T.
1951 *The Social System.* New York: Free Press.

Peräkylä, A.
1991 Hope work in the care of seriously ill patients. *Qualitative Health Research* 1, 407–433.
1995 *AIDS Counseling: Institutional Interaction and Clinical Practice.* Cambridge: Cambridge University Press.
1997 Conversation analysis: A new model of research in physician–patient communication. *Journal of the Royal Society of Medicine* 90, 205–208.
1998 Authority and accountability: The delivery of diagnosis in primary health care. *Social Psychology Quarterly* 6, 301–320.

Pomerantz, A.
1980 Telling my side? Limited access as a fishing device. *Sociological Inquiry* 50, 186–198.
1984a Pursuing a response. In Atkinson, J. M. and J. Heritage (eds.), *Structures of Social Action: Studies in Conversation Analysis.* Cambridge: Cambridge University Press, 152–163.
1984b Agreeing and disagreeing with assessments: Some features of preferred/dispreferred turn shapes. In Atkinson, J. M. and J. Heritage (eds.), *Structures of Social Action: Studies in Conversation Analysis.* Cambridge: Cambridge University Press, 57–101.
1988 Offering a candidate answer: An information seeking strategy. *Communication Monographs* 55, 360–373.

Roberts, F.
2000 The interactional construction of asymmetry: The medical agenda as a resource for delaying response to patient questions. *Sociological Quarterly* 41, 151–174.
Robinson, J. D.
1998 Getting down to business: Talk, gaze, and body orientation during openings of physician–patient consultations. *Human Communication Research* 25, 97–123.
2001 Asymmetry in action: Sequential resources in the negotiation of a prescription request. *Text* 21(1/2), 19–54.
Sacks, H.
1992 *Lectures on Conversation: Volumes I and II* (G. Jefferson, ed.). Oxford: Blackwell.
Sacks, H., E. A. Schegloff, and G. Jefferson
1974 A simplest systematics for the organization of turn-taking in conversation. *Language* 50, 702–735.
Schegloff, E. A.
1972 Notes on a conversational practice: Formulating place. In Sudnow, D. (ed.), *Studies in Social Interaction*. New York: Free Press, 75–119.
1980 Preliminaries to preliminaries: "Can I ask you a question?" *Sociological Inquiry* 50, 104–152.
Sorjonen, M. L. and J. Heritage
1991 "And"-prefacing as a feature of question design. In Laitinen, L., P. Nuolijarvi, and M. Saari (eds.), *Asennonvaihtoja [Changes in footing]: Essays in Honor of Auli Hakulinen*. Helsinki: Vastapaino, 68–84.
Stivers, T.
2002 Presenting the problem in pediatric encounters: "Symptoms only" versus "candidate diagnosis" presentations. *Health Communication* 14, 299–338.
Stivers, T. and J. Heritage
2001 Breaking the sequential mold: Answering "more than the question" during comprehensive history taking. *Text* 21(1/2), 151–185.
ten Have, P.
1989 The consultation as a genre. In Torode, B. (ed.), *Text and Talk as Social Practice: Discourse Difference and Division in Speech and Writing*. Providence, RI: Foris, 115–135.
1991a Talk and institution: A reconsideration of the "asymmetry" of physician–patient interaction. In Boden, D. and D. Zimmerman (eds.), *Talk and Social Structure: Studies in Ethnomethodology and Conversation Analysis*. Cambridge, UK: Polity, 138–163.
1991b The physician is silent: Observations on episodes without vocal receipt during medical consultations. In Conein, B., M. de Fornel, and L. Quere (eds.), *Les formes de la conversation, Vol. 2*. Issy les Moilineaux: CNET, 55–76.
2001 Lay diagnosis in interaction. *Text* 21(1/2), 251–260.
Todd, A. D.
1983 A diagnosis of physician–patient discourse in the prescription of contraception. In Fisher, S. and A. D. Todd (eds.), *The Social Organization of Physi-*

*cian-Patient Communication.* Washington, DC: Center for Applied Linguistics, 159–187.

Treichler, P. A., R. M. Frankel, C. Kramarae, K. Zoppi, and H. B. Beckman
1984 Problems and problems: Power relationships in a medical encounter. In Kramarae, C., M. Schulz, and W. O'Barr (eds.), *Language and Power.* Beverly Hills: Sage, 62–88.

Uhlmann, R. F., T. S. Inui, and W. B. Carter
1984 Patient requests and expectations: Definitions and clinical applications. *Medical Care* 22, 681–685.

West, C.
1983 "Ask me no questions ..." An analysis of queries and replies in physician–patient dialogues. In Fisher, S. and A. Dundas (eds.), *The Social Organization of Physician-Patient Communication.* Washington, DC: Center for Applied Linguistics, 75–106.
1984 *Routine Complications: Troubles with Talk between Physicians and Patients.* Bloomington: Indiana University Press.

West, C. and R. M. Frankel
1991 Miscommunication in medicine. In Coupland, N., H. Giles, and J. Wiemann (eds.), *Miscommunication and Problematic Talk.* Newbury Park, CA: Sage, 210–228.

Winefield, H., M. Chandler, and D. Bassett.
1989 Tag questions and powerfulness: Quantitative and qualitative analysis of a course of psychotherapy. *Language in Society* 18, 77–86.

# Chapter 7
# Aggravated resistance to problem formulations in therapy

*G. H. Morris*

*G. H. Morris offers yet another view of expert authoritarianism. In this case, the expert is a psychotherapist who is trying to work with a couple to formulate the sources of dissatisfaction in their marriage. What is remarkable about this interaction is that the expert is unable to direct discourse in ways that he intends. The couple does not assume a cooperative stance, and the attempts by interactants to identify or diagnose the problems are "torpedoed." Morris explores what may have caused the aggravated resistance and drives home the crucial notion that successful diagnosis is a negotiation between the diagnostician and those diagnosed.*

The description and formulation of problems define consultation (Weick and Browning 1991) and are a central occupation in therapeutic interaction (Buttny 1993, 1996; Buttny and Jensen 1995; Jones and Beach 1995). When couples seek therapists' help, they first describe their problems (Wodak 1981) and then receive reformulations (Davis 1986) of their problems. Therapists' reformulations conceptualize problems in ways that encapsulate insight and/or reframe the meaning of described actions in therapeutically useful ways (Watzlawick, Weakland, and Fisch 1974; Weick and Browning 1991). However, participants in therapy sometimes express differing viewpoints about the correct interpretation of the couple's problem, its cause, and what may or should be done about it. These differences may give rise to efforts by clients to resist therapeutic ascriptions as well as attempts by therapists to overcome clients' resistance (Labov and Fanshel 1977) by engaging in persuasion with clients (Buttny 1996). Useful consultation depends partly on how well clients and therapists manage to negotiate differing interpretations of problems in and through therapeutic interaction (Bergmann 1992; Ferrara 1994).

This project is a single case analysis (Phillipsen 1982; Stake 1994) of a spectacularly unsuccessful negotiation of the problem during a Marriage and Family Therapy (MFT) session. Whereas clients usually mitigate (Cody and McLaughlin 1985; Labov and Fanshel 1977) the extent of their disagreements, participants in this session pursued resistance to the therapist's formulation of their problem in an extremely aggravated way. Because it diverges so radically from what ordinarily happens in therapy sessions, this interaction provides a glimpse of some of the preconditions and limits of therapeutic sensemaking. After reviewing how therapists and clients typically formulate problems in therapy sessions, I analyze how disagreements were handled in this case. The analysis focuses on the "aggravated resistance" the husband raised and its consequences for ensuing interaction in the session. Concluding discussion addresses a few theoretical and practical implications of the analysis.

## 1. Formulating problems in marriage and family therapy

The process of problem formulation begins as clients describe their own understandings of the situations that led them to seek therapy. Therapists acquaint themselves with the couple's situation by probing for additional, clarifying information (Jones and Beach 1995) and by utilizing "information eliciting tellings" (Bergmann 1992; Buttny 1996; Pomerantz 1980). That is, therapists bring up information they already know about clients' stories, prompting elaboration from clients. Therapists manage the interaction in such a way that both individuals may tell their side of the story and therapists avoid the perception of siding with either individual. This may involve deferring one member's contributions to the encounter until the other has taken his or her turn (Jones and Beach 1995).

As participants tell about their problems, therapists also observe clients' interaction; their observations may provide evidence for their interpretations of clients' problems. Jones and Beach (1995: 53) overview the process as follows:

> Narrative descriptions provide an opportunity for therapists to directly observe how family members interact with one another during the session. By integrating information of externalized events produced through the narrative, and data apparent in the ways family members produce these narratives in real-time therapy sessions, the "raw material for the therapeutic work" (Labov and Fanshel 1977, p. 35) is made available.

Based upon their inquiries and observations, therapists eventually propound a version of the clients' problem (Davis 1986). As with any formulation (Heritage and Watson 1979; Pomerantz 1986), therapists' reformulations entail choice from among alternative ways of describing a situation. Psychotherapists may formulate problems as individual failings (Davis 1986) for example. In MFT, reformulations generally define problems as interactional in nature rather than ascribing blame to an individual. For example, instead of formulating a problem as one person's failure to express his or her emotions, the therapist might construe it as a breakdown of communication between individuals.

Clients' confirming/disconfirming orientation to how the therapist has formulated the problem is displayed in their uptake (i.e., their "evaluation") (Buttny 1993; 1996). Clients typically confirm therapists' formulations, but this is not necessarily the case. Because individuals often come to therapy believing their partners' actions are the problem, a formulation of the problem as interactional may not resonate well with individuals' understandings. Individuals or couples may perceive the therapist's formulation as obvious, irrelevant or absurd and, therefore, unhelpful (Morris and Morris 1997; Weick 1979).

The unmarked, structurally preferred alternative is for clients to confirm the problem formulation. The following instance shows a therapist's understanding of a husband's view of the problem and the husband's confirmatory response:

(1) T: You sound almost a little puzzled.
H: I am puzzled. I don't- all I've ever done is to try to- every ounce of my energy has been toward our family, and I'm sort of puzzled at why all the hostility directed at me ...

Note that the husband confirms and specifies his puzzlement at his wife's comportment. By contrast, one or both clients may display a lack of full alignment in orientation. For example,

(2) T: Sounds like to me you sound thirsty
(.) sort of (.) thirsty for some
W: I'm very restless. I'm ready to walk.
I've thought about it

In this instance, the wife upgrades the seriousness of the problem, treating it as more urgent or acute than does the therapist. Not only does she desire something beyond what she's getting, she is ready to exit the relationship. Note, however, that her version of the problem is not built as disagreement with the therapist's formulation, but only as a restatement that more accurately reflects her perspective. The same upgrading restatement is displayed in the following instance:

(3) (Adapted from Gale, Odell, and Nagireddy 1995: 116)
T: You know what, it sounds almost more like a roommate relationship=
W: =Yes, that's what (.) in fact (.) that's I tell him=
T: =than a marital relationship, a little bit?
W: Well, I'll tell you another thing too. We haven't slept together in probably about a year, so it is a roommate-in fact, I tell him he's my roommate.

In this instance, the wife agrees immediately but goes on to upgrade the seriousness of the situation. Although she agrees with the formulation, she treats it as one she herself has reached and discussed previously, not as a new, insightful conceptualization.

In summary, therapists offer problem formulations after hearing couples describe problems. Couples display their confirming/disconfirming orientation to what therapists tell them. Generally, couples avoid explicitly disagreeing with problem formulations.

## 2. Mitigating disagreement with a problem formulation

When clients do disagree with therapists' problem formulations, their disagreements are usually managed to avoid bald and on-record disagreement. In rare instances, however, individuals or couples may disagree explicitly and directly with a therapist's formulation (Buttny 1996). In the following instance, disagreement surfaced by one party and seconded by another becomes the occasion for correcting a therapist's misunderstanding:

| (4) | Couple (adapted from Buttny 1996: 131) | |
|---|---|---|
| 4 | T: | Ah::: (0.6) and that may:: (3.^ >create some problems< |
| 5 | | pt ah (.) indeed therapy create some problems, yeah? |
| 6 | W: | Um huh |
| 7 | T: | An ah ^if I understand correctly individual therapy |
| 8 | | created some problems in the couple that you are |
| 9 | | trying to solve (.) ^and reasonably so by means |
| 10 | | of ah of ah: ah::: (0.9) bringing Larry into (.) ah: couple |
| 11 | | therapy in which case ah both of your can tune up a bit |
| 12 | | (0.8) |
| 13 | W: | Uh huh |
| 14 | T: | Uhm |
| 15 | | (1.3) |
| 16 | H: | I don't think that individual therapy created problems |
| 17 | | be[tween us |
| 18 | W: | [>It didn't< Yeah, it didn't create the problems but it |
| 19 | | just made us more aware (.) of problems |
| 20 | | (1.3) |
| 21 | W: | The problems were already there (.) so they weren't |
| 22 | | crea[ted-they weren't created by the individual therapy but |
| 23 | T: | [( ) |
| 24 | T: | What kind of problems were there? |

Here, the husband's explicit disagreement (lines 16–17) is taken up by the wife in overlap (line 18). Rather than attributing the cause of their problems to her individual therapy, she credits the individual therapy for making her more aware of previously existing problems (lines 18–19). Hearing no uptake from either other individual (line 20), she restated her objection (lines 22–23) to the therapist's formulation. The therapist appears to defer to their version of the situation as he proceeds to inquire about the previously existing problems.

Notice how participants managed to mitigate disagreements in these examples. In instances two and three, clients offer a reformulation based upon the therapist's but modifying it by upgrading it in seriousness. In instance two, the therapist's version ("you seem thirsty") is modified into a more urgent one ("I'm ready to walk"). In instance three, the therapist's version ("It seems like a roommate relationship") is modified into a more severe and unusual one ("We've had no sex in about a year"). In the last instance, clients rejected the therapist's formulation (i.e., that individual therapy caused the couple's problems) in favor of one they treat as more accurate (i.e., that in actuality, problems preceded the individual therapy). Nevertheless, the husband's disagreement is mitigated. It was not volunteered, but seems to have been offered after being specifically provided for by the therapist. Even though the wife had concurred with his formulation (in line 13), the therapist's minimal utterance (at line 14) followed by a significant gap (line 15) suggests he waited for the husband to comment. When he did, his reply was hedged ("I don't think ...") rather than declaimed more forcefully. In each case, clients' replies seem to be in the service of arriving at a slightly more accurate understanding of their situation. Corrections of therapists' versions are handled with some delicacy. In turn, as Buttny (1996) argues, therapists utilize clients' responses to design subsequent formulations and/or to convince clients to accept their own views.

Overall, clients and therapists mitigate disagreements and cooperate to arrive jointly at a workable problem formulation (Buttny 1996).

## 3. Aggravated resistance to a problem formulation

The clients in this case study were a husband and wife who were in the midst of a multiple-session course of therapy to overcome their dissatisfactions with their marriage. The session was conducted by a therapist in a university clinic and was audiotape recorded, with the couple's permission, for teaching and research purposes. The therapist employed a style of systemic therapy influenced by both the Milan Style (Selvini-Palazzoli, Boscolo, Checchin, and Prata 1978) and the MRI Style (Watzlawick, Weakland, and Fisch 1974).

In the very beginning of the session, the husband (designated as "H" in excerpts) began to tell the therapist about an argument the couple had the previous evening. As the husband's and wife's (designated as "W" in excerpts) sides of the story started to diverge, they began to argue within the session about what had been said in their previous argument. This escalated rapidly and led to the husband severely disparaging his wife in a mean-spirited way the therapist recognized as typical of their interaction. In short, the first part of the session was a fight. It was brought to closure by the husband and wife with no attempt by the therapist to intervene. As the fight concluded, the stage was set for an observation of some kind by the therapist, presumably one that would make use of what he had just observed to conceptualize the couple's difficulties for them in a new way.

The therapist, in fact, did seek at that moment to formulate the couple's problem, as follows:

(5) "There is no making up"
133 T: you know one of uh ((sniff))
134 we were‹ ta:lking?
135 earlier today?
136 (2.7)
137 couple my colleagues and I
138 and uh (.)
139 ˙hhh
140 we were discussin some cases
141 and we ›we were discussin‹ you guys.
142 (2.3)
143 ˙hhh
144 and uh
145 (2.4)
146 one reason uh
147 ›that you guys probly like to argue‹
148 or somethin ›you know there's‹
149 ˙hhh there's still somethin missin
150 but uh *he* stated that uh
151 *some* people like to
152 (.)
153 ˙hh ARgue becu:zsss
154 there's th- there's a *pas*sion
155 in arguing
156 (.)
157 there's the *pas*sion in
158 in ˙hh the marriage when people argue
159 (1.2)
160 u:m
161 ›whether it's you‹ guys or not
162 if you stopped arguin?
163 that may just be::
164 ›you know‹ cut the passion
165 completely out of your marriage

The therapist's formulation was stated in a format typical of how diagnostic information, particularly "bad news," is often delivered. First, it is attributed to a third party, not to the therapist himself. Because the bad news could be discrediting, the therapist distances himself from having authored it (Maynard 1998). Second, it is presented in a syllogistic format (Maynard 1998). The logic presented is that some couples argue to generate passion, this couple argues, so perhaps they argue to generate passion. Third, it is qualified (Bergmann 1992; Buttny 1996) as not providing a full account of the situation. It is proposed as "one reason," not *the* reason for the couple's difficulties and is acknowledged to be incomplete (i.e., "there's still somethin missin") and tentative ("that *may* just ..."). Consistent with Buttny's (1996) description of how therapists reveal possible futures/consequences of a problem, the formulation uses if-then conditional syntax to unveil a possible future that would be unfortunate. This future is constructed as an extreme case (Pomerantz 1986) in which passion is cut *completely* out of the marriage. (See Beach 1996, Ch. 3 for an extensive analysis of extreme case formulations used to amplify the seriousness of problems in another health care setting.) Finally, the problem formulation was not said accusingly, but was rather stated in a mild, provisional, diagnostic, consultative way.

Because the therapist's formulation was pronounced so casually and hesitatingly, its artful design as a therapeutic move may be obscure. As a potentially therapeutic contribution – seen from within the MFT paradigm within which he was working – it has a number of virtues. The therapist avoided endorsing or failing to endorse the husband's formulation of their problem, which is that his wife is to blame for their difficulties. Instead, he made an observation about the manner of interacting the couple had just exhibited--having an argument – and the function it may serve in their relationship. The therapist's formulation reframed their recurrent arguments as jointly constructed and functional; the couple were invited to see their intense hostile outbursts as expressions of passion for each other. Presumably, if they were able to find alternative ways to express their passion, their interaction would be less problematic for them.

Even though the therapeutic logic of the therapist's contribution may be evident, it could not be construed as providing a "good hearing" of the husband's telling of the problem, and it is conceivable that this oversight may have lessened the husband's receptivity to the therapist's idea. Moreover, entailed in the therapist's formulation is an assumption that other forms of passion are not present for the couple. To accept the therapist's problem formulation would be to accede to a description of their relationship as devoid of passion, except for the passion in argument. This pill may not be very easy to swallow.

Clients undergoing this kind of therapy are capable, as we have seen, of disagreeing with problem formulations in ways that result in refinements in them. The husband's reply to the problem formulation seems to go beyond what would have been necessary to contest what he took to be an inadequate understanding of their problem:

| | | | |
|---|---|---|---|
| (6) | 166 | | ((rubbing of sleeves on upholstered furniture)) |
| | 167 | | (1.2) |
| | 168 | H: | OH |
| | 169 | | I disagree with *tha:t*? |
| | 170 | T: | YO[U DO? ] |
| | 171 | H: | [I MEAN ]THAT IS SO |
| | 172 | | FAR OFF BASE? WHOEVER TOLD YOU THA:T?= |
| | 173 | W: | =hh heh huh |
| | 174 | T: | is– |
| | 175 | H: | good[ness gra- ] |
| | 176 | T: | [completely off the wall?] |
| | 177 | H: | AHOH *TOTALLY O:FF* THE *WA:LL* |
| | 178 | W: | (mm?) |

The husband's evaluation of the formulation treats it as having no merit whatsoever. Rather than any kind of provisional acceptance, mild agreement with a grain of truth, polite disagreement, or mere silence, the husband states his disagreement explicitly and directly ("I disagree with *tha:t*?") and casts what the therapist says as wrong in the extreme ("SO FAR OFF BASE?"). He next begins loudly to disparage the originator of the idea ("WHOEVER TOLD YOU THA:T?="). In apparent preference to continuing into part two of this disparagement, he instead expels a derisive exclamation ("goodness gra-"). Obligingly, the therapist completes the denunciation in overlap, supplying the characterization ("is completely off the wall?"). Notably, he does so with question intonation. By asking if the originator of the idea is completely off the wall, the therapist exposed the possibility that there may be some shred of usefulness in the idea, that it is not completely mistaken. This possibility is foreclosed by the husband's reply. Going beyond mere ratification of the assessment that the originator of the idea is completely off the wall, the husband upgrades it loudly and with a derisive, haughty tone and exaggerated cadence ("AHOH *TOTALLY O:FF* THE *WA:LL*").

The husband's response can be considered to be aggravated resistance because it rejects the idea in its entirety, casts the therapist's formulation as extreme, casts aspersions on the originator of the idea, and is voiced in a loud and aggressive tone. This overbuilt display of indignation (Drew 1998) symbolizes the husband's orientation toward the possibilities and purposes of the therapeutic encounter. To accept provisionally the therapist's formulation or oppose it civilly would suggest he respects the therapist's prerogative to make therapeutically relevant observations about the couple's behavior. By contrast to this stance, what he actually said and did seems to strike at the foundations of the therapeutic relationship and calls into question the extent to which he truly seeks an improvement in his relationship with his spouse.

The wife's contributions to this part of the encounter are so minimal as to defy confident analysis. Given that the therapist's formulation of their problem is more flattering of her than is the husband's, we might expect that she would try to agree with, defend, or even extend the therapist's interpretation. This is not what happens. Her responses are minimal, but her laughter in line 173 is not disaffiliative with the line her husband has just taken. She may be siding with her husband in denouncing the therapist's formulation; displaying her enjoyment of the husband's aggressive vocalizations toward the therapist; or expressing some relief that the therapist, not she, is presently the victim of her husband's denunciation. Regardless, her failure to offer support for the therapist's formulation is evident.

Of what consequence is the husband's immediate, visceral opposition for the progress of therapeutic sensemaking in the encounter? Had he not deferred judgment momentarily, he might have learned earlier and before committing himself to an assessment that he had misunderstood the therapist:

| | | | |
|---|---|---|---|
| (7) | 179 | H: | listen that's just out– |
| | 180 | T: | Wull ›wull *why* is he‹ off the wall |
| | 181 | H: | Well ›*I* don't see any‹ compassion |
| | 182 | | at all in that at a:ll |
| | 183 | | (.) |
| | 184 | T: | you [don't see any compassion in your marriage?] |
| | 185 | W: | [no he doesn't mean compa:ssion |
| | 186 | H: | [UR *PASSION* |

Line 185 is a correction of the husband's substitution of "compassion" for what the therapist had actually said, "passion." It indeed seems far-fetched that arguing is compassionate, and if this was the husband's understanding, it is unsurprising that he failed to support it. But his over-vigorous denunciation of the idea is not reversible at this point. He fails to credit the possibility that arguing constitutes passion "*I* don't see any‹ (PASSION) at all in that at a:ll." His misunderstanding occasioned the therapist's question in line 184 "you don't see any compassion in your marriage?" which is not treated as an accurate formulation of what the husband had said.

Had the husband's denunciation not been so complete and extreme, the therapist might have been able to further explain his reasoning, to try to get the couple to better appreciate how this observation about what happens in some couples might also apply to them. Instead, he offers a series of questions which serve only to confirm that the analysis he has offered does not fit. The first of these occurred in line 184: "you don't see any compassion in your marriage?". This question was answered incredulously in line 190:

| | | | |
|---|---|---|---|
| (8) | 187 | T: | ER |
| | 188 | | (.) |
| | 189 | | you know– |
| | 190 | M: | in in in *ar*guing? |

The therapist treated "in in in *ar*guing" straightforwardly as eliciting clarification, rather than as an incredulous negative reply. Accordingly, he asks the husband to confirm that he does not see arguing as part of his marriage:

| | | | |
|---|---|---|---|
| (9) | 191 | | (.2) |
| | 192 | T: | um hmm |
| | 193 | | (.) |
| | 194 | | you don't see that as part of your marri[age? ]. |

In reply, the husband offers evidence to illustrate that their arguments are violent, not passionate:

| | | | |
|---|---|---|---|
| (10) | 195 | H: | [listen? ] |
| | 196 | | you oughta see the *raz*or marks on the my |
| | 197 | | *back* |
| | 198 | | (.) |
| | 199 | | an (hh) I(h)'m not jus kid(h)din |
| | 200 | | heh- heh- heh- heh- heh- |
| | 201 | | ˙hhh |

The laughter the husband supplies in lines 199 and 200 is not responsive to something the therapist has said, but rather comprises laughing at the therapist. The evidence, razor marks, is treated as showing that the therapist's formulation is not only off target, but also ludicrous. Speculatively, it could also work to counter the suggestion that there is no passion in their relationship aside from arguing. He has battle scars to prove his wife's passion for him.

After this, the husband's disparagement of the idea is compounded in a still more derisive and conclusive form:

| | | | |
|---|---|---|---|
| (11) | 202 | | I disagree with that whole heartally |
| | 203 | | that's that is [just |
| | 204 | T: | [SO |
| | 205 | H: | Preposter- I just don't ›bleve that at all‹ |

His disagreement is upgraded to wholehearted disagreement and the idea is denounced as outrageous or "Preposter(ous)," as completely without credence ("I just don't ›bleve that at all‹").

It is one thing to propose that the couple argues to generate passion and another to formulate their problem as a complete absence of passion. Things appear to go from bad to worse (in terms of the severity of the problem being ascribed to the couple) as the therapist reformulates the meaning of the husband's contention:

| | | | |
|---|---|---|---|
| (12) | 206 | T: | SO YER, THE passion in yer marriage |
| | 207 | | is nonexistent. |

The suggestion that passion is absent has more dire consequences for the relationship than the previous formulation of their problem. If they find passion in arguing but this has negative consequences the couple wants to overcome, then a path toward solutions is evident. They can be helped to learn how to express their passion more constructively. On the other hand, if there is no passion, perhaps there is no basis upon which to build a sustainable, satisfying relationship. The husband's reply to this reformulated problem, also a disconfirmation, leaves open the possibility that there is passion somewhere in the relationship:

| | | | |
|---|---|---|---|
| (13) | 208 | M: | ˙hhh it's not in *a:r*guments |
| | 209 | | (1.7) |
| | 210 | H: | I kin tell you that= |
| | 211 | T: | =But= |
| | 212 | H: | =*right*^ now |

Here the husband denies explicitly that arguments provide the passion in their marriage. If arguments do not comprise passion for the couple, then they cannot be arguing to generate passion and their problem has not been adequately understood. But a more encompassing view of the pattern of their interaction, including arguing and making up recurrently, offers a way to redeem the original problem formulation without making it necessary for the couple to disavow any passion in their relationship. The therapist next proposed:

| | | | |
|---|---|---|---|
| (14) | 213 | T: | [but] in the making up |
| | 214 | | ((four plus one taps on the table in rapid succession)) |
| | 215 | W: | There *is* no making up. |

Again in this instance, the therapist's formulation (i.e., that the couple generates passion when they "make up" after having fought) is disconfirmed, this time by the wife. If there is no making up, there can be no passion generated in the way proposed:

| | | | |
|---|---|---|---|
| (15) | 216 | T: | °Oh it's just°- ((shuffling)) |
| | 217 | | it's the time out and then |
| | 218 | | that's it |
| | 219 | | (1.4) ((one plus three taps)) |
| | 220 | H: | No |
| | 221 | | ((two more taps)) |

With this attempted formulation, the therapist seeks confirmation that the couple simply fight and fall silent. This would mean, evidently, that after arguing they leave their disputes unresolved rather than doing anything to rectify the harm they may have done to each other. As before, this formulation is resisted by the husband (line 220), though it seems worth noticing that he does not offer any alternative description of the aftermath of their arguments. Perhaps this is why the wife next elicits his viewpoint about whether they make up or not:

| | | | |
|---|---|---|---|
| (16) | 222 | | (5.0) |
| | 223 | W: | Is there making up? .hhh |
| | 224 | H: | uh no (2.6) umhmm |
| | 225 | | (5.0) |
| | 226 | H: | And that's on both sides |
| | 227 | | (3.5) |
| | 228 | T: | So neither one of you- you both have |
| | 229 | | a hard time makin up then |

Here is the fifth and last of the therapist's formulations of their problem. That they do not make up after arguments is reformulated as *having difficulty* making up, a difficulty expressly attributed to both partners. This occasions a lengthy sequence during which the therapist explains what he means by making up (namely, "Giving each other a hug or a kiss, saying 'I'm sorry,' I didn't mean to, you're right ..."), and the couple confirm that they never do this. Reflexively, this may in fact confirm the therapist's contention that both of them have trouble making up.

To summarize: After the initial observation was given and then rejected, the therapist adapted his conceptualization of the problem through three subsequent versions which were also disconfirmed. Eventually, working with the therapist's fifth formulation, the parties seem to uncover a deeper, more difficult to resolve problem, which is that they "have a hard time making up." Rather than recurrently cycling around bouts of arguments and making up, they are mired in their arguments and seem not to know how to transcend them.

If the first and last problem formulation are compared, it appears that the first formulation had the advantage of providing an explanation for the couple's continual arguments, namely, that the arguments constituted passion for each other. The last formulation, that they have trouble making up, lacks such an explanation. It is still an open issue why this couple do not interact in a more satisfying fashion, and no means of resolving the couple's problems is apparent. Overall, then, the husband's aggravated resistance thwarted the achievement of therapeutic sense-making in the session.

The manner in which resistance was pursued is noticeably uncivil. Unlike in ordinary social interaction and therapy talk, where parties who disconfirm formulations generally provide alternative ones, in this context the therapist proposes and the husband denounces. When it is clear the husband has misunderstood ("compassion" for "passion"), there is no effort to acknowledge the error and correct for its consequences. Whereas people tend to avoid "bald, on record" disparagement of their fellow interactants and show each other some degree of deference (Goffman 1967), in the session the therapist, his colleagues, and his ideas were belittled. The husband's response to the therapist exhibits such a lack of consideration for the therapeutic process or appreciation for the attempt to better understand their situation that it calls the therapeutic relationship into question.

## 4. Conclusion

There could be any number of explanations for why this couple's therapy did not progress and, more particularly, why this definition of the problem did not have purchase in the therapeutic system. Perhaps the problem formulation was ill-timed since it came right after another very heated moment in interaction. It might just have been a poor idea. Some might fault the therapist's clumsy manner of delivery. This case analysis suggests that the husband's mean-spirited contributions to the process of coming to an understanding of the problem thwarted progress toward a consensual definition of the problem and thereby forestalled resolution of the couple's difficulties.

By highlighting an extreme case in which cooperation was absent and resistance was pursued malignantly, one limit on the capacity of a therapeutic system to make progress has been brought into focus. Attaining a viable understanding of clients' problems is contingent upon the character of the interaction as parties negotiate. Clients are usually capable of engaging in a process of therapeutic interaction which involves describing situations, making proposals about problems, and refining these proposals through polite, respectful disagreement and reformulation. It is possible, however, for clients to adopt and pursue a malignant style of communication that derogates others and their ideas in an extreme way. Negotiations of problems may degenerate into impasse when aggravated resistance forecloses therapeutic possibilities. In such cases, clients' ability to interact cooperatively may need to be bolstered before problems specific to a relationship can be addressed productively.

Reconceptualizing problems is an integral part of the therapeutic process that epitomizes the skills therapists and other consultants may possess (Weick and Browning 1991). But no matter how brilliant a counselor's formulation of a problem may be, it can be torpedoed by a client's aggravated resistance. Applied communication practitioners, in general, need on occasion to create an interactional context that permits the civil exchange of ideas before progress can be made toward understanding and resolving clients' problems.

## *References*

Beach, Wayne
1996 *Conversations about Illness: Family Preoccupations with Bulima.* Mahwah, NJ: Erlbaum.

Bergmann, J. R.
1992 Veiled morality: Notes on discretion in psychiatry. In Drew, P. and J. Heritage (eds.), *Talk at Work.* Cambridge, UK: Cambridge University Press, 137–162.

Buttny, R.
1993 *Social Accountability in Communication.* London: Sage.
1996 Clients' and therapist's joint construction of the clients' problems. *Research on Language and Social Interaction* 29, 125–153.

Buttny, R. and A. Jensen
1995 Telling problems in an initial family therapy session: The hierarchical organization of problem-talk. In Morris, G. H. and R. J. Chenail (eds.), *The Talk of the Clinic: Explorations in the Analysis of Medical and Therapeutic Discourse.* Hillsdale, NJ: Erlbaum, 19–48.

Cody, M. J. and M. L. Mclaughlin
1985 Models for the sequential construction of accounting episodes: Situational and interactional constraints on message selection and evaluation. In Street, R. L. and J. N. Cappella (eds.), *Sequence and Pattern in Communicative Behaviour.* Baltimore: Edward Arnold, 50–69.

Davis, K.
1986 The process of problem (re)formulation in psychotherapy. *Sociology of Health and Illness* 8, 44–74.

Drew, P.
1998 Complaints about transgressions and misconduct. *Research on Language and Social Interaction* 31, 295–326.

Ferrara, K. W.
1994 *Therapeutic Ways with Words.* New York: Oxford University Press.

Gale, J., M. Odell, and C. Nagireddy
1995 Marital therapy and self-reflexive research: Research and/as intervention. In Morris, G. H. and R. J. Chenail (eds.), *The Talk of the Clinic: Explorations in the Analysis of Medical and Therapeutic Discourse.* Hillsdale, NJ: Erlbaum, 105–129.

Goffman, Erving
1967 *Interaction Ritual.* New York: Pantheon.

Heritage, John and D. R. Watson
1979 Formulations as conversational objects. In Psathas, G. (ed.), *Everyday Language: Studies in Ethnomethodology.* New York: Irvington, 123–162.

Jones, C. and Wayne Beach
1995 Therapists' techniques for responding to unsolicited contributions by family members. In Morris, G. H. and R. J. Chenail (eds.), *The Talk of the Clinic: Explorations in the Analysis of Medical and Therapeutic Discourse.* Hillsdale, NJ: Erlbaum, 49–71.

Labov, William and D. Fanshel
1977 *Therapeutic Discourse: Psychotherapy as Conversation.* New York: Academic Press.
Maynard, Douglas W.
1998 Praising versus blaming the messenger: Moral issues in deliveries of good and bad news. *Research on Language and Social Interaction* 31, 359–395.
Morris, G. H. and P. K. Morris
1997 Beyond the communication breakdown: Conceptualizing problematic interaction in therapy. Paper presented at the International Communication Association Annual Convention, Montreal, May, 1997.
Phillipsen, G.
1982 The qualitative case study as a strategy in communication inquiry. *The Communicator* 12, 4–17.
Pomerantz, Anita
1980 Telling my side: "Limited access" as a "fishing" device. *Sociological Inquiry* 50, 186–198.
1986 Extreme case formulations: A way of legitimizing claims. *Human Studies* 9, 219–229.
Selvini-Palazzoli, M., L. Boscolo, G. Cecchin, and G. Prata
1978 *Paradox and Counterparadox.* New York: Jason Aronson.
Stake, R. E.
1994 Case studies. In Denzin, N. K. and Y. S. Lincoln (eds.), *Handbook of Qualitative Research.* Thousand Oaks, CA: Sage, 236–247.
Watzlawick, P., J. Weakland, and R. Fisch
1974 *Change: Principles of Problem Formulation and Problem Resolution.* New York: W. W. Norton.
Weick, K. E.
1979 *The Social Psychology of Organizing.* Menlo Park, CA: Addison-Wesley.
Weick, K. E. and L. D. Browning
1991 Fixing with the voice: A research agenda for applied communication. *Journal of Applied Communication Research* 19, 1–19.
Wodak, R.
1981 How do I put my problem? Problem presentation in therapy and interview. *Text* 1, 191–213.

# Chapter 8
# Learning to diagnose: Production of diagnostic hypotheses in problem-based learning tutorials

*Phillip Glenn and Timothy Koschmann*

*In this chapter Phil Glenn and Timothy Koschman study medical students as they become enculturated into the ways of doing diagnosis. They show how alternative diagnoses become accepted or rejected by the group and argue convincingly that the act of doing diagnoses, whether by professionals or lay people, is best understood as a relatively unstable action affected by and embedded in interactional, sequential events.*

In the current Western model for medical practice, a patient with symptoms sees a health care provider who provides a diagnosis and some recommended intervention. Diagnosis provides the link between symptoms and cure. Physicians must learn to diagnose with a fairly high degree of accuracy in order to provide effective treatment and maintain a basis for invoking and instantiating the difference in expertise between physician and layperson.[1] Although it may be tempting to think of diagnosing as solely or primarily a cognitive activity, recent research (including several chapters in this book) shows that diagnosing is in fundamental ways a communicative process. Whatever happens in the mind of someone coming up with a diagnosis, it gets constituted through language-in-interaction, produced in and for social contexts that may involve judgments of the competence or expertise of the diagnoser. Combining these two observations – that diagnosing is learned and that diagnosing is communicative – invites research into communicative dimensions of how professionals learn to diagnose.

In this chapter we analyze instances of medical students learning to diagnose. Specifically, we will show some discursive practices through which medical students occasion, produce, and respond to possible diagnoses. What these students constitute as a diagnosis is not solely based on the semantic content of utterances but upon interactional features such as sequential location, context, and understandings displayed. In other words, instead of analyzing diagnosis as a thing to be understood somewhat independent of the context in which it occurs, we examine *diagnosing* as a communicative practice that is socially constructed through interaction. At the same time, the actions through which students discuss possible diagnoses reflect and constitute their pedagogical context. These are learning activities, and participant actions are subject to evaluation as evidence of their developing knowledge and expertise. These themes will be developed in the analysis and returned to in the closing discussion.

Our data come from video recordings of tutorial meetings in a problem-based learning (PBL) curriculum. Originally developed for use in professional schools (Barrows and Tamblyn 1980), PBL now is widely employed in a variety of undergraduate disciplines and in secondary education. In this PBL curriculum, groups of six students, working closely with a faculty tutor, collaboratively explore a sequence of clinical cases. In each case they diagnose and prescribe treatment for patients whom they encounter in the form of a photograph or video of the actual patient or of an actor; either way, the simulation is based on details of an actual case. The tutorial groups regularly schedule meetings to discuss these clinical problems, recessing between meetings for periods of self-directed study. Typically, the students devote two or three meetings of two or three hours' duration to each case. Participants in these meetings produce, test, and evaluate diagnostic hypotheses concerning the problem under study (Barrows 1994; Koschmann, Kelson, Feltovich, and Barrows 1996). The students generate a number of diagnostic hypotheses, and then follow a deductive inquiry process in obtaining the information needed to determine the correct hypothesis(es). In determining what should count as an hypothesis students are instructed, "hypotheses should refer to anatomical locations, pathophysiological (or disease) processes, psychophysiological process, etiological mechanisms – as appropriate to guide investigation into the patient's problem" (SIU School of Medicine 1994: 1). The faculty Tutor (sometimes called "Coach") participating in the meetings does not provide answers but steers the group toward effective reasoning and identification of learning issues (see Koschmann, Glenn, and Conlee 2000). Students have access to a case book containing information and patient statements from the medical examination plus test results, all organized according to questions the students may ask (Distlehorst and Barrows 1982). Students do not read through everything in this text, but instead consult it only to look up those items about which they happen to think to ask. This restriction is designed to achieve greater parallel between the simulation and actual medical examinations (Barrows 1990). One student takes the role of *reader*, looking up items in the casebook as group members think of them. Another student takes the role of *scribe*, writing symptoms, hypotheses, learning issues, and other information on the board.

Early in the process, the students review the patient's initial complaints and generate hypotheses (tentative diagnoses). They discuss the case, consulting the casebook at times. They identify tests they want run on the patient. They also identify learning issues and divide up research tasks to pursue these. The group members meet again after they have had time to research the learning issues. After sharing what they have found, they discuss the case, consult the casebook, refine hypotheses, order any further tests, and identify additional learning issues. During early portions of the process, group members are expected to produce many hypotheses. They make use of these to generate discussion, learning issues, and other hypotheses. Eventually (typically in a third meeting) they "solve" the case by agreeing on a diagnosis. They consult the casebook to learn what was actually diagnosed and what treatment was done in the case. Finally, they summarize the learning issues, evaluate the process, and discuss what they have learned.

The research presented here reflects assumptions and methods of ethnomethodological conversation analysis (for recent treatments see Psathas 1995; Pomerantz and Fehr 1997; ten Have 1999). This naturalistic research enterprise involves describing and interpreting people's procedures for organizing and accomplishing everyday interaction in various casual and institutional settings. With close attention to the sequential organization of talk, conversation analytic (CA) research characterizes recurrent combinations of actions that make up interactions. Sacks (1992: 339) proposed that "the idea is to take singular sequences of conversation and tear them apart in such a way as to find rules, techniques, procedures, methods, maxims ... which ... can be used to generate the orderly features we find in the conversations we examine." According to Clayman and Maynard (1995: 14), Sacks' principle of sequential organization "embodies investigatable practices through which parties to an interaction precisely time and place their talk so as to both demonstrate one's heed for another's activity and to claim other's attention to one's own in the collaborative building of a course of action." In that these PBL participants are expected to generate diagnostic hypotheses, and know they are to do so, analysts may examine their interactions to discern their methods for accomplishing this task. The method, then, involves explicating and interpreting participant methods for generating social order in and through interaction.

Diagnostic hypotheses come about through complex courses of action across many turns at talk. In the presentation of data that follows we find it useful to begin with sections focusing separately on how participants *occasion*, *present*, and *respond to* hypotheses. We then present an extended case study showing how these three activities combine organically as participants jointly constitute hypotheses. In the closing discussion, we will return to considering participant orientation to the constraints of the pedagogical context and to social interactional dimensions of their process.

# 1. Occasioning diagnostic hypotheses

## *1.1. Soliciting hypotheses*

Upon opening a new case, the PBL process requires students to "generate a number of hypotheses to explain the patient problem" (SIU School of Medicine 1994: 1). The group member assigned to be scribe records diagnostic hypotheses on the board. Although the formal structure of the PBL process makes this an expected activity, participants must still provide for the sequential relevance of producing hypotheses at particular moments in the talk. Routinely, the faculty coach or one of the group members will provide first pair parts (Schegloff and Sacks 1984) such as questions or prompts that work to solicit hypotheses in response.

In the instance below, the Coach invites the students to explain symptoms that he summarizes in his question. One of the students provides a possible explanation:

(1) Coach: So why would a twenty-five year old person after surgery (.)
or a woman •hh after surgery develop numbness and tingling in the
↑hands (0.8) and difficulty moving the ↑arms is that what it says?=
Han: Uh the only thing I can come up with is ahh (0.8) maybe a
nerve or something.

Rather than solicit hypotheses from the group as a whole, the coach may query one particular student:

(2) (#91-002; # 1, 10:50)
Coach: Well what's *wrong* with him Norman?
(0.5)
Norman: £Stroke slash TIA type of pathology£

Solicitations also come from the students themselves. In this instance, one student's question prompts group members to stop viewing a video tape and move into hypothesis generation:

(3) (#95-004.1; # 1, 1:08:40)
Vickie: Are we- are we gonna do hypotheses? (.) also?
Coach: °Sure°
John: Yeah
((distorted sound from monitor))
Vickie: Stop it for a second- *stop* °stop°
[
(male: Yeah
Coach: Stop
Todd): Huh hh
Vickie: I'm sure we *all* are thinking of things=

### *1.2. Volunteering hypotheses*

Although group members generate many of their hypotheses in the early stages of deliberation, they may introduce additional ones later in the process. Students are instructed to "Review hypotheses, inquiry, and synthesis in the progress of [the] problem solving process as new information, or lack of helpful information, may dictate" (SIU School of Medicine 1994: 1). New hypotheses may be developed, therefore, as part of an explicit re-evaluation of the hypothesis list or when new information about the case is revealed. For example, the hypothesis below is generated in the context of evaluating the hypothesis list:

(4) (#00-005.1; 1:33:00)
Ben: Well one thing fff it could be Hashimotos beginning or
the beginning of Hashimotos so
(0.3)
Laura: That's true.
(0.2)

Here, a student proposes a new hypothesis following the emergence of a significant clinical finding:

(5) (00-001.2; 0:06:??)
Chuck: ((*Reading*)) Patient underwent a right thyroid lobectomy one
week ago.
(3.1)
Chuck: Can I put up another hypothesis?
(1.0)
Sissie: ((typing))One (.) week (.) ago (.) okay?
(0.6)
(?): hmm-
(0.9)
Chuck: Hypocalcemia.

The PBL group process allows for, and encourages, volunteered hypotheses to be introduced in the course of ongoing discussions. Soliciting hypotheses is more common in early, brainstorming phases. Next we consider the structure of turns which get constituted as hypotheses.

## 2. Presenting diagnostic hypotheses

### *2.1. Forming an acceptable hypothesis*

A diagnostic hypothesis may consist simply of a word or phrase naming a medical condition:

(6) (#91-001; beginning)
Betty: Stroke

(7) (#00-001.2; 0:07:21)
Ben: Ovarian cyst or somethin like that.

(8) (#91-001; beginning)
Lill: Senile dementia Hhh

(9) (#95-014; 1:28:00)
Barb: Could it be renal stenosis?

In other cases, a diagnostic theory might be more extensively elaborated as in this example:[2]

(10) (#91-002; 0:21:38)
Betty: My other theory is that if it was- I- I- if it's not a
vascular lesion but a space occupying lesion if it was
(.) right there ((points to chart)) in the area we were
pointing to it would be like in a posterior limb of the
internal capsule which would be where (.) the corticospinals
to the leg would be going through that part.

Through their interaction, participants in a PBL tutorial display a criterial basis for what might constitute an acceptable diagnostic proposition. In general, in order to serve as an acceptable diagnosis, the proposition must name a pathological (i.e., abnormal) condition. The examples provided above satisfy this simple condition. However, supplying something other than the name of a pathological condition can in certain circumstances also serve as an acceptable hypothesis. Consider the following example:

(11) (#95-004.1; 1:08:51)
Vickie: I'm sure we all are thinking of things=
Todd: =Yeah↓ well?
Jane: Hun uh •hh
Todd: Don't know hh •hh hh (.) I'm thinking amygdala
tha(h)t's all huh uh •uhh huh hh=
Jane: =Hypothesis amygdala

Amygdala is a region of the brain. On first glance it would not seem to meet the criterion of specifying a pathological state or condition. In part it is hearable here as a hypothesis because of the way in which Todd ties it to Vickie's previous talk. Vickie calls on the group to produce hypotheses, then adds that she is sure they all are "thinking of things." Todd's use of the verb "thinking" ties "I'm thinking amygdala" to her previous "thinking of things." In the turn that follows, Jane confirms acceptance of "amygdala" as an hypothesis by other members of the group.

There are further criteria for what can serve as an acceptable diagnostic hypothesis. Not just any pathological condition will suffice. The proposed condition must account for at least some of the known symptoms. There is a need, therefore, for students to coordinate their theories with the facts of the case. Evidence that students are orienting to this criterion can be seen in situations in which a proposed diagnostic theory is challenged. For example, the following hypothesis was proposed in jest:

(12) (#00-001.2: 0:06:??)
Ben: Patient is forlorn.
(0.7)
Coach: Seems to be sitting.=
Laura: Heh-heh-↑heh-↑heh-[↑heh
Sissie: [Yeah
(2.7)
Ben: That's classic forlorn.
(0.8)
Coach: What's what's that?=
Han: =He-he-↑he-↑he-↑he
Coach: Forlorn?
Ben: Yes.
Coach: You wanna put that up as a hypothesis?=
Han: =•he[hh
(Sissie): [heh-heh-heh-heh-he=
Ben: =No: that's an obvious diagnosis.

Ben's proposition works as a joke precisely because "forlorn" fails as an hypothesis – it doesn't explain any of the patient's symptoms. As another example, consider the response to Betty's theory (shown earlier) of a "space-occupying lesion." Her proposition draws challenges first from Maria, and then from the Coach:

(13) (#91-002; 0:21:53)
Maria: [Wouldn't you expect to [see a lot=
Norman: | [*khh* hh huh hh
Coach: [Whao [kay

Maria: ⌊greater in-⌈volvement if you got
Norman: ⌊hh hh yeah
Maria: internal capsule?=

A moment later Coach adds:

(14) Coach: So why do the leg findings go away?
(1.0)

Maria challenges Betty's diagnostic theory on the grounds that the patient's symptoms were not as severe as one might expect, given Betty's theory. Coach, on the other hand, calls into question Betty's proposition that the symptoms were the result of a "space occupying lesion" on the grounds that the patient's symptoms appear and then go away.

Diagnoses can vary in terms of specificity: lesion of the amygdala, for example, is more specific than brain tumor, which, in turn, is more specific than neurological problem. Not only does a diagnostic theory have to name a pathological condition, one that is consistent with the known symptoms, but it must also provide at least as much specificity as previously provided and related theories. In the following, Vickie's "brain tumor" theory draws disaffiliative laughter from Jane, self-deprecating criticism by Vickie herself, and (moments later) criticism from the Coach:

(15) (#95-004.1; 1:08:53)
Vickie: ( ) I'm thinking (.) brain tumor
Jane: Huh huh ha
Vickie: Real specific there.
((six lines omitted))
Coach: =Brain tumor is pretty *vague*.=

Vickie's theory does name a pathological condition and it is a condition that is implicated by the known features of the patient's illness. Her proposition follows after Todd's proposition of a lesion in the region of the amygdala, however, and is less specific than his. The responses treat this hypothesis as inadequate.

### 2.2. *Marking stance with regard to a diagnostic theory*

Routinely, speakers mark their relative confidence in, or commitment to, the hypotheses they are producing. PBL members can and do produce hypotheses with declarative intonation and no tentativeness:

(16 [=6]) (#91-001; #1, beginning)
Betty: Stroke

More commonly in these data, however, speakers produce hypotheses with markers of uncertainty, tentativeness, or possible nonseriousness. An hypothesis may be marked as tentative through interrogative intonational contour:

(17) (#91-001; # 1, beginning)
Maria: Encepha*lo*pathy?

It may be presented in a questioning syntactic format:

(18) (#95-004.1; # 1, 1:08:40)
Jane: How about neurologic lesion?

(19) (#95-014; #4. 1:28)
Barb: Could it be renal stenosis?

It may be produced with linguistic or syntactic uncertainty markers, such as a modal verb ("Could" in the preceding example) or conditional adverb ("Maybe" in the example below):

(20) (91-001; # 2, 57:00)
Betty: Maybe he's got a cancer that's (.) growin' upstairs.

In the case below, the speaker uses the subjunctive mood in suggesting that another diagnosis be added to the list:

(21) (95-004.1; # 2, 1:28:45)
Suzi: I'd add dorsal column (0.5) lesion.

An hypothesis may be produced with laughter or other indication of nonseriousness. In the following example, Norman produces two closely-related diagnostic possibilities – "stroke" and "TIA" (transient ischemic attack) – with a smile and a near-laughing vocal quality (indicated on the transcript [IT2] by the "£" signs):

(22) (91-002; # 1, 10:50)
Norman: £Stroke slash TIA type of pathology£

Within a span of a few seconds, Lill offers two possible diagnostic hypotheses, following each with brief laughter:

(23) (91-001; #1, beginning)
Lill: Alzheimers hh hh

(24) (91-001; #1, beginning)
Lill: Senile dementia Hhh

Several of these features can work in combination. In Todd's proposition of "amygdala," discussed earlier, he marks uncertainty through a disclaimer ("don't know"); overt reference to mental process ("I'm thinking") which could mark uncertainty regarding what he is saying; a minimizer ("that's all"); and laughter:

(25) 95-004; # 1, 1:08:40)

Todd: Don't know hh •hh hh (.) I'm thinking amygdala
tha(h)t's all huh uh •uhh huh hh=

As these examples illustrate, the medical students produce hypotheses in ways that mark their *stance* relative to the hypotheses; that is, their certainty about, commitment to, confidence in, or seriousness about the diagnosis proposed.[3] Producing hypotheses with varying degrees of uncertainty provides interactive resources that interactants may draw upon in subsequent talk. Not coincidentally, these same ways to mark stance also constitute the hypothesis-utterance as performing different actions: making a proposition, joking, etc. It may be that an hypothesis marked as highly uncertain more readily makes disagreement or modification relevant than one produced without such marking.

## 3. Responding to diagnostic hypotheses

The PBL process calls for all hypotheses to be written on the board for further study and consideration. This provides a tangible indicator of what items group members have accepted as hypotheses. Group members respond to possible hypotheses as propositions making relevant subsequent actions culminating in acceptance or rejection. At its simplest, this can consist of a proposed hypothesis getting written on the board with no additional talk.

(26) (91-001, #1, 0:01:15)

Coach: Just- (0.4) ⌈(Put up stuff)
Norman: ⌊St⌈roke
(Betty): ⌊Stroke

In other cases, group members respond to hypothesis with actions such as repair, challenge, or agreement/disagreement. However long treatment of a single proposed hypothesis may continue, it culminates in the item being written on the board (accepted) or not (rejected).

### *3.1. Repair and correction*

Participants may forward the gist or central idea of a hypothesis while initiating repair (Schegloff, Jefferson, and Sacks 1977) or providing correction (Jefferson 1987) of the term or formulation of the idea. In the next example, Lill proposes hypothyroidism as an hypothesis then begins to formulate a question linking it to the symptoms. Betty reproduces the prefix slightly changed, with a questioning intonation that invites confirmation or correction. Lill repeats "hypo" thus declining the repair. This interlude serves as a side sequence (Jefferson 1972) after which participants discuss the proposed hypothesis (shown in the next section).

(27) (91-001 # 2, 57:00)
Lill: How about hypothyroidism (.) does that cause
Betty: Hyper?
Lill: Hypo

In the next example one group member presents an hypothesis of cancer with the colloquial expression "growin' upstairs" to indicate its location in the brain. Several turns later (the intervening talk is not about this hypothesis), Maria – the scribe who is standing at the board, marker in hand – returns to this hypothesis, restating it as "metastatic"; that is, as having originated elsewhere in the body and then developed in the brain. She does so with a questioning intonation that marks it as subject to confirmation. Betty accepts this correction, repeating "metastatic" and adding "CA" (abbreviation for cancer):

(28) (91-001; 0:57:00)
Betty: Maybe he's got a cancer that's (.) growin' upstairs.
((20 lines omitted))
Maria Metastatic?
Betty: Yeah maybe a metastatic CA.

Repair may work to clarify wording or move the proposed hypothesis to greater specificity or to technical language.

### *3.2. Question or challenge*

Participants (the Coach or the students) may question or challenge the hypothesis by calling on its producer to provide an explanation for it. In the following example, Chuck proposes a new hypothesis. He provides only a single word with no elaboration. After a pause, the Coach asks him to explain, and he offers his reasoning:

(29) (00-001.2; 0:06:??)
Chuck: Can I put up another hypothesis?
(1.0)
Sissie: ((typing))One (.) week (.) ago (.) okay?
(0.6)
(?): hmm-
(0.9)
Chuck: Hypocalcemia.
(1.2)
Coach: Wanna talk about that?
(0.7)
Ben: (Move) your on ⌈learning issues there
Laura: ⌊OH you're righ:⌈t!
(Sissie): ⌊•HHH
Laura: ((whispered)) Parathyroid ⌈gland!
Chuck: ⌊Coulda also cut out the
parathy:roid hh (0.7) I'm guessing and it caused
hypocalcemia.

Here, students respond to the Coach's call for evidence to back up their diagnosis of atherosclerosis:

(30) (#91-002; 0: 58:10)
Coach: What evidence do you have for it.
Maria: U:m hypertension? history of hypertension?
(1.0) high cholesterol high fat diet um
(1.0) long time history of smo⌈king fifty two
Norman: ⌊Smoking
Maria: years (and um) alcohol

### *3.3. Agreement or disagreement*

When one student presents an hypothesis, others may mark their agreement or disagreement with it. Here, John offers "Alzheimers"; after a pause, Jane first points out a problem with this theory (specifically, that the patient is "young," while Alzheimer's typically is ascribed to older patients), then gives tentative acceptance of it (although we cannot hear all of her words).

(31) (#95-004; 1:15:37)
John: What about Alzheimers (0.5) °Alzheimers°?
(1.0)
Jane: She's young but I guess you ((remainder unintelligible))

In the "hypothyroidism" example (also shown earlier), Betty implies disagreement by raising an objection (although we cannot fully understand what she is saying, the word "though" at the end of her turn displays it as disagreeing with the prior). May then asks a question containing a "candidate answer" (Pomerantz 1988) that may challenge the basis for Betty's preceding disagreement. Following this, Betty agrees with May and an account that allows for Lill's proposition to stand as an exception to a regular pattern ("it could present really weird"). Then without pause, Betty evaluates this theory as "a good possibility":[4]

| | | |
|---|---|---|
| (32) | (91-001 # 2, 57:00) | |
| | Lill: | How about hypothy[roidism (.) does that cause |
| | Maria: | [Yeah |
| | Betty: | Hyper? |
| | Lill: | Hypo |
| | Betty: | Usually (it ) chunky though. |
| | May: | I'n't that in the old (   ) I mean |
| | Betty: | Yeah it could present really weird. |
| | | Yeah that's a good possibility |
| | Lill: | >Cause I was just looking at his heart rate< |
| | Betty: | I think that should go up there in the hypotheses: |

Following her suggestion, the scribe adds it to the list of hypotheses on the board.

## *3.4. Proposing a test to confirm or disconfirm an hypothesis*

One way of responding to an articulated diagnostic theory is to propose a test to more conclusively rule in or rule out the theory. In the fragment that follows, the group is reviewing the list of previously proposed hypotheses. Several of the theories (e.g., Graves syndrome, hyperthyroidism, thyroid carcinoma) implicate the thyroid gland, but they realized at this point that they had not performed the relevant examination:

| | | |
|---|---|---|
| (33) | (#00-005.1; 1:36:00) | |
| | Chuck: | There are a couple of things we need to do |
| | | [right off the bat.] |
| | Sissie: | [We did not        ] do:: (0.5) a thyroid exam (0.4) |
| | | we did we looked at her eyes that's the only thing we did. |
| | Han: | Yeah we didn't do exams yet. |
| | Ben: | Yeah we haven't done exams. |

In a study of scientific reasoning, Okada and Simon (1997) described how one way of responding to a theory proposition is to propose an experiment to test the theory. In the PBL tutorials we have been analyzing, a parallel action involves turning to the casebook to find information from the patient's case history or medical examination. In this instance, the students consulted the casebook to determine the results of a thyroid exam.

The elements reviewed in list fashion above – ways that hypotheses are occasioned, produced, and responded to – become more meaningful when seen in combination as unfolding in their sequential contexts, in holistic hypothesis episodes. How speakers occasion hypotheses influences how they are produced recognizably as such; how they are produced guides and constrains how they are treated. Through these elements in combination, PBL members go about the business of creating and constituting diagnostic hypotheses.

## 4. The components working together: Interactive production of multiple diagnostic hypotheses

In this section we show excerpts from several minutes early in a PBL tutorial in which occasioning, producing, and responding to hypotheses work jointly as the participants generate a list of possible diagnoses to pursue. This interval of interaction is highly relevant to the topic of hypothesis generation because all of the diagnostic theories proposed by the group were proposed here, even though the group's deliberations with respect to this case went on for an additional five and a half hours segmented into three meetings.[5] The transcript fragment begins with Betty reading aloud the reasons for which the patient had come to the clinic (i.e., "the presenting situation"). After a request to repeat some information, some laughter, and a bit of digressive talk, the Coach *solicits* hypothesizing. He asks a question that prompts students to connect the symptoms they have just heard to possible explanations.

(34) (SIUC PBL 91-001; #1, beginning)
Betty: Sixty-five year old white male (2.0) explains
he has had recent problems with his memory and with quote
expressing himself
(5.0)
Norman: (white gentleman)
Coach: (          pathological part) huh is the proper way of
putting that hhh
Norman: °huh huh huh° What's he got?
(Lill): [(Explain it again)
Betty: [He's had recent problems with his memory and with
expressing himself.
(Maria): We had this (guy before) (.) didn't we (          )
Betty: The hemi:paresis?
(Lill): [Heah huh hh
(Betty): [(hah huh)

May: (In other [words how res )]
Coach: [So what does that make ]you think of.

In close succession, two students *present* a possible hypothesis via a single word, “stroke.” The Coach *responds to* this hypothesis with an “okay” (see Beach 1993) that shows acceptance of it; following a pause, he provides another *occasioning* prompt:

(35) Coach: Just- (0.4) [(Put up stuff)
Norman: [St[roke
(Betty): [Stroke
(0.8)
Coach: Okay
(1.2)
Coach: Anything else?

This “Anything else?” question is important not only for what it solicits but for what it does not solicit; specifically, it directs talk away from further discussion of “stroke” which might lead to premature acceptance or rejection of that hypothesis. By this move the Coach displays that it is relevant now (in this brainstorming phase of the process) to produce more than one possibility before accepting or rejecting the first one. In response to the Coach’s prompt, Lill *produces* the diagnostic hypothesis “Alzheimers.” After a pause, Norman *responds* with a question clarifying whether Lill is suggesting a recent onset of Alzheimers as an hypothesis. She does not answer the question (perhaps orienting to this as the brainstorming phase of their process) but chuckles briefly then *produces* another candidate hypothesis, first stated as “kidney problems” then self-corrected to “hyperuricemia.” Norman *responds* to this hypothesis by assessing it positively (“I can buy that”). Coach repeats the diagnostic term with questioning intonation, possibly initiating *repair* on it.

(36) Lill: Alzheimers hh hh
(0.5)
Norman: Recent?
Lill: °hh hh •hh° um kidney problems (.)
hyperuricemia
(1.0)
Norman: I can buy that
Coach: Hyperuricemia?

However, group talk digresses to joking and process clarification for several turns (not shown). Moments later, the scribe (Maria) is writing hypotheses on the board. After writing “stroke” she turns to Lill, asks Lill to confirm, and repeats the term "hyperuricemia." Thus this hypothesis is re-topicalized. Lill does not speak, although she may display affirmation visually (she is off camera). Betty *responds* to this hypothesis by soliciting an explanation from Lill. The adverbial phrase "a little bit," which projects what sort of answer is to be provided, may show Betty's orientation to this phase of the group process: that this is not the time for protracted discussion, but for brief accounting for the hypothesis. It may also display that Betty does not see yet see this candidate hypothesis as self-evidently related to the symptoms. Lill jokingly declines to account; Maria gives what may be an alternative way to express this hypothesis:

(37) Maria: What did you say? hyperuricemia?
(0.5)
Betty: Could you explain that a little bit.
Lill: °No°
(?): Huh hah [huh
Maria: [Some kind of encephalopath[y: for kidney
(Lill): [Yeah
Maria: failure.

Coach invites correction of the name. Lill begins to produce a corrected version. Someone else in the group offers a candidate repair and asks Lill for confirmation, which she provides. Norman, Betty, and Maria repeat the corrected version of the hypothesis, and the Coach *responds* with an "Okay" that shows acceptance of this term:

(38) Coach: Is there a better name for that.
Lill: Hyper:=
(?): Hyperuremia is that whatchyou mean?=
Lill: =Yeah.
Norman: Yeah Hyperuremia
Betty: Hyperuremia
Coach: Okay

This instance demonstrates several ways PBL participants treat hypotheses early in the group process. The Coach *occasions* hypotheses and shapes the talk to minimize critical discussion of them. The students *produce* hypotheses in simple versions. Their *responses* such as clarifying questions and assessments mark the degree to which they accept the hypotheses as candidates worthy of further consideration. Correction and repair initiation raise possibilities for preserving the sense of an hypothesis but providing an alternative label which may prove more accurate or helpful. Calling for and providing preliminary explanations of hypotheses allows for topicalizing the reasoning and evidence that underlie their suggestion.

Having the student scribe (in this case, Maria) *write* possible hypotheses on the board provides a procedure for disambiguating whether or not these initial suggestions are to be considered further. When the Coach responds to hypotheses with an "Okay," his "acceptance" does not mean it is *the* correct diagnosis, but that it is an acceptable *candidate* hypothesis, which the scribe can add to the list. Other actions such as repeating or initiating repair on a candidate hypothesis precede its getting written on the board.

## 5. Constituting diagnostic hypotheses in interaction: Two contrasting cases

The preceding examples show the range of lexical items within various turns at talk that group members treat as diagnostic hypotheses. Hypotheses may appear vague or partial rather than well-formed, complete statements. Items gain or fail to gain tacit acceptance as candidate hypotheses through interactive processes. Participants may treat quite similar lexical items as a hypothesis in one situation and not so in another. The following two examples, both drawn from the same interaction shown in the preceding section, provide illustrative contrast.

The group's discussion proceeds with various students posing questions and Betty (in her role as reader) reading information from the casebook. At one point she reads a long response from the patient's wife which suggests that the patient may have an alcohol abuse problem. Although a history of alcohol abuse has not yet been established, Maria proposes a new diagnostic hypothesis based on this possibility:

(39) Maria: It could be that (0.2) ↑thiamine deficiency thing that Wernicke's?

Betty overlaps Maria's turn at talk to produce what sounds like a process suggestion for the group, disattending Maria's utterance in progress and potentially moving the talk in some different direction. Maria continues her utterance, however, by naming the syndrome she believes to be the result of thiamine deficiency ("Wernicke's"). The Coach begins a query presumably relevant to Maria's proposition, and another question from Norman overlaps the coach's question. It is the latter to which Maria's "No" responds:

(40) Betty: We should see (0.1) we should just
Coach: When is that ⌈( )⌉
Norman: ⌊Is that an⌋ acute onset though?
(0.8)
Maria: No.

Though stated as a query, Norman's utterance represents a challenge to Maria's candidate hypothesis by raising an implication that would stand at odds with the information they have on the case. Maria replies to Norman's question by providing a link between her proposed hypothesis and the drinking symptom just reported:

| | | |
|---|---|---|
| (41) | Maria: | If [he's been ] drinking you know? |
| | Norman: | [(more common)] |

The Coach asks Maria the mechanism by which thiamine deficiency could produce the symptoms seen in the patient. After an extended discussion in which Maria, Lill, and May attempt to construct such an account,[6] Coach invites Maria to add her theory to the list of hypotheses on the board:

| | | |
|---|---|---|
| (42) | Coach: | What is it? |
| | | (0.5) |
| | Coach: | What causes Wernicke's? |
| | | (0.9) |
| | Maria: | Thiamine deficiency. |
| | | (1.5) |
| | Coach: | And why do you think he might have a thiamine deficiency? |
| | | (0.6) |
| | Maria: | Cuz he's an alcoholic maybe. |
| | Coach: | Okay then you want to add that to your list of encephalopathic conditions? ((*waves hand toward board*)) |

Maria's suggestion gets added to the hypothesis list on the board – that is, jointly constituted by the group as an hypothesis – through the ways other members of the group, most particularly Betty, Norman, and Coach, respond to it. Each offers challenges to Maria's theory. Betty suggests that they wait on advancing such a theory until they have firm data to support it, Norman argues that Maria's hypothesis is inconsistent with the clinical presentation, and Coach presses the group to provide a mechanism that would justify including Maria's hypothesis as a diagnostic theory. While perhaps showing skepticism to her idea, the others treat it seriously, engaging in the "hypothesis space" it puts forward. Critical questions and challenges are among the range of actions made "procedurally relevant" (Schegloff 1991) by such a proposition.

The following example shows quite different treatment of a possible hypothesis. Somewhat earlier in the segment, Betty had observed that the patient's responses in the book are written in such a way as to suggest that the patient had some form of speech dysfluency. Norman and Maria offer two ways of accounting for this fact:

(43) Norman: Memory
Maria: That means he can't speak
Norman: or: ⌈( ) memory
Betty: ⌊So that might be related to=
Maria: =expressive aphasia

This discussion went no further. Following this, Lill made a humorous suggestion to Betty about her readings of the patient's responses and Betty shifted topic to discussing other cases in which the patient's responses were written in unusual ways. No one responded to "expressive aphasia" as if it were a hypothesis proposition, and Maria did not record it on the board. However, it appears to offer an explanation for the patient's symptoms and thus conceivably could earn hypothesis status. Why doesn't it?

To one not familiar with medical terminology, "expressive aphasia" might seem like something that could serve as a diagnostic theory in the same way that "Wernicke's syndrome" apparently did. There is a large difference between the two, however, in terms of their usefulness as objects "to guide investigation into the patient's problem." Maria's proposition of Wernicke's syndrome introduces a pathophysiological mechanism to account for the patient's symptoms. The assertion that the patient suffered from expressive aphasia, on the other hand, does nothing more than supply a technical name for what she had already observed, namely that the patient "can't speak." Similarly, no one orients to Norman's proclamation of "Memory" as a diagnostic theory. The other members of the group treat both of these contributions as descriptions (not explanations) of symptoms and proceed with their business accordingly. What we see here then are two semantic entities, "Wernicke's syndrome" and "expressive aphasia," one treated interactionally as a hypothesis, the other treated interactionally as a non-hypothesis.

## 6. Discussion

An hypothesis is not a stable, independent social fact; rather, social actors jointly produce and constitute some lexical item as an hypothesis through their actions embedded within ongoing sequential activities. Its meaning – i.e., the action(s) that it accomplishes, and the activity(ies) of which it is part – gets shaped in part by how participants occasion it, produce it, and respond to it. PBL members (including the coach) solicit hypotheses explicitly, particularly at certain points in the deliberative process. At other times, members volunteer hypotheses, marking them as having been touched off by the talk. The lexical items that constitute an hypothesis, and production features that shape what actions it accomplishes and mark the speaker's stance towards it, also contribute to its emergent sense and status.

Although some items get placed on the hypothesis list immediately after they are uttered, with little or no discussion, routinely substantive talk occurs between the first mention of the hypothesis and its appearance on the board. Corrections and repair, questioning and challenging, agreeing or disagreeing, and testing, are ways to develop an hypothesis topically and interactionally. In the PBL process, the medical students are expected to generate lists of hypotheses, and a candidate item attains formal status as a hypothesis when the scribe writes it on the board. It remains there until students decide to revise it, discard it, or select it as the best diagnosis for the case.

How group members occasion, produce, and respond to hypotheses directly orients to (and in turn helps constitute) the phase of the group process in which the hypothesizing occurs. During early portions of the process, group members are expected to produce many hypotheses in brainstorming fashion. They invoke and orient to these to generate discussion, learning issues, and other hypotheses. Group members do not evaluate hypotheses against each other in order to select one or more as "correct." To do so would make relevant closing down talk on topic, thereby precluding possibilities for learning and identifying learning issues which are central purposes of PBL. However, hypotheses do get treated critically.

Diagnosing as a cognitive and interactive process occurs in countless situations, both institutional and casual. These data provide snapshots of students in transition from laypersons to expert diagnosticians; along the way they must learn the cognitive and communicative processes necessary to achieving acceptable diagnoses. Diagnosing is crucial to effective practice, at least as conceived of in the Western medical model.[7] Diagnosing is a central activity in problem-based learning, and developing diagnosing skills is a central purpose for the PBL curriculum. The students' diagnostic work approximates its "real life" parallels, yet there are fundamental differences. They come up with diagnoses outside or out of earshot of patients or clients, and in this way their practices perhaps are more like what physicians do "backstage" (consulting with other medical professionals, writing, studying) than what they do when consulting with a patient. When talking directly to patients, medical care providers must orient to role expectations, time constraints, and other factors that shape how diagnosing gets communicatively accomplished.

Despite the absence of a patient or client, however, the students' diagnostic work is absolutely "on stage." These participants face real pressures to perform well, such performance being the basis for medical school evaluations and social judgments. Stance markers, for example, show speakers orienting to the social and evaluative environment. It is understood that second-year medical students have much yet to learn; it is understood that they must come to recognize clearly their own knowledge deficiencies. They are encouraged to make evident their knowledge deficiencies and uncertainties. Accordingly, there are good reasons to offer "bad" hypotheses. However, it may be important to display to co-participants that one *understands* one's talk to be ignorant, wrong, insufficient, etc. Just as Shakespeare teaches us that the wise man knows he is a fool, so the wise PBL student will let other participants know that his or her idea may be way off base, or that it isn't worded properly, or that it is incomplete. To fail to do so risks being proven wrong or judged as not knowing any better. On the other hand, students are expected to develop confidence along the way in their abilities to diagnose, and it is conceivable that marking distance from one's hypotheses could also lead to participants questioning one's competence.

Consider, for example, two hypothesis presentations shown earlier in this paper:

(44) (#91-002; 0:21:38)
Betty: My other theory is that if it was- I- I- if it's not a
vascular lesion but a space occupying lesion if it was
(.) right there ((points to chart)) in the area we were
pointing to it would be like in a posterior limb of the
internal capsule which would be where (.) the
corticospinals to the leg would be going through that part.
(1.0)

This candidate diagnosis – Betty calls it a "theory" – of a "space occupying lesion" is located within an argument showing how it would account for the patient's symptoms. Although it draws critical questioning from other group members, it is treated as a serious possibility. Perhaps it is wrong, but it is informedly so; it shows a reasonable reasoning process, that of ruling out plausible alternative explanations. In contrast, the stance markers accompanying the hypothesis below, whatever else they may be doing, might leave its speaker open to judgments of lack of confidence or competence.

(45) (95-004; # 1, 1:08:40)
Todd: Don't know hh •hh hh (.) I'm thinking amygdala
tha(h)t's all huh uh •uhh huh hh=

It is clear which of the two examples above "sounds" more like a doctor (and, probably, which of the two most us would want to hear from our doctors!). Perhaps the medical school educational process provides a systematic basis for inculcating the kind of strong confidence doctors sometimes show that gets read as egotistical or arrogant.[8] These social considerations impact and are impacted by the turn-by-turn unfolding of interactions. We note their importance while deferring formal analysis of them for future research.

In this analysis we eschew critical evaluation of the hypothesizing process in favor of descriptive and interpretive analysis of members' displayed reasoning procedures. We do not claim that the participants got it right; it might be that medical experts viewing this interaction would find fault with the reasoning, the knowledge invoked, or the outcome. Nevertheless, these data provide a glimpse into the kinds of diagnostic work students do while learning to diagnose as doctors. They offer a valuable resource for characterizing diagnosis as a communicative achievement. Identifying means by which participants in any environment interactively constitute diagnostic hypotheses will provide a richer picture of how people accomplish "interpretation in sequential terms" (Sacks 1992: 134).

## *Acknowledgments*

An abbreviated version of this paper was presented at the 1999 Annual Meeting of the American Education Research Association (AERA) in a symposium entitled, "Learning Environments for Exploring Hypothesis Generation, Reasoning, and Argumentation." Portions of this paper were first presented at the LSI in Communication Disorders Roundtable, University of Rhode Island, June, 1998. The analysis has profited from discussions at the Roundtable and in Department of Speech Communication data sessions at Southern Illinois University, Carbondale. Mindy Conlee, Elizabeth Gullickson-Tolman, Jane McGuire, and Stephanie Poole-Martinez provided capable transcription assistance. Dana Kovarsky and an anonymous reviewer provided helpful feedback. Finally, we wish to thank the Abbott Fund for its continued support of our research program.

## *Appendix A. Transcribing symbols*

(Developed by Gail Jefferson; see J. M. Atkinson and J. Heritage (eds.) 1984, *Structures of Social Action; Studies in Conversation Analysis.* pp. ix–xvi. Cambridge University Press)

| | |
|---|---|
| [ ] | Brackets indicate overlapping utterances. |
| = | Equal marks indicate contiguous utterances, or continuation of the same utterance to the next line. |
| ( . ) | Period within parentheses indicates micropause. |
| (2.0) | Indicates timed pause in approximate seconds. |
| ye:s | Colon indicates stretching of sound it follows. |
| yes. | Period indicates falling intonation. |
| yes, | Comma indicates relatively constant intonation. |
| yes? | Question mark indicates upward intonation. |
| yes! | Exclamation indicates animated tone. |
| yes- | Single dash indicates abrupt sound cutoff. |

| | |
|---|---|
| *yes* | Italics indicate emphasis. |
| YES | Capital letters indicate increased volume. |
| °yes° | Degree marks indicate decreased volume of talk between them. |
| hhh | Indicates audible aspiration, possibly laughter. |
| •hhh | Superscript period indicates inbreath audible aspiration, possibly laughter. |
| ye(hh)s | Indicates within-speech aspiration, possibly laughter. |
| ((cough)) | Items within double parentheses indicate some sound or feature of the talk which is not easily transcribable. |
| (yes) | Parentheses indicate transcriber doubt about hearing of passage. |
| ↑yes ↓yes | Arrow indicates marked change in intonation. |
| £yes£ | Pound signs indicate "smile voice" delivery. |

## Notes

1. This may be undergoing some change of late. An article in *New York* (Kaufman, 15 October 2001) makes the case that increased availability of medical information on the internet leads more patients to present their own diagnoses to health care providers. According to the article, doctors do not necessarily welcome this trend.
2. For an analysis of this instance see Glenn, Koschmann, and Conlee (1999).
3. In his explication of the notion of *footing,* Goffman (1981: 144–147) deconstructs the notion of *speaker* to suggest the possibility that a person uttering some talk may but need not necessarily also be a "principal," that is, someone who is committed to the idea expressed. By marking uncertainty, these medical students continue as (in Goffman's terms) "animators" and "authors" of the diagnostic hypotheses, but reduce their stance as principals wholly committed to the ideas. See also Schiffrin (1990) for application of these notions to arguments and stories.
4. Betty's use of the word "Yeah" parallels instances described by Pomerantz (1984: 68–69) of speakers responding to first assessments with second assessments. In such uses, "Yeah" shows agreement but often is followed by disagreement such that Pomerantz characterizes it as a way to show downgraded or "weak" agreement. Similarly here, "Yeah" is a way for Betty to support Lill's proposal while showing skepticism.
5. The emergence of multiple diagnostic theories during this period was summarized in Conlee and Koschmann (1997).
6. We are not well enough versed in alternative models to offer informed commentary. However, it is difficult to imagine any health or medical treatment practice that does not rely in some fashion on explaining or accounting for physical conditions, i.e., on diagnosing.
7. This claim forwards the ethnomethodological preference for eschewing judgment of

the quality of participant actions in favor of careful description and interpretation of how they are doing what they do in the first place. The ironical use of "bad" here is meant to imply that such features as lay wording, incomplete utterances, and stance markers of uncertainty, which might tempt one to question the competence of these students, are all methodical in their usages; they are ways to accomplish social actions in interaction. For a parallel, see Harold Garfinkel's (1967) "Good organizational reasons for 'bad' clinic records."

8. Thanks to an anonymous reviewer for suggesting this point.

## References

Atkinson, J. Maxwell and John Heritage
1984 *Structures of Social Action; Studies in Conversation Analysis*. New York: Cambridge University Press.

Barrows, Howard S.
1990 Inquiry: The pedagogical importance of a skill central to clinical practice. *Journal of Medical Education* 24, 3–5.
1994 *Practice-Based Learning: Problem-Based Learning Applied to Medical Education*. Springfield, IL: Southern Illinois University School of Medicine.

Barrows, Howard S. and R. Tamblyn
1980 *Problem-based Learning; An Approach to Medical Education*. New York: Springer.

Beach, Wayne
1993 Transitional regularities for 'casual' 'Okay' usages. *Journal of Pragmatics* 19, 225–252.

Clayman, S. and Douglas Maynard
1995 Ethnomethodology and conversation analysis. In ten Have, P. and G. Psathas (eds.), *Situated Order: Studies in the Social Organization of Talk and Embodied Activities*. Washington, D.C.: University Press of America, 1–30.

Conlee, M. and Timothy Koschmann
1997 Representations of clinical reasoning in a PBL meeting: The Inquiry Trace. *Teaching and Learning in Medicine* 9, 51–55.

Distlehorst, L. and Howard S. Barrows
1982 A new tool for problem-based self-directed learning. *Journal of Medical Education* 57, 466–488.

Garfinkel, Harold
1967 Good organizational reasons for 'bad' clinic records. In *Studies in Ethnomethodology*. Englewood Cliffs, NJ: Prentice-Hall, 186–207.

Glenn, Phillip J.
1998 Medical students' interactive diagnosing in a problem-based learning group. Sixth International Pragmatics Conference, Reims, France, July, 1998.

Glenn, Phillip, Timothy Koschmann, and M. Conlee
1999 Theory presentation and assessment in a problem-based learning group. *Discourse Processes* 27, 119–133.

Goffman, Erving
1981 Footing. In Goffman E., *Forms of Talk*. Philadelphia: University of Pennsylvania Press, 124–159.
Jefferson, Gail
1987 On exposed and embedded correction in conversation. In Button, G. and J. R. E. Lee (eds.), *Talk and Social Organization*. Clevedon: Multilingual Matters, 86–100.
1972 Side sequences. In Sudnow, D. (ed.), *Studies in Social Interaction*. New York: The Free Press, 294–338.
Kaufman, J.
2001 Click and cure. *New York*, 15 October, 40–42.
Koschmann, Timothy, Phillip Glenn, and M Conlee
2000 When is a problem-based tutorial not tutorial? Analyzing the tutor's role in the emergence of a learning issue. In Hmelo, C. and D. Evensen (eds.), *Problem-based Learning: Gaining Insights on Learning Interactions through Multiple Methods of Inquiry*. Mahwah, NJ: Lawrence Erlbaum, 53–74.
Koschmann, Timothy, A. C. Kelson, P. J. Feltovich, and Howard Barrows
1996 Computer-supported problem-based learning: A principled approach to the use of computers in collaborative learning. In Koschmann, T. D. (ed.), *CSCL: Theory and Practice of an Emerging Paradigm*. Hillsdale, NJ: Lawrence Erlbaum, 83–124.
Okada, T. and Herbert Simon
1997 Collaborative discovery in a scientific domain. *Cognitive Science* 21, 109–146.
Pomerantz, Anita
1984 Agreeing and disagreeing with assessments: Some features of preferred/dispreferred turn shapes. In Atkinson, J. and J. Heritage (eds), *Structures of Social Action; Studies in Conversation Analysis*. Cambridge: Cambridge University Press, 57–101.
1988 Offering a candidate answer: An information seeking strategy. *Communication Monographs* 55, 360–373.
Pomerantz, Anita and B. J. Fehr
1997 Conversation analysis: An approach to the study of social action as sense making practices. In van Dijk, T. A. (ed.), *Discourse as Social Interaction*. Thousand Oaks, CA: Sage, 64–91.
Psathas, George
1995 *Conversation Analysis; The Study of Talk-in-Interaction*. Thousand Oaks, CA: Sage.
Sacks, Harvey
1992 *Lectures on Conversation, Volume II*. (G. Jefferson, ed.). Oxford, UK: Blackwell.
Schegloff, Emmanuel
1991 Reflections on talk and social structure. In Boden, D and D. Zimmerman (eds), *Talk and Social Structure*. Berkeley: University of California Press, 44–70.
Schegloff, Emmanuel, Gail Jefferson, and Harvey Sacks
1977 The preference for self-correction in the organization of repair in conversation. *Language* 53, 361–382.

Schegloff, Emanuel and Harvey Sacks
1984 Opening up closings. In Baugh, J. and J. Sherzer (eds.), *Reading in Sociolinguistics; Studies in Language in Use,* 66–69.
Schiffrin, Deborah
1990 The management of a cooperative self during argument: The role of opinions and stories. In Grimshaw, A. D. (ed.), *Conflict Talk: Sociolinguistic Investigations of Arguments in Conversations.* Cambridge, UK: Cambridge University Press, 241–259.
Southern Illinois University School of Medicine
1994 Unit 10 document: Nervous system, psychiatry, and the musculo-skeletal system. Unpublished curricular document: Southern Illinois University, Springfield, IL.
ten Have, Paul
1999 *Doing Conversation Analysis; A Practical Guide.* London: Sage.

# Chapter 9
# Emotion and objectivity in medical diagnosis

*Dana Kovarsky, Linda K. Snelling, and Elaine Meyer*

*Kovarsky, Snelling, and Meyer take a look at the emotional side of discourse among physicians and between physicians and their patients. While physicians' discussions of emotion are usually suppressed in face-to-face interactions with patients, these authors find that emotion sometimes comes to the surface in private meetings among physicians. The authors argue from their discourse analysis that dealing with feelings not only deepens the diagnostic discourse, but also legitimizes the emotional reactions of physicians who are trying to come to grips with the life-world realities associated with the death of their patients. In group discussions among physicians themselves, the voice of medicine is interpenetrated by their emotional response to illness and death.*

Reflecting on her own medical training in pediatrics, Remen (1996) described the following difficult experience:

> The second day of my internship in pediatrics I went with my senior resident to tell some young parents that the automobile accident from which they had escaped without a scratch had killed their only child. Very new to this doctor thing, when they cried, I had cried with them. After it was over, the resident took me aside and told me that I had behaved very unprofessionally. "These people are counting on our strength," he said. I had let them down. I took this criticism very much to heart. By the time I was a senior resident, I hadn't cried in years. During that [senior residency year] a two-year-old baby, left unattended only for a moment, drowned in a bathtub. We fought to bring him back but after an hour we had to concede defeat. Taking the intern with me, I went to tell these parents that we had not been able to save their child. Overwhelmed, they began to sob. After a time, the father looked at me standing there, strong and silent in my white coat, the shaken intern by my side. "I'm sorry, Doctor," he said. "I'll get ahold of myself in a minute." I remember this man, his face wet with a father's tears, and I think of his apology with shame. Convinced by then that my grief was a useless, self-indulgent waste of time, I had made myself into the sort of person to who one could apologize for being in pain. (Remen 1996: 53–54)

From popular films like Patch Adams to the autobiographical account presented by Remen, there is a cultural sense that traditional medical training practices in North America require physicians to develop an objective professional "voice" while subordinating their own subjective, emotional responses to the expressed concerns, experiences, and worries of patients. Over the past three decades, however, there has been a growing concern that a lack of attentiveness to the patient's subjective lifeworld can lead to missed opportunities for appropriate medical diagnosis and treatment (Ainsworth-Vaughn 1998; Barton 1999; Fisher and Todd 1993; Korsh and Negrete 1972; Mishler 1984). When there is an exclusive focus on diagnostic categories without attending to the emotional experience of illness, valuable information needed to care for patients may be lost (Remen 1994: 224).

Clearly, physicians face a daunting challenge. Their biomedical expertise is greatly valued and needed to appropriately diagnose and treat patients. At the same time, they must also seek to apprehend the values, feelings, and experiences of patients in ways that often are not part of their medical training. In short, physicians must learn to exercise the authority and power associated with objective medical expertise in ways that incorporate human experiences with illness; experiences that are not only biomedical, but also social and emotional.

Given the vast store of biomedical knowledge that modern physicians must acquire, it is not surprising that far less attention has been paid to the intersubjective side of medical training: a side that would require physicians to develop a medical voice that integrates their own personal experiences, concerns, and values with those of their patients. This chapter describes a special type of speech event within the practice of medical training called psychosocial rounds in which efforts are made by professionals to integrate the objective and intersubjective aspects of diagnosis. During these rounds, physicians-in-training would meet as a group with the Chief of the Pediatric Intensive Care Unit (PICU) to discuss difficult cases. Here, the Chief would encourage these physicians to examine their own emotional reactions to ongoing diagnosis and treatment within the PICU.

As data were collected and examined, we became interested in how the "voice of medicine" (Mishler 1984) was related to the experienced emotional reactions expressed by the participants in the meetings. Mishler described the voice of medicine as a "structure of meanings" (1984: 103) characterized by "disinterested" observers operating in "objective space and time" according to the principles of "scientific rationality and formal logic" (1984: 122). This medical voice is grounded in the use of medical terminology, objective descriptions of physical symptoms, and the classification of these ailments within a reductionist biomedical model for the purpose of diagnosis and treatment. Mishler contrasted the medical voice with that of the patient lifeworld in which "the self is the center of space and time coordinates [and] ... events take on relevance from their relationship to acting subjects' interests, purposes, and plans" (1984: 122). This voice is expressed in the use of non-technical discourse about the subjective experience of illness in relation to the patient's social relationships and the everyday world.

Based upon an analysis of first time, doctor–patient visits, Mishler found that these two voices were in constant conflict with one another: "the medical interview may be viewed as an arena of struggle between the natural attitude with its common sense lifeworld and the scientific attitude with its objectified world of abstract logic and rationality" (1984: 123). In his view, the medical voice was not only dominant, but it also served to disrupt and disorganize the voice from the patient's lifeworld. While patients "try and gain some control over the communicative space of the medical interview to enhance possibilities to present their experiences, understandings, and aims; [physicians] try to control topics and direct the interview course so as to accomplish their clinical tasks as systematically as possible" (Hyden and Mishler 1999: 178).

In pursuit of biomedical signs and symptoms of disease, patients' narrative accounts of their lived experiences with illness are disrupted and minimized or ignored. Because these socially grounded accounts of experienced illness are viewed as a significant source of data in medical decision-making (Brody 1987; Kleinman 1988), the loss of such information is not trivial: "clinical practitioners must become versed" in their patients' socially situated accounts of experienced illness, "not only for correct diagnoses, but also to develop treatment plans that are acceptable to patients and more likely to result in compliance" (Hyden and Mishler 1999: 180). In short, there are calls for a new voice of medicine that moves beyond traditional biomedical notions of diagnosis and treatment to account for the phenomenologically grounded, lived experience of illness.

In the present investigation, we sought an alternative vantage point from which to examine the voice of medicine; one that afforded us at least a partial glimpse into the lifeworld of the physicians themselves. We focused on interactions among physicians as they participated in psychosocial rounds, a context one-step removed from directed doctor–patient contact. Our analysis of this context revealed that the voice of medicine did not stand in opposition to the voice of the patient lifeworld. Not only did the expressed emotional reactions of professionals to the subjective experiences of patients and colleagues provide impetus for medical diagnosis and treatment, these reactions also served a didactic function as physicians-in-training acquired biomedical information.

We begin by describing the manner in which data were collected and analyzed in the PICU. Next, background information on the nature and purpose of psychosocial rounds is presented. Following this, transcribed excerpts from the rounds are used to illustrate the relationships between the reported emotional experiences of physicians-in-training and their medical diagnoses. In short, not only did emotion appear to be an inescapable aspect of professional life for those who worked in the PICU, one that could fuel the search for biomedical diagnoses, the reported emotional experiences also served an important didactic function within the context of psychosocial rounds.

## 1. Data collection and analysis

The data reported on here were part of a larger, ongoing investigation into the everyday medical practices of a PICU affiliated with an urban teaching hospital. As part of this larger project, undergraduate and graduate student fieldworkers observed activities within the "pod" – a unit with its own separate physical space for addressing the needs of critically ill infants, children, and adolescents. Within the pod, fieldworkers would locate themselves both inside and outside the rooms of patients. This included the observation of traditional hospital rounds where attending physicians were accompanied by physicians-in-training as they went from room to room to discuss and monitor patient progress.

One common observation among fieldworkers was the lack of intense emotional display on the part of the medical staff within the PICU. This apparent lack of emotional display stood in stark contrast to the devastating events in the lives of children and families that were playing themselves out on a daily basis. As one fieldworker noted in a journal entry:

> ... out on the unit, [emotions] are never shown, or at least not in any manner that an outsider would be able to pick up on. I have only witnessed one outward expression of grief and sadness on the unit and that was this morning when the nurse came out of [a child's] room. [At those times when feelings are expressed], the emotion seems to be dictated by the presence of devastated family members ... For the most part, a front is put up of a collected, calm caretaker who is simply doing [her/his] job. (7-9-98)

While strong affective displays of grief and sadness did not appear frequently among the medical staff, there was a sense that these difficult, critical care circumstances did have an emotional impact upon them. A sense that has been supported by the writings of others detailing the emotional stresses facing critical care clinicians who work with critically ill children in hospital settings (Beardslee and DeMaso 1982; Chesla and Stannard 1997; Remen 1996).

The psychosocial rounds described here occurred inside the PICU, in a private conference room with closed doors; the topics to be discussed were not to be overheard by those who were out in the pod. These rounds were convened by the Chief of the PICU and attended by physicians-in-training. In addition, depending upon their availability and interests, other attending physicians, psychiatrists and/or nurses might also participate. For the most part, discussions were directed toward the emotional and personal experiences of physicians-in-training as they sought to provide pediatric critical care. Thus, these meetings provided a rare window for viewing their reported emotional experiences in relation to diagnosis and treatment. In fact, after a fieldworker observed a psychosocial round's meeting, she reported "It is the most emotion I have seen from the group of residents in all my observations. I am blown away by all the feelings that are coming out."

Each of the two psychosocial rounds to be reported on here lasted from 45 to 60 minutes and was audio-recorded. Written transcriptions were then made for the purpose of further analysis. From these transcripts, it became apparent that two different types of talk ran adjacent to one another: talk about emotion and talk about biomedical diagnosis and treatment. Because these two types of talk were embedded in one another, they formed a single unit of analysis for examining the relationship between reported emotional experiences and medical diagnosis. Whereas Mishler's (1984) analysis "focused on the distinction between the voices of the lifeworld and of medicine as representing different and incompatible ways of organizing and thinking about experience" (p. 138), our analytic lens changed to reflect a more positive, symbiotic relationship between these two voices.

With written transcripts in hand, the three authors also met to replay and review audio-taped psychosocial rounds meetings. The reviewers would stop the tape at any point of interest and discuss it. One of the reviewers (LKS) was the Chief of the PICU and led the psychosocial round discussions. These review meetings were also audio-taped and transcribed for further analysis.

## 2. The nature and purpose of psychosocial rounds

Although not standard within the scope of traditional medical training practices, beginning about 6 years ago, psychosocial rounds were held periodically by the Chief of the PICU. The rounds were initiated, in part, based upon her earlier positive experiences with similar forums as a medical resident:

> When I was a resident, we had a resident support group. Nobody had a bias against that term and that's what we called it. It was really helpful. [Later] when I was at [a university hospital], one of the social workers held one almost every week. It was very valuable to me individually ... There was and is resistance to considering these psychosocial things important. So depending on the biases of the attending physician, the residents will follow.

Here, psychosocial rounds were viewed as part of a process for training physicians to be more family-centered: from treating parental concerns as valuable diagnostic input, to gathering case history information. From the Chief's perspective:

> We really have to listen to what parents are saying. If they are saying that their kid is not right, we better consider that this is a diagnosis, not just parents venting

> their emotions. It's not just that you politely pat them on the back and say "I understand, I understand." If I came by and said to a resident "this kid is not right," he would not dismiss that as venting ... The mother who says "my child is not right" is still viewed as someone who needs to be tolerated and allowed to vent, instead of a diagnostician. It's as if the parents are not considered reliable. They're a third party to their child's own illness. (reviewer discussion, 9-98)

With this desire to construct a context that gave parental concerns a more legitimate voice in medical diagnosis, it was explained that certain kinds of case discussions were likely to be privileged over others during psychosocial rounds. That is, the patients who were discussed tended not to have complicated diagnoses that required "lots of tests and very fined tuned medicines and fluids." Rather, those cases mentioned aroused "a lot of emotions in the people who came to rounds." The cases were difficult "because the exchange with the family was difficult, or it was a tragic situation, or those patients were dying." As these situations were discussed during psychosocial rounds, the Chief reported that there was a tendency among the discussants to react negatively to families when they behaved in ways that were deemed inappropriate:

> [The psychosocial round discussants would say] it was a bad mother, or it's a hostile father, or the parents are tense, or they're not being good parents, or they're too loving, or they're not loving enough. They're there too much. They're not there enough. Whatever the criticisms, the parents don't fit the expectations, or they demand a lot from the staff. And the staff feel uncomfortable about it. (reviewer discussion, 9-98)

Within this setting, the purpose of psychosocial rounds was twofold: to integrate the emotional reactions of patients, their families, and physicians into the process of medical diagnosis and treatment; and to have the physicians move from reflecting on the emotions of others to reflecting on their own emotions. In what follows, each is discussed briefly.

## *2.1. To integrate emotional reactions into medical diagnosis and treatment*

The Chief of the PICU was concerned about "a bias" that existed in medicine whereby "emotion was viewed as something that was bothersome and that needed to be squelched; that emotion made you less objective." In contrast, she believed that "emotion is a huge area of data that can make you a more astute physician. If you just squelch it, or you just tolerate it, but don't use it, you cast away a lot of the data that you have about the patient." From her point of view, emotional responses constituted a source of data every bit as legitimate and real as those physical symptoms associated with traditional, objective medical diagnosis.

### *2.2. To reflect upon the emotions of others and the self*

Psychosocial rounds were viewed as a learning context that, over time, would encourage physicians to be more accepting of and reflective about their own emotions, and those of their patients and families. The Chief indicated that "some physicians may need to spend many sessions before they're able to even acknowledge that they have feelings about their patients." Initially, people might attend psychosocial rounds in order to "feel better" about themselves. However, later they would realize that rounds were "a way to develop self-understanding and self-awareness about their own feelings." As physicians-in-training began to talk about and evaluate the perspectives of their patients and families, it was hoped they would begin to incorporate these lifeworld perspectives into a diagnostic process that was often steeped in devastating emotional circumstances.

## 3. Emotional force and psychosocial rounds

In trying to apprehend the grief and rage that impelled Ilongot men from the Philippines to head hunt, as well as the tragic loss of his own wife, Rosaldo (1989) noted that the cultural analysis of emotion required an understanding of emotional force: "The notion of force involves both affective intensity and significant consequences that unfold over time" (1989: 20).

The intense type of emotional force described by Rosaldo was always present in the PICU. As hospital staff sought to provide life saving medical diagnosis and treatment, they were in constant, personal contact with emotionally forceful and devastating circumstances, as is illustrated by the excerpts to be presented here from two different psychosocial round meetings. Across both meetings, four different patients and their families, who were all given fictitious names for the purpose of this paper, were discussed. Three patients are presented here. Danny was an eighteen-year-old who died after a year-long illness. Billy was a youngster who came into the hospital in a reasonably healthy state and then died unexpectedly. Joshua was an eleven-year-old boy who died accidentally through drowning. The emotional force that these situations carried for the discussants revealed itself in their comments during psychosocial rounds. For example, Jim, a resident in emergency medicine doing a rotation in the PICU, described his experiences with Danny, the terminally ill eighteen-year-old:

> Oh yeah like he [Danny] was completely alert and stable. He had a Dunkin Donuts ice coffee. He had some soup. We talked about football like a good 45 minutes. He was telling me about how he just graduated from high school and he was proud of himself for doin' that. He was completely with it all day. And you know it was almost a blessing. He just arrested. He was sleeping and he just arrested.

According to Tannen (1986), it is through the description of concrete images like having "Dunkin Donuts ice coffee," and "soup," and concrete activities like playing "football" and graduating "from high school" that the force of Danny's eventual death is communicated more powerfully:

> The particularity and familiarity of details make it possible for both speakers and hearers to refer to their memories and construct images of scenes: people in relation to each other engaged in recognizable activities ... It is in large part through the creation of a shared world of images that ideas are communicated and understanding is achieved. (1986: 135–136)

Jill, a medical student and sub intern, discussed her reactions to activities surrounding the medical diagnosis and treatment of the boy (Billy) who died unexpectedly and of unknown causes:

> I think what was hard about that situation was that there was so much tension figuring out what was goin' on. It was so much intellectual energy and just feeling like "what is going on with this kid?" And *then* you have this whole other component which is just this raw emotion of these parents who of course are completely out of control. Just upset, angry, scared, yelling. I had to stand like all the way on the other side of the room when he actually died. I had been standing closer to the father before and I looked over at him and I he was a fuse ready to blow. And I just, like I didn't want to breathe in the wrong direction because I was I was scared. When he was standing there, I just really stayed still. I just didn't do anything and then he walked away. In another situation if I felt there was a parent just feeling down or a sad situation, I might try to reach and be consoling in some way. I just I just didn't want to because I I didn't know how it would be perceived. That's one situation where I felt there was really nothing I could say. Even saying anything was going to set him off, so I just sat there. We were all just incredibly quiet because I think that was just right after they were doing chest compressions and then he had already died.

Here, Jill had described a situation highly charged with emotional force not only because medical diagnosis and treatment were failing, but also because she perceived the father's reaction to be a potential threat to her own well being; a threat great enough that she responded by not consoling him after the boy had died. As this discussion progressed, Lisa (an intern) commiserated "unfortunately, I was here in January and we had like six or seven deaths."

These intersubjectively grounded, narrative recountings of diagnosing and treating illness in emotionally charged contexts with patients and families were characterized by an "epistemology of [the] character[s]" who were being described according to their "perceptions, thoughts, knowledge, intentions, goals, and other psychological attributes" (Bruder and Wiebe 1995: 342): "he was a fuse ready to blow," or "parents who are completely out of control. Just upset, angry, scared, yelling." In contrast, as will be noted subsequently, comments more characteristic of an objective voice of medicine manifested themselves differently as the participants ruminated over the medical facts and physical symptoms surrounding diagnosis and treatment: "the first thing they noted [was] very dark urine and ... then there was no urine output for several hours and then the pressures went down" (utterance #36, p. 25).

## 4. The relationship between emotional and medical talk

As emotionally charged experiences, such as those described previously, were being recounted by residents and interns, at least three different relationships between emotion and medical diagnostic talk emerged. First, the recountings of emotional experience served as a catalyst for talk about objective, medical diagnosis. At the same time, talk of objective medical diagnosis functioned as a mechanism through which the discussants could reflect upon the emotional perspectives of themselves and others. Third, the emotional circumstances described by the residents and interns were used by the medical director as an occasion to impart information relevant to medical diagnosis and treatment.

## 5. Emotion as impetus for diagnosis

Prior to audio taping the rounds, a small group of medical residents and interns were interviewed, among other things, about communicative practices within the PICU when diagnosis and treatment were being conducted under life threatening circumstances. Jim, a resident from emergency medicine doing a rotation through the PICU, replied that "if things run the way they are supposed to, people should remain calm and people shouldn't be yelling orders and such. Obviously, people get emotionally charged or anxious, but you try to avoid chaos and go about things in a team effort." Paul, a third year resident in pediatrics, added that "it's usually not people running around yelling and such. We try to avoid that kind of confusion."

When illustrating a circumstance in which confusion reigned, Jim described a situation in which the medical staff struggled frantically to save the life of a young boy who came into the hospital on his own to be treated after a relatively minor accident. The discussion began when the Chief of the unit (K), who had been away during the previous week, asked what had happened during her absence:

| | | | |
|---|---|---|---|
| (1) | 1 | K: | What happened last week? |
| | 2 | Jim: | Yeah you missed a pretty crazy week um especially with that one child dying. |

3 K: The boy that [fell]?

4 Jim: Yeah and it was pretty stressful. I was actually thinking it almost woulda been nice to have had you here because no one ever said anything or communicated anything. I mean there was just a lot of emotion. Just a feeling of being out of control. I think all the way up to the attendings just feeling like "I think I had no idea what was goin' on." And really being helpless to try and figure out what was going on. There was a lot of anger and emotional upset. It was pretty nuts.

5 Jill: And we never got a chance to talk about it afterwards. We all pretended like "oh that's kind of terrible" and we kinda moved on. I think we have a lot of unresolved ya know kind of intellectually "well what happened?" I think there's an M and M [morbidity and mortality conference] today. A surgical M and M about him. So I want to go just to see like whatev- I don't know ((pause)) kind of put it into perspective and see what happened 'cause it was so crazy and stressful ya know. You kind of want to see what was going on and if you could help out. But then there was just such a high emotional energy going on just because you were in the way and so it was just tough. You know we were on call that night and=

6 K: =The next mor[ning

7 Jill: [Yeah then we never talked about what happened to the child.

8 K: So you were on call when he was still alive?

9 Jim: Yeah he di[ed that morning.

10 Jill: [He died the next morning on rounds at 8 o'clock.

In response to the Chief's question, Jim said that it had been a "crazy week" in which all the physicians, including the most senior "attendings," could not generate a diagnosis to help explain the boy's failing medical condition. Not only was the staff helpless, angry, and upset with a medical situation that was out of control, both Jim and Jill (a sub-intern), indicated that after the child died, none of the senior physicians communicated with anyone about what had transpired. In fact, Jill expressed her interest in attending a morbidity and mortality conference within the hospital in an effort to learn more about the medical cause of death in the face of such a "stressful" situation.

The quotation marks in turns 4 and 5 mark the appearance of constructed dialogue – where the thoughts and speech of others and the self are quoted or reported (Tannen 1989: 98–133). Here, reported speech served to highlight their emotional sense of diagnostic helplessness both before and after the child's death:

(2) Jim: .all the way up to attendings just feeling like "I think I had no idea what was goin' on"

Jill: .We all pretend like "oh that's kind of terrible" and we kinda moved on . "well what happened?"

After indicating that they had both witnessed the efforts made to save the boy's life, Jim and Jill went on to jointly reconstruct the sequence of events in more detail:

(3) 17 Jim: There was just a lot of people in the room. They had like renal consults. They had like everyone under the sun coming in trying to brainstorm and figure out=

18 Jill: =And they ran him to angiography and then he came back and the cardiologists were here and the neurologists were here=

19 Jim: =Everyone from neurosurgery saw him.

20 Jill: I think there were at least ten people in the room at all times.

21 K: Wow.

22 Jill: And then they had to dialyze him and then they had that going and so there was so much activity that ya know I was trying to pay attention to see what was going on. But it really nobody knew what was going on ((pause)) you know kind of putting [it] together. And Paul [a third year resident] was there kind of checking labs and running running back and forth.

23 Jim: I think it woulda been kinda good if someone coulda like stepped back for just one minute. One of the attendings xx. Everyone was just jumping in with their two cents and then they'd run this way and do this you know=

24 K: =Right.

25 Jim: Neurosurgery came in and said "oh well why don't you get an angiogram" you know. It was highly unlikely that anything was the matter with the vessels. "Go do that." So they rushed him off to do an angiogram. Then he [the patient] comes back and he [the physician] says "well we gotta right away do dialysis." I thought it was pretty chaotic ((pause)) ya know. And once again I like like you know people were just grabbing at things 'cause no one had any idea what was goin' on. As far as I- it's probably actually probably one of the I mean it's definitely I mean I feel like a almost a cause of this kid dying. A young healthy kid otherwise. Ya know a previously young healthy kid coming in and as far as we know no reason to die. That's very xx.

26 K: XXX (intercom noise)

| | | |
|---|---|---|
| 27 | Jim: | No not at all. |
| 28 | Jill: | He walked in you know. My understanding was that he was injured and he kind of got up and was like "oh I better go to the emergency room just to make sure everything's okay" and then he died two days later. |
| 29 | K: | So you never really talked about it then. What's your understanding of why he died? |

Through a sequence of latched turns, or pairs of utterances with minimal junctures between them (O'Donnell 1990: 229), Jim and Jill described a situation in which neurologists, cardiologists and renal consultants were all seeking to apprehend the medical cause of the boy's failing condition: "they had like everyone under the sun coming in trying to brainstorm and figure out" what was wrong. "I think there were at least ten people in the room at all times."

In the midst of this chaotic situation where "everyone was jumping in with their two cents" and issuing orders for medical procedures of questionable value, ranging from an angiogram to dialysis, Jim expressed a desire for someone to "step back" and organize the diagnostic process. Through a series of hedged phrases – "actually, probably, I feel like almost" – Jim revealed his fear that their treatment caused the death of this child who had come to the hospital with survivable injuries.

Echoing this sentiment more forcefully in a piece of constructed dialogue, Jill assumed the child's voice and expressed his reasoning after being injured in a bicycle accident: "oh I better go to the emergency room just to make sure everything's okay." The use of constructed dialogue not only adds authenticity to the concerns being expressed (Hill and Irvine 1993: 11), but, as Tannen (1989) notes, "the animation of voices" (p. 102) helps create a heightened sense of emotional involvement among the audience as they become actively involved in "interpreting the significance of the character and the action" (p. 124).

As a result of his decision to seek treatment at the hospital, a decision that would be viewed positively by adults as the mature response to an injury, "he died what two days later." In response the Chief reiterated the group's previous concern about the lack of discussion about this case and asked them to provide a diagnosis regarding the cause of death. Jill replied by constructing a tentative biological explanation based upon her reading of the medical literature:

| | | |
|---|---|---|
| (4) 30 | Jill: | It's my understanding just from doing this kind of reading on my own from articles that had been circulating more with the nursing staff about this. This was a response to [a drug]. And just through the case studies that I've read what happened with him mirrors almost exactly what's happened with these other children in the past who've had this rhabdomyolysis [destruction of muscle tissue] from a |

[drug reaction]. So you know that to me it makes sense but I wouldn't bet the farm on it. You know I really don't ((pause)). There could be any other thing. There could've been some underlying enzymatic deficiency that was brought out by something that we did. But I think we all just kind of feel the same way. If he had just gone home he would be fine today.

31 Jim: I think that fortunately you know when they get the histology back from the uh post mortem hopefully they'll give some answers as far as about not a true answer. But at least point you in the right direction of you know whether he had small microemboli everywhere or was it uh you know some evidence of why he went into such organ failure.

32 Jim: I don't know I mean what do you think.

33 K: I don't I only heard a little bit about it. I think I'd have to really look at the record the progression.

34 Jim: Well it seems like first he went into renal failure. His urine output went down apparently the day before. No one thought much of it. He actually probably started first on rhabdomyolisis and then went into renal failure secondary to that. And then what looked like next the liver went and then [uh

35 Jill: [Well didn't his blood pressure I mean I don't really know but did didn't didn't his blood pressure and perfusion drop off early in the morning.

36 Jim: It did but if you look first. The first thing that was noted is they actually write very dark urine noted and you know then there was no urine output for several hours and then pressures went down and everything sorta just uh ((pause))

37 Jill: Creatinine jumped in like two hours three points.

38 K: How come uh how come nobody ever talked about it?

39 Jim: I think we talked about it like amongst the residents. It seems like none of the attendings or anyone else wanted to talk about it heh heh. They were all just so aghast from the situation that happened that no one felt comfortable talking about it. Certainly everyone was like "okay he's dead that was horrible" and sweep it under the carpet and that was it.

40 Jill: And th- just went to xray rounds and ((pause))

41 K: That was it huh?

42 Jim: And [they] never mentioned it again.

43 Jill: And it was never brought up again as a group.

44 Lisa: Unfortunately I was here in January and we had like six or seven deaths and it was so busy. And I kind of felt the same way. Like you know there was nobody there. But I feel like we had to talk to get out the emotions.

Much of this final stretch of talk was a clear illustration of the biological voice of medicine that residents and interns appropriate as they learn to present themselves in front of their peers and more senior physicians in a manner deemed competent: "in an ideal case presentation (from the student point of view) clear description of symptoms is followed by a definite and correct diagnosis" (Erickson 1999: 113). Although this was not an ideal situation because further test results were needed to clarify the cause of death, it was through the synthesis of various pieces of objective biological information that potential diagnoses were formulated.

Jill began by providing an explanation that, from a medical point of view, was both logical and coherent. A drug used to treat the boy's injury triggered a rare and unexpected reaction that resulted in the destruction of muscle tissue (rhabdomyolysis). Within this same turn, after expressing her uncertainty about this diagnosis and suggesting an alternative enzymatic deficiency, she reiterated her subjective reaction to the entire situation forcefully by speaking for the entire group of interns and residents: "But I think we all just kind of feel the same way. If he had just gone home, he would be fine today."

Jill's sense of diagnostic uncertainty in the face of this catastrophic outcome was also expressed by Jim who not only hoped more would be known after additional test results were available, but asked the Chief for her explanation regarding the cause of death. When the Chief indicated that she lacked sufficient information about the progression of the boy's illness, Jim and Jill offered their versions of the progression of symptoms.

Instead of offering a potential diagnosis or requesting additional information or clarification regarding the biological symptoms, the Chief asked the group to speculate about why none of the senior physicians had talked about this case.

In a training context designed to provide apprentices with hands-on medical information from the experts, it was notable when the senior physicians were reportedly reluctant to discuss the medical facts of the case. Simply put, the medical circumstances of the case, coupled with the perceived reticence of the senior physicians, provided a context for discussing potential emotional reactions to diagnosis and treatment: emotion not only provided impetus in searching for a medical diagnosis, but the objective medical facts of the case provided a warrant for reflecting on the emotional reactions of the physicians who were involved in this case.

Jim believed that while everyone "felt horrible," the senior physicians were intentionally not talking because of their lack of comfort about what had taken place. Lisa, an intern, indicated that she had noted this same reaction on the part of physicians when other individuals had died and that it was distressing. In short, the residents and interns reacted negatively to the perceived unwillingness of senior physicians to discuss the case with them and to provide their retrospective diagnoses.

When taken in its entirety, this diagnostic story revealed a bi-directional, symbiotic relationship between discussed emotional reactions and medical diagnosis. More specifically, the disturbing experiences recounted by the residents and interns fed their continuing search for a biological explanation for the child's death. When faced with a chaotic situation in which the treatment of a relatively healthy child ended in death rather than recovery, there was an expressed desire for a biomedical diagnosis that would put the entire experience into emotional perspective. At the same time, the medical circumstances surrounding the cause of death served to fuel a discussion of the emotional and communicative reactions among the physicians involved in diagnosis and treatment.

## 6. Experienced emotion and teachable moments

Along with instances where emotions propelled the search for a medical diagnosis, there were also times when presented emotional reactions served a didactic function. During these teachable moments, pertinent medical information about the diagnosis and treatment of other patients was introduced. Jim, for example, recounted another situation in which he witnessed an attending physician who "was crying like crazy" and "had horrible remorse" after resuscitating a child being treated for a drowning accident in an emergency room:

| | | |
|---|---|---|
| (5) 1 | Jim: | When I went on transfer to pick him up it was quite a highly emotionally charged scenario in the emergency department at [the hospital]. And the attending there was really crying like crying like crazy. And he said that he had "horrible remorse" that he actually resuscitated the child. |
| 2 | K: | The EMT (emergency medical technician)? |
| 3 | Jim: | No the attending physician. He was like tears streaming down his face saying "it was such a bad thing that I resuscitated this kid. We shoulda just called the code and now look at all of the grief we are putting the parents through." It was really something. It was ((pause)) incredibly overwhelming with the emotions I've had. Everyone was just beyond themselves. I think a lot of people felt like "oh well this happened to the kid. Oh how horrible." It was very emotionally charged trying to resuscitate him for a long period of time. And they finally got him back saying "why did we bring this kid back? He's obviously brain dead. Look how the parents are just that much more anguished seeing him resuscitated. We sort of gave them false hope maybe thinking something is going to happen." It's like they let the parents watch resuscitation [and gave them] a false hope. We know that maybe they felt |

| | | |
|---|---|---|
| | | some hope by the time they got back a heart beat. They didn't truly understand the severity of the. |
| 4 | K: | It's actually commendable that they would resuscitate him while the parents were there. |
| 5 | Jim: | Yeah. |
| 6 | K: | Actually usually that's something that occurs in places where you have a lot of discussion about it. Here it was quite a big deal the first time having parents stay and so that's commendable. |
| 7 | K: | But why do you think they felt that they shouldn't have resuscitated him? |

Through the use of constructed dialogue, Jim described the emotional reaction of an attending physician who sought to save the child's life: "why did we bring him back? He's obviously brain dead. Look at how the parents are just that much more anguished seeing him resuscitated. We sort of gave them false hope thinking something was going to happen."

In what followed, K expressed her concern for the clinical reasoning underlying this reported reaction on two counts. First, from her perspective, the medical staff were to be commended for allowing the parents to view life saving efforts made on behalf of their child. Second, beginning with turn 7, K initiated what was to be a series of quiz questions about the appropriateness and inappropriateness of resuscitation. In response, Jim explained that the child was already dead by the time he arrived at the hospital:

| | | |
|---|---|---|
| (6) 8 | Jim: | I guess that they just felt that you know that he was pretty much by all means dead when he arrived. And that even if you were able to stabilize him that it was such an insult to his brain that it would never function normally except for the organ donation. We talked about the only bright side was allowing the family to grieve. |
| 9 | K: | Does anyone else think that we shouldn't have resuscitated him when he came in? |
| 10 | Jim: | I think he should have been resuscitated. But I guess twice it got a heart beat back. Then it stopped and it went on like this for a good twenty minutes. He probably should've called it then. He said he actually went outside of the protocol and gave double the amount of epi (epinephrine) with each dose. |
| 11 | K: | What's that? |
| 12 | Jim: | It finally brought him back. So he said he "I really went beyond the means to bring this kid back and I wonder why." |
| 13 | Mona: | How though did he know at the time? Because I thought the first story that we had heard was the kid might have been |

down for a five minutes um and did he know?

14 Jim: Yeah he said when he first came in he got an idea that it was pretty bad. I mean his pupils were fixed and dilated. He was ((pause)) um it was pretty grim just by coming in. He didn't respond very quickly to resuscitation initially you know. But we got him back and he went down again. And we decided let's try everything possible we can think of to try and to bring him back.

15 K: Is it irrational [to try and bring him back.

16 Jim: [No I don't think it's irrational no no. Not at all=

17 K: =I mean some of it actually may be a little of a knowledge deficit cause about fifteen percent of the kids who show up with pupils fixed and dilated walk out normal.

18 Jim: Yeah no no I I I I want to base i[t

19 K: [It's a significant number.

20 Jim: No I want to base it upon what I was just saying. I think they they all felt a lot of grief when they saw them resuscitate this child. They felt you know he was not that not what they did anything wrong or anything like that. They were just like completely overwhelmed by the fact that this kid this young healthy kid. It was such a horrible thing and the family was there the whole time. I mean I felt uncomfortable just thinking XX. The mom this mother was appropriately grieving but really wailing and screaming "don't let my baby die. Wake up. Wake up. When are you going to wake up? It's okay to wake up." It's hard to sit there.

In turns 7 through 20, the Chief kept pursuing a response: "But why do you think they felt they shouldn't have resuscitated him?" "Does anyone else think we shouldn't have resuscitated him when he came in?" "Is it irrational to try and bring him back?" Jim first explained that irrespective of whether or not the child's condition was "stabilized," "he would never function normally." By immediately following Jim's response with a question to the entire group, asking them to either agree or disagree with his explanation, the Chief's request not only functioned as a potential negative evaluation of Jim's account, but also highlighted the importance of this particular topic.

When no one else in the group responded, Jim went on to clarify his position. He believed that the child "should have been resuscitated."

However, life saving efforts should have ceased after twenty minutes, instead of going "outside of the protocol" by giving the boy an unusually high dose of epinephrine. Jim continued to support his position by revoicing the words of the attending physician: "I really went beyond the means to bring this kid back and I wonder why."

Interestingly, the Chief's question in turn 11 ("what's that") was not responded to or pursued further in the group discussion. However, during a review of the audio tape, the Chief revealed that she was asking Jim and the group to consider what it meant to go "outside the protocol" in life threatening circumstances. She explained that "in very extreme situations" where the diagnosis is certain death without some type of radical intervention, "there is no protocol. You simply try different things that may have a reasonable chance of saving someone's life." In such a circumstance, doubling the typical dose of epinephrine is a legitimate course of medical action.

It was, however, at this point in the psychosocial rounds group discussion that Mona (a first year intern) asked for clarification regarding the length of time the child had been underwater. With Mona's question, this particular didactic point concerning the boundaries of the protocol was never made a topic for public discussion among the group members.

However, Jim's description of the boy's pupils being "fixed and dilated" did result in a publicly displayed teachable moment in which the Chief sought to redress a potential "knowledge deficit" on the part of these less experienced physicians: "about fifteen percent of the kids who show up with pupils fixed and dilated walk out normal." From the Chief's perspective, an understanding of this diagnostic fact warranted the pursuit of treatment beyond the boundaries of any preconceived protocol for administering epinephrine or other procedures.

At this point, Jim responded by saying there was nothing wrong with the medical treatment per se. Rather, it was the context of treatment that made this a difficult situation to observe: there was "this young healthy kid," "the family was there the whole time," and the mother was "wailing and screaming. It's just hard to sit there."

In sum, it was Jim's recounted experience of watching a distraught attending physician attempt to save the life of a drowning victim that initiated a discussion regarding the appropriate medical assessment and treatment of drowning victims. The Chief's pursuit of a response to a question of when to stop resuscitation and her eventual answer both reflected the importance of the information being conveyed. As Sorlie, Forde, Lindseth, and Norberg (2001) revealed through their analysis of narratives among experienced and inexperienced physicians in pediatric critical care situations, "less experienced physicians" are searching for "criteria" that can "tell them when to stop treatment, and they expect the more experienced physicians to be able to teach them about such things" (p. 657).

When taken together, the emotional reactions and diagnostic information discussed by the physicians-in-training were related in three distinguishable ways. First, emotions provided a catalyst for seeking further information regarding the biological cause of illness and death. Second, the search for biological diagnoses served to distance these physicians from their devastating, work related experiences with life and death, potentially helping them to regain their emotional perspective. Third, their presented emotional reactions and diagnostic commentary provided the Chief of the unit with an opportunity to impart new medical information regarding the evaluation and treatment of children, and to reflect publicly upon the handling of emotional reactions to children in critical care situations. In the ensuing discussion, the implications of these findings will be considered.

## 7. Discussion

There were several motivations for the present investigation. To begin with, we desired to move beyond traditional studies of medical discourse that, until recently, have focused almost exclusively on the analysis of dyadic, doctor–patient encounters. Given that the discursive practices of many professionals, physicians included, are far more complex than any one type of speech event can reveal, we wanted to examine alternate contexts of talk that informed the construction of medical diagnosis and treatment. As Atkinson (1999) has suggested:

> There is a distinct value orientation among many researchers that leads them to celebrate the spoken actions of patients, while being critical of the equivalent work of the professional practitioner ... an overtly ideological commitment to patients and other underdogs should not relieve us of the methodological imperative of symmetry ... It is not enough to dismiss the work of medical practitioners as bureaucratic, or dehumanising, or disempowering, while celebrating the lay perspectives of their clients. The obsessive gaze that has been directed towards the dyadic consultation has yielded a micro-politics of medical encounters, but only a partial exploration of the forms and functions of spoken discourse in medical settings ... A great deal of organized medical work goes on at one or more removes from the patient. The consulting-room and the patient's bedside are not the only arenas in which medical histories are recounted, investigations discussed, differential diagnoses considered, or treatments explored. (Atkinson 1999: 75–76)

By examining meetings where novice physicians at different levels of training discussed their own experienced reactions to diagnosis and treatment with an expert (the Chief), we were able to further illuminate the practitioner's perspective on medical care.

Within this context, we were also interested in apprehending Mishler's (1984) contrast between the two conflicting "voices" of medicine that was based upon his analysis of face-to-face, doctor–patient encounters: the biomedical and the lifeworld of the patient. The former is realized in the physician's search for physiological symptoms that can point to underlying etiologies and potential courses of treatment. In the biomedical voice, as physicians seek to diagnose patients, primary emphasis is placed on the objective description of reality in terms of its physical features. As Kleinman describes (1995: 30):

> Biology is made visible as the ultimate basis of reality which can be viewed, under the microscope if need be, as a more basic substance than complaints or narratives of sickness with their psychological and social entailments. The psychological, social, and moral are only so many superficial layers of epiphenomenal cover that disguise the bedrock of truth, the ultimately natural substance in pathology and therapy, the real stuff: biology as an architectural structure and its chemical associates. The other orders of reality are by definition questionable.

On the other hand, the voice from the lifeworld manifests itself "when patients refer to the personal and social contexts of their problems" (Mishler 1984: 95). This lifeworld becomes visible as patients express contextually-grounded and emotional experiences and problems in their lives. The meanings of these expressions are "dependent on the patient's biographical situation and position in the social world" (Mishler 1984: 104). In his analysis of face-to-face encounters between physicians and patients, these two modes of discourse were in constant conflict with one another to the detriment of both diagnosis and treatment.

Examination of psychosocial rounds, a speech event once removed from direct contact between doctors and patients and intended explicitly to bring the emotional experiences of physicians-in-training and patients to the foreground, revealed that these two voices were not necessarily in opposition to one another. Whereas Mishler's analysis of doctor–patient encounters found "the struggle between these voices" to represent "different and incompatible ways of organizing and thinking about experience" (p. 138), our examination of these two discourses in a different context of medical practice revealed a symbiotic relationship between them. This may be because psychosocial rounds were comprised of health care professionals who were not functioning in the observable presence of patients; practitioners who were encouraged to ruminate on their emotional responses to medical diagnosis and treatment.

As physicians revealed their own emotional reactions to the devastating lifeworld experiences of their patients through communicative devices such as constructed dialogue, valuable biomedical information was integrated into their discussions of diagnosis and treatment. Not only did the emotional reactivity of physicians fuel the search for a biomedical diagnosis and provide opportunities for teaching valuable medical information, but diagnosis served as a means for coping with the emotional force of particularly traumatic cases.

Our observations are not intended to diminish the ground-breaking work of Mishler (1984). Instead, by extending our analysis beyond the confines of face-to-face, doctor–patient interaction, we have sought to deepen our understanding of the communicative practices associated with medical diagnosis from the perspective of physicians. In doing this, we discovered that the voice of medicine was interpenetrated in constructive ways by concerns for the intersubjective experience of illness in the context of providing critical care. Here, when allowed an expression within the discursive context of psychosocial rounds, both voices served important, positive functions. Hyden and Mishler (1999) suggest that "the dominant discourse of medicine is undergoing radical change, invaded by new definitions and theories of health and illness, and alternative forms of practice" (p. 190). From this perspective, it may be that psychosocial rounds bear witness to a developing discursive practice for an evolving voice of medicine.

## *References*


Ainsworth-Vaughn, Nancy
1998 *Claiming Power in Doctor–Patient Talk.* Oxford, UK: Oxford University Press.

Atkinson, Paul
1999 Medical discourse, evidentiality and the construction of professional responsibility. In Sarangi, S. and C. Roberts (eds.), *Talk, Work and Institutional Order.* Berlin/New York: Mouton de Gruyter, 75–108.

Barton, Ellen
1999 The social work of diagnosis: Evidence for judgments of competence and incompetence. In Kovarsky, D., J. Duchan, and M. Maxwell (eds.), *Constructing (In)Competence: Disabling Evaluations in Clinical and Social Interaction.* Mahwah, NJ: Erlbaum, 257–290.

Beardslee, William R. and David R. DeMaso
1982 Staff groups in a pediatric hospital: Content and coping. *American Journal of Orthopsychiatry* 52(4), 712–718.

Brody, Howard
1987 *Stories of Sickness.* New Haven: Yale University Press.

Bruder, Gail A. and Janyce Wiebe
1995 Recognizing subjectivity and identifying subjective characters in third-person fictional narrative. In Duchan, J., G. Bruder, and L. Hewitt (eds.), *Deixis in Narrative.* Hillsdale, NJ: Erlbaum, 341–356.

Chesla, Catherine A. and Daphne Stannard
1997 Breakdown in the nursing care of families in the ICU. *American Journal of Critical Care* 6(1), 64–71.

Erickson, Fred
1999 Appropriation of voice and presentation of self as a fellow physician. In Sarangi, S. and C. Roberts (eds.), *Talk, Work and Institutional Order.* Berlin/New York: Mouton de Gruyter, 109–143.

Fisher, Sue and Alexandra Todd (eds.)
1993 *The Social Organization of Doctor–Patient Communication.* Norwood, NJ: Ablex.

Hill, Jane H. and Judith T. Irvine
1993 Introduction. In Hill, J. H. and J. T. Irvine (eds.), *Responsibility and Evidence in Oral Discourse.* Cambridge: Cambridge University Press, 1–23.
Hyden, Lars-Christer and Elliot G. Mishler
1999 Language and medicine. *Annual Review of Applied Linguistics* 19, 174–192.
Kleinman, Arthur
1988 *The Illness Narratives. Suffering, Healing, and the Human Condition.* New York: Basic Books.
1995 *Writing at the Margin: Discourse between Anthropology and Medicine.* Berkeley: University of California Press.
Korsh, Barbara M. and Vida F. Negrete
1972 Doctor–patient communication. *Scientific American* 227(2), 66–74.
Mishler, Eliot
1984 *The Discourse of Medicine: Dialectics of Medical Interviews.* Norwood, NJ: Ablex.
O'Donnell, Katherine
1990 Difference and dominance: How labor and management talk conflict. In Grimshaw, A. (ed.), *Conflict Talk.* Cambridge: Cambridge University Press, 210–240.
Remen, Naomi
1996 *Kitchen Table Wisdom.* New York: Riverhead Books.
Rosaldo, Renato
1989 *Culture and Truth.* Boston, MA: Beacon Press.
Sorlie, V., R. Forde, A. Lindseth, and A. Norberg
2001 Male physicians' narratives about being in ethically difficult care situations in paediatrics. *Social Science and Medicine* 53, 657–667.
Tannen, Deborah
1989 *Talking Voices.* Cambridge: Cambridge University Press.

# Chapter 10
# The diagnostic practices of Speech-Language Pathologists in America over the last century

*Judith Felson Duchan*

*Judith Duchan takes a look at how cultural conditions can influence the way professionals go about doing diagnosis. She examines various historical contexts in the field of speech-language pathology and their impact on the diagnostic endeavor. Her story begins in the pre-professional period of the late 1800s, when experts provided diagnostic-free speech therapy in the United States. Other cultural influences on the diagnostic practices of speech-language pathologists were the testing movement of the early 1900s, the normative research in the 1920s, and the impact of the Second World War.*

In this chapter, I want to take a step back in time and examine the role and activity of diagnosis by describing some diagnostic practices of clinicians practicing and writing in the 19$^{th}$ and 20$^{th}$ centuries. This broad backward sweep will allow us to see how diagnostic practices are not only influenced by current interactional contexts in the here and now, as has been demonstrated so vividly by other authors of this volume, but also how such practices are influenced by the frameworks within which those current acts of diagnosis are embedded. A contextualized view of the diagnostic process such as this runs counter to the view held by many diagnosticians who see their diagnostic activities as objective, decontextualized, scientific matters of fact.

My aim in this chapter is to show that speech-language pathologists diagnosing a communication disorder are engaged in a cultural practice of social construction as much as they would be if they were to go to a Jewish bar mitzvah or a Mexican Day-of-the-Dead celebration. I will use two sorts of evidence to argue for this culturalized and situated construction of diagnosis: a broad historical examination of how changes in society influenced diagnostic practices of speech-language pathologists in the 19$^{th}$ and early 20$^{th}$ centuries, and a more detailed examination of the writings of later 20$^{th}$ century speech pathologists about their diagnostic practices.

The social and cultural construction of diagnosis will be shown to tie closely to the widespread cultural use in the 19$^{th}$ century of the medical model, in which a diagnosis is used to name a condition causing problematic symptoms. The aim of a professional working within the medical model then and now is to diagnose a condition so that its course can be predicted and its symptoms treated (Duchan 2004; Thagard 1999). The diagnosis, intended to explain and classify a set of symptoms, is often used as a way to classify those diagnosed. He is deaf; she is retarded; they are mentally ill.

In the medical model the "condition" being named by the diagnostic term is construed to be a cluster of "presenting" symptoms, some of which are used as criteria for the diagnosis. For example, hearing loss is seen as a symptom required for ascribing a diagnosis of hearing impairment or deafness.

## 1. Political and intellectual contexts for construing a diagnosis

Those doing speech therapy did not always apply the medical model to their work. In the early part of the 19th century, those carrying out speech therapy saw themselves as teachers rather than clinicians and construed their jobs as speech improvement rather than speech therapy. They called themselves elocutionists (Simon 1953), and their activities included improving the delivery of actors, singers, and "platform readers" for public performances as well as those with speech problems. Alexander Graham Bell, a latecomer in this group, focused more on the defects side, as is indicated by his advertisement of his new clinic in Boston as one that was devoted to "the correction of defects of utterance" (Bell 1872).

The emphasis of Bell and his fellow elocutionists was not on diagnosis but on designing methods to improve both normal and abnormal performance in the areas of speech, voice, and movement. Also, their teaching methods did not call for categorizing people into diagnostic groups since they tended to do use the same methods to teach all their "pupils." Bell, for example, taught the same course to everyone, regardless of their "defects of utterance." His course consisted primarily of teaching sound production based on the "visible speech" system, a phonetic system developed by his father. Visible speech was a pictographic display of the articulatory positions needed to produce different speech sounds (Duchan 2005).

It was later in the 19th and early 20th centuries that those doing speech therapy began to incorporate diagnoses in their practices. This dramatic change coincided, not incidentally, with the emergence of the scientific method in medicine. Physicians in America began studying with medical researchers in Germany who were conducting biological experiments in their laboratories to discover the biomedical origins of disease (Bonner 1963). Speech therapists, some of whom were physicians, followed this lead, incorporating the medical model, i.e. diagnostic methods, into their practices (see Potter 1882, for a review and example of this new diagnostic focus.)

These medically-based speech professionals took their diagnostic categories from the medical literature. Greek and Latin based terms were taken from medical dictionaries of the time (e.g., Dunglison 1874). Twentieth century American authors in the field of speech-pathology spent considerable time outlining the various diagnostic categories related to speech disorders (e.g., Stinchfield [1933] and Robbins and Stinchfield [1931]).

At the same time that speech-language pathology was being established as a separate profession in the US, the testing movement was evolving in America. This movement offered its proponents another framework for constructing diagnoses. Rather than just using the presence or absence of criterial symptoms as criteria for a diagnosis, diagnosticians began using test norms as a guide classifying people into diagnostic groups. Below average performance on standardized tests was taken as evidence of a problem.

Children, for example were being given individual intelligence tests, diagnosed as retarded, and placed in special education classes or newly established state-institutions for the mentally retarded (Trent 1994).[1] Other children were given hearing tests, diagnosed as deaf, and sent to state-subsidized residential schools for the deaf, a number of which had been established in the 50 year period between 1817–1867 (Moores 1978). Adults, who were being recruited into the military to serve in the First World War, were given paper and pencil multiple choice intelligence tests. Recruits who obtained high scores qualified for officer training and those with lower scores were either assigned to labor forces or disqualified based on mental incompetence (for more detail, see Hanson 1993: 211).

A substantial portion of the clinical manuals in speech language pathology from the 1920s were made up of descriptions of standardized and informal tests and how to administer them. The tests were designed to obtain objective measures (mostly numerical) that went into the factors used to diagnose speech disorders in children and adults. West in his 1936 "Clinical Manual of Methods and Apparatus" says:

> Diagnosis comes from the Greek verb "to distinguish" which in turn was made up of two common Greek words meaning to "know through and through." In the field of speech correction it is very important to make a diagnosis in that old sense (dia–gnosis), since to classify disorders of speech on the basis of their speech symptoms is often meaningless. No real diagnosis can be arrived at in this field without arriving at the causes. So every test described in this book is included because the author has found it helpful in this business of looking through the superficial symptoms of a case into its real etiology. (West 1936: 1)

Tests have offered clinicians comparison measures with a cohort group. In order to interpret a score obtained on a rapid movement test, for example, one needs to compare it with ordinary performance. So, collecting normative data has been a central activity for those involved in developing diagnostic instruments. This gathering of norms was part of a general trend in the US following World War I toward educational measurement and scientism (Cremin 1988).

In the 1920s educational researchers in a newly founded Bureau of Educational Experiments (Johnson 1928) as well child development researchers in research stations at universities across the nation (all supported by John D. Rockefeller funds) were busily engaged in collecting data on the physical, mental, emotional, and social growth of young children (Bradbury 1937). The product of these efforts was a series of published studies that were used by professionals and parents throughout America to evaluate children's development. Arnold Gesell's norms were the best known. He published a series of books that offered lists of developmental norms that were used by parents to assess their children's developmental progress (Gesell 1925, 1928, 1929, 1949).

Speech correctionists, as they called themselves at the time, focused on the subset of these norms having to do with speech and language development in children. In 1946 Dorothea McCarthy, a researcher who had been working in the University of Iowa Child Development Station, gathered the research studies on speech and language development in a summary article (McCarthy 1946). McCarthy's article and the research it was based upon provided speech-correctionists in the 1930s on with comparison data to determine whether their children's speech and language performance was normal or not. It also offered clinicians new areas and approaches for their information gathering in the course of diagnostic evaluations.

The Second World War also had a profound influence on the practice of speech correction in the United States. Clinicians and researchers worked in newly established military clinics throughout the United States servicing soldiers with articulation problems caused by gunshot wounds of the head and neck (Peacher 1948), with hearing losses, and with aphasia due to head trauma. It was during these years that the field of audiology came into its own with a particular emphasis on aural rehabilitation for soldiers with hearing losses. Mark Ross a well-known audiologist today, comments on his experience in a military hospital as a soldier with a hearing impairment:

> By all accounts, the audiology profession had its genesis in WW II as an outgrowth of the aural rehabilitation programs provided for servicemen who lost hearing in the war... My first experience with the field of audiology [was] when I entered Walter Reed Hospital ... as a patient. ... I am not sure if the staff used the term "audiologist" to describe themselves... but what they did in the next two months was what I came to think that audiology was all about... .(Ross n.d. web site)

As a function of the war, a new diagnostic category was discussed in the literature – that of malingering. Clinicians were alerted to the possibility that their clients were feigning poor performance on their speech or hearing tests in order to avoid military service (Morley 1941). The national organization established a committee on tests and measurements to develop special tests for speech malingering, differential diagnosis, and surveys (Morley 1941).

Perhaps the greatest impact of the Second World War on diagnosis of communication disabilities in the United States was the immigration to the United States of well-established diagnosticians. Included were Kurt Goldstein, Emil Froeschels, and Deso Weiss, all of whom were to influence clinical practices in the US. Among their contributions to diagnosis were Goldstein's "abstract attitude" associated with aphasia, and "word deafness" associated with childhood language disorders (Goldstein 1948). Froeschels and Weiss introduced the diagnostic category of "cluttering" as a form of stuttering that was language based and involved rapid, dysfluent speech (Froeschels 1946; Weiss 1964).

These researchers/clinicians also introduced diagnostic methods used in Europe and the United States. Goldstein had been a director of a hospital clinic that was engaged in serving the war wounded (Goldstein 1942). Froeschels reviewed current clinical practices going on in Europe for the American speech-pathology community (e.g., Froeschels 1943, 1948).

In the 1960s in America, professional practices in diagnosis were strongly impacted by the civil rights movement. Prior to that time, speech-language pathologists were misdiagnosing children and adults with dialect differences, treating the difference as a disorder. The sensitivities gained from the civil rights struggles both outside and within the profession led to methods for making what came to be known as the deficit/difference distinction. Diagnostic methods were developed to avoid diagnosing individuals with speech or language dialects as speech or language disordered (e.g., Taylor 1986).

Recent clinical practices in speech-language pathology have been directly influenced by changes in the health care system. Managed care practices developed by health insurance companies have led to the regulation of services provided by speech-language pathologists. This regulation is especially true for clinicians working in hospitals and agencies that provide services to adults with communication disorders. Diagnostic categories are now influenced by insurance codes that are often dictated by those associated with medical practices. For example, in order to be paid by insurance companies for their services, speech-pathologists must use diagnostic codes of the World Health Organization as indicated in their International Classification of Diseases.

This cursory sweep of two centuries of practices in the field of speech-language pathology has shown how clinical practices in this field have been very much part of cultural zeitgeist in the United States and how the practices have led to different constructions of the need for diagnosis, how to go about it, and the very categories used.

Early therapies administered by elocutionists were not based on diagnoses. It was only later, when clinicians began to work within the medical model, that speech-language pathologists placed diagnosis at center stage. Diagnostic categories provided clinicians with the vocabulary for classifying their clients. The tests and developmental norms provided as a result of the intelligence testing and child study movement in the US gave them standards for comparison, as they sought answers to whether their clients were abnormal enough to deserve a diagnostic label. The Second World War provided them new diagnostic categories and a new discipline within their field, audiology. And the Civil rights Movement gave them the sensitivity to be able to distinguish dialect differences from speech or language disorders. Finally, managed care is dictating a new set of diagnostic categories, ones that govern insurance payments for speech and language services.

## 2. Diagnostic categories and diagnostic logic used over the years

Even before there were professionals who called themselves speech clinicians, there were diagnostic manuals about speech disorders. Throughout the $20^{th}$ century, manuals as well as the basic textbooks of the times, have provided information and outlined procedures for doing diagnosis. Most diagnostic manuals had a section on physical aspects of speech production; all offered a taxonomy of speech problems, and a list of tests to give to diagnose them. Some also provided a section on therapy including a description of approaches and materials for remediating the different types of problems. My attention here will be on the taxonomy of disorders that provide clinicians with their diagnostic categories. (See Table 1 for a chronological listing of the books used in this review.)

*Table 1.* A chronological list of popular diagnostic handbooks and foundational texts in speech correction and speech-language pathology

| | |
|---|---|
| Samuel Potter | *Speech and its Defects* (1882) |
| Samuel Robbins, Sara Stinchfield | *Dictionary of Speech Terminology* (1931) |
| Lee Edward Travis | *Speech Pathology* (1931) |
| Mildred Berry, Jon Eisenson (1942) | *The Defective in Speech* (1942) |
| Wendell Johnson, Fred Darley, D. C. Spreistersbach | *Diagnostic Manual in Speech Correction* (1952) |
| Helmer Myklebust | *Auditory Disorders in Children* (1954) |
| Lee Edward Travis | *Handbook of Speech Pathology and Audiology* (1971) |
| James Nation, Dorothy Aram | *Diagnosis of Speech and Language Disorders* (1977) |

| | |
|---|---|
| Fred Darley, D.C. Spriestersbach | *Diagnostic Methods in Speech Pathology* (1978) |
| James Nation, Dorothy Aram | *Diagnosis of Speech and Language Disorders* (1984) |
| Norman Lass, Leija McReynolds, Jerry Northern, David Yoder | *Handbook of Speech-Language Pathology and Audiology* (1988) |
| J. Bruce Tomblin, Hugh Morris, D. C. Spriestersbach | *Diagnosis in Speech-Language Pathology* (1994) |
| J. Bruce Tomblin, Hugh Morris, D. C. Spriestersbach | *Diagnosis in Speech-Language Pathology* (2000) |
| American Psychiatric Association | *Diagnostic and Statistical Manual IV-T*R (2000) |
| World Health Organization | *International Classification of Disease* (9th revision) Clinical Modification (2001) |

Samuel Potter, who wrote the first known handbook on "Speech and its Defects" wrote the book for his fellow physicians who, he lamented, knew nothing of speech defects (Potter 1882). Drawing from the European "speech doctors," especially those in Germany in the mid 1800s, and from his medical dictionary (Dunglison 1874), Potter provided his colleagues with a broad typology of speech-defects that included four main diagnostic categories (see Table 2). For each of the four types of problem, Potter specified a biological cause. In fact, he placed the cause at the heart of the diagnostic definition. Two of the conditions are caused by problems in the brain (psychical alalia and paralytic alalia), one involves problems in the muscles (paralalia) and one originates in the nerves (dyslalia).

*Table 2.* Potter's typology of speech defects (Potter 1882)

*Alalia*: The psychical defects. Due to cerebral lesions or disorder of the higher centers governing written or spoken language. Includes aphasia, agraphia, amnesia, agraphia, paraphrasia, paragraphia.

*Alalia*: Paralytic impairment of articulation. Due to lesions of the medulla oblongata, disordered motor cortex or other diseases such as posterior spinal sclerosis and cretinism.

*Paralalia:* Defective speech and pronunciation. A failure in the action of certain muscles of articulation. Its divisions are as follows: lalling (/l/ substituted for other sounds; lambdacisms (/r/ for /l/), blaesites (hard consonants are softened eg, /m/ for /p/; or soft consonants for hard e.g., /f/ for /v/) gammacism, t/k, d/g; iotacism (z/ch), rhinism (nasal twang), uraniscophia or palatining (h/k due to fissure to hole in palate), rhotacism (/r/ problem), and sigmatism (frontal lisping).

*Dyslalia:* Stuttering. A spasm implicating "deranged nerve-functions." (Potter: 76). Difficult, interrupted speech (spasmodic hesitation, clonic spasm of articulation, tonoid spasm of articulation).

Potter's biologically based taxonomy may have been the first effort of someone in the United States to create a system dedicated to identifying and diagnosing individuals with communication disorders. Samuel Robbins and Sara Stinchfield, following in Potter's footsteps some 40 years later, created another, more extensive set of categories to be used by speech clinicians in America. The two college professors worked with a committee of the fledgling American Speech Correction Association, to establish a sanctioned list of categories for classifying or diagnosing communication disorders (Robbins and Stinchfield 1931). Their list, published by the organization that was to grow into today's American Speech-Language and Hearing Association, included a set of general categories and a much larger list of subcategories under each. There were seven general speech problem types, 42 disorders associated with them, and 106 subtypes associated with the 42 disorders. For example, they named articulation disorders dyslalia and described alalia (mutism) as one of its sybtypes. Under alalia they listed delayed speech.

Robbins and Stinchfield's subtypes included: dysarthria (defects of articulation due to lesions of the nervous system), dyslalia (functional and organic defects in articulation), dyslogia (difficulty in the expression of ideas by speech, due to psychoses), dysphasia (impairment of language due to weakened mental imagery through disease, shock, or injury), dysphemia (variable disorders of speech due to psychoneuroses), dysphonia (disorders of voice), and dysrhythmia (defects of rhythm). Their seven-category typology differed from Potter's in that its categories were not only physically caused (dysarthria, organic articulation), but also psychologically caused (dysphasia, dysphemia). They also offered descriptive categories for disorders whose causes were not known (functional articulation, rhythm), as well as disorders that had multiple causes, both physical and psychological (voice). Robbins and Stinchfield depict dysphasia, for example, as a problem with a psychological cause (weakened mental imagery) that was, in turn, caused a more basic physical problem (disease, shock or injury).

This causal chain concept associated with doing diagnoses is a common one in the diagnostic literature and has been from the birth of the profession in the US. When there are several causes that are arranged in a diagnostic chain, it is typically the case that the first or primary causes, the ones considered fundamental (West et al. 1947), are the biological causes. For example, a common depiction of learning disabilities, a modern day diagnosis, is that it originates with a neurological condition that eventuates in a psychological problem (a psycholinguistic delay or difficulty or a learning problem) that leads to academic difficulties.

West, and his colleagues, in their classic text that went through four popular editions (1937, 1947, 1957, 1968), adopt the taxonomy of Robbins and Stinchfield but add deafness as a category. The textbook was called, somewhat long windedly, *The Rehabilitation of Speech: A Textbook of Diagnostic and Corrective Pro-*

*cedures Based upon a Critical Study of Speech Disorders.* In the 1947 edition, West reflects on the difference between diagnosis and description:

> After we have definitely decided that the only possible cause of a given speech defect is a real pathology or abnormality, then, and only then, do we venture to undertake what can properly be called a *diagnosis.* When we *describe* a case of speech defect, we think in terms of the several *abilities* necessary to speech; when we diagnose it, we think in terms of causes. The two studies, description and diagnosis, differ largely in approach. Description is concerned with the *phenomenology* of the case being studied, diagnosis with its *etiology.* The one deals with the condition of the patient's speech as we observe it today; the other deals with the development of that condition in the past, and traces it, if possible, to its beginning and its fundamental cause. (West, Kennedy, and Carr 1947: 61)

West also describes what he sees as the difference between primary and secondary causes, when he talks about diagnosis. Primary disorders are physiogenic (what I have been referring to as biological). Secondary disorders may be either physiogenic or psychogenic (what I have been calling psychological). West explains what he means by physiogenic and psychogenic as follows:

> A disorder is physiogenic when its chief and original cause was (or is) some defect in the physical machinery used in the utterance of speech, in the nervous tissue controlling it, in the sensory end organs guiding it, or in the blood tissues supporting its several processes. A disorder is psychogenic when the chief and original cause was (or is) none of the defects mentioned under physiogenic disorders, but rather a mental reaction of the individual to some factor of his social or physical environment or to some physical characteristic or condition of his own body that could not of itself directly cause a defect of speech. (West, Ansberry, and Carr 1957: 8)

The speech-pathology profession, at that time, focused their diagnostic taxonomies on disorders of speech production. This left little room for diagnosing and evaluating the abilities of individuals who were not yet speaking. (The cases of nonverbal individuals in West et al, were ones who had once spoken and lost their speech, not those who had not yet developed it.) (See Book III, case histories in West et al. 1947.) Also the early taxonomic systems tended to focus on peripheral mechanism of speech – voice, articulation, fluency – failing to venture into the terrain of the mental. To do so would require hypothesizing gaps in knowledge or processes that were not directly observable, a rationalist approach to theorizing about speech disorders that was not the way the empiricist founders of speech pathology were thinking. Finally, early diagnosticians working early in the 20th century, assigned greater worth to the more observable biological causes than the psychological ones.

Some things changed in the profession's middle years, between 1940 and 1970. Others things stayed the same. The old and new are nicely represented in a book called *The Defective in Speech*, published in 1942, by Mildred Berry and Jon Eisenson (Berry and Eisenson 1942). These authors included in their category list some of the old terms – dysphasia, stuttering – but changed other old terms to be more English sounding (articulation rather than dyslalia, voice disorders rather than dysphonia). They also added blindness as a diagnostic condition associated with defective speech.

The effort of Berry and Eisenson was to avoid the technical terminology of diagnosis used in the early years of the profession and to make their diagnoses more understandable to others. As expressed in the editor's foreword "It [the book] tells a straight-forward story throughout and is free of all unnecessary technicalities and overly elaborate nomenclature" (Berry and Eisenson 1942: vii). This aim toward simplicity and accessibility was also expressed and enacted by West, in the later editions of his handbook, and by others of this period who wrote new handbooks on methods of diagnosing those with speech and language problems. The days of the detailed diagnostic taxonomies involving Greek and Latin terminology were left behind.

Interestingly, Berry and Eisenson struggled with the distinction between biologically and psychologically caused disorders. They deemphasized a distinction between organic and functional causes, providing the following rationale for doing so:

> Most of those who have worked for any time in the field of speech correction soon realize that it is difficult to assign any specific organic disturbance as being the sole basic cause for a specific speech disorder. Nor is it enough to say that if no organic anomaly is present or discovered, the speech deviation is functional in origin. Patients with defective speech may or may not have discernible or organic defects, and two persons with comparable organic defects do not necessarily manifest the same speech disturbance. (Berry and Eisenson 1942: ix)

In 1954 Helmer Myklebust published a more specialized book on doing diagnosis, called: *Auditory Disorders in Children: A Manual for Differential Diagnosis* (Myklebust 1954). Unlike the taxonomies of earlier authors, this book emphasized the speech perception side of communication disorders rather than speech production. It was also different from prior handbooks in that it was focused primarily on the communication difficulties of children rather than adults.

Myklebust, in the preface of his text, argued for broadening the diagnostic domain of auditory disorders to include not only deaf or hearing-impaired children, but also "children with psychic deafness, aphasic children, and the mentally deficient, who are presumed to have hearing impairment" (Myklebust 1954: xii). The aim of the diagnosis, as he portrayed it, was to differentiate the source of a particular condition from the other possibilities (differential diagnosis) so as to identify and isolate a single cause of the child's auditory and speech and language symptoms.

Johnson, Darley, and Spriestersbach, published a handbook in 1952, that was to be revised twice (Johnson, Darley and Spriestersbach 1963; Darley and Spriestersbach 1978). In the later editions of their handbook, the authors emphasize the difference between what they call "appraisal" and "diagnosis."

Although the terms *appraisal* and *diagnosis* are often used together, they are not synonymous. When a clinician specifies the presenting aspects of a problem and says something about their relative severity, he is appraising the problem... It is not to be thought of as the complete diagnostic process, for in diagnosis the clinician evaluates the description of present status – the appraisal – in light of what the case history reveals about the past status. The goal is to reach a conclusion about the characteristics of the person or of his or her environment that may be responsible for the occurrence and continuation of the disorder. Having reached a conclusion regarding etiology, the clinician proceeds to formulate therapy and to make a prognosis thereby fulfilling – at least for the first round – the responsibility undertaken.

All three versions of the Darley handbooks were widely used in diagnostic courses of their time. The diagnostic categories included in all versions of this handbook called *Diagnostic Methods in Speech Pathology* were: articulation disorders, voice disorders, and speech retardation. The 1963 version added language disorders, and the 1978 version added hearing disorders and acquired motor speech disorders. These additions coincided with the changes going on in other disciplines – a development of the fields of language acquisition, psycholinguistics, and psychoacoustics, as well as a conceptual shifting from behavioral to rationalist theorizing that was to become the hallmark of the next period in the development of speech-language pathology in America.

The last three decades of the 20th century brought with them considerable specialization in the field of speech pathology accompanied by dramatic shifts in diagnostic categories and practices. A proliferation of handbooks on particular diagnostic domains began to emerge in the 1970s (see Table 3). The field became one of specialty experts with researchers and clinicians focusing on particular diagnostic domains. The national organization is now providing clinicians with specialty certificates to acknowledge the specialty expertise of particular clinicians. So today's speech-language pathologists can obtain specialty recognition in the fields of neurogenics, childhood language disorders, and stuttering.

Characteristic of the profession in these last 30 years has been an elaboration of information processing frameworks that serve as models of how a person interprets speech and language (see Duchan 2004, for examples). These models were first developed to represent adult language and cognitive knowledge systems (e.g., Osgood and Miron 1963; Wepman 1960). They were later adapted by clinicians to structure their diagnostic approaches and to pose and answer their assessment questions (Bishop 1997; Nation and Aram 1984). The models depicted linguistic levels in separate boxes that included phonology, morphology, syntax, and semantics. A new pragmatics box was added in the 1970s to represent a newly developing diagnostic/assessment domain having to do with the contextual understandings of communication (see Duchan 1984 for a review of this development).

*Table 3.* New handbooks and textbooks on diagnostic methods for specific communication disorders (1970 to 1985)

| The specific disorder | Texts covering the specific disorder |
|---|---|
| Central auditory processing disorders | Keith 1977 |
| Language disorders in children | Berry 1969<br>Bloom and Lahey 1978<br>Miller 1981<br>Aram and Nation 1982 |
| Motor speech disorders | Darley, Aronson, and Brown 1975<br>Johns 1978 |
| Phonological disorders | Ingram 1976 |
| Stuttering | Bloodstein (five editions from 1969 to 1995) |
| Swallowing (dysphagia) | Logemann 1983<br>Groher 1984 |
| Voice disorders | Moore 1971<br>Aronson 1980 |

Researchers and clinicians working within the linguistic model paid considerable attention to the error patterns in their client's spoken language. Methods for analyzing samples of an individual's spoken language were developed or borrowed from those used in researching normal children's language (e.g., Bloom and Lahey 1978; Ingram 1976; Miller 1981). Language sampling analyses allowed clinicians to discover the patterns produced at each of the levels. (For reviews of these approaches see Lund and Duchan 1993; Owens 1999; Paul 2001).

These linguistic methods, referred to as "language assessment approaches," resembled what had previously been designated as appraisals (Darley and Spriestersbach 1978). The analytic methods were used both to assess the patterns at various levels of language performance as well as to identify knowledge differences that "caused" the problems. This notion of "deep structure" or internal causality allowed the new approaches to serve as a kind of soft diagnosis – one that was knowledge-based rather than biologically based.

Underlying rules were portrayed as being the source of an individual's communication difficulties. Children's articulatory substitutions of, say, /t/ for /d/ and /k/ for /g/, were caused by their rule of devoicing. Such linguistic rules were occasionally used by clinicians not only to describe the problem, but also to explain it. Children's phonological errors were caused by their deep structure misconceptions. Just as cleft palates or motor speech disorders can cause misarticulations, phonological deficits can cause misarticulations.

The most common characterization for underlying rules, however, was that they are descriptive, not causal. Indeed, the name of the approach or model has been called "descriptive-developmental" to emphasize this new focus (see Paul 2001). Arguments in favor of a descriptive approach have involved making a case against the search for etiological causes for language disorders. Lahey (1988), for example, argues in favor of descriptive approaches because it is often impossible to find out the cause for a child's language disorder and that descriptions resulting from assessment offer a better entré into intervention than etiologies, since they describe the details of the individual's knowledge deficits. Knowing that a person has aphasia does not necessarily help clinicians develop language goals for the client.

Emerging alongside the knowledge models in the 1980s were processing models. In processing models the focus was on how information was processed, rather than on how it was represented. A diagnostician working with a processing model might test an individual's short-term memory abilities, one working with a knowledge representation model might assess syntax abilities. The various abilities evaluated in the processing models are sometimes seen as separable processing modules, just as they are for the knowledge models. For example, each may be evaluated separately and different diagnoses made for the different areas of difficulty.

Nation and Aram (1977, 1984) developed a blended model containing elements of both knowledge and processing models (see Figure 1). They offer their model as a guide to diagnosing speech and language disorders and describe what sorts of tests might be given for each level of the model to determine whether it is normal or not.

Following close on the heels of Nation and Aram's second edition was a 1988 publication of a *Handbook of Speech-Language Pathology and Audiology* by Norman Lass and his colleagues. The handbook contained several twists on previous taxonomies. They rename the organic vs. function distinction as diagnoses with known or unknown etiologies. They refer, for example, to articulation disorders as being neurogenic or of unknown etiology. They also express relationships between primary and secondary diagnoses indirectly. For instance, they treat hearing impairment as being "related" to certain speech and language disorders. Their diagnostic taxonomy, judging from the primary sections of the book, include articulation disorders, fluency disorders, language disorders, and voice disorders. Under a miscellaneous section entitled "special populations" are speech and language disorders related to hearing impairment, speech and writing disorders in the learning disabled student, communication problems in the autistic client, and dysphagia (swallowing disorders) associated with speech problems.

An end of the century handbook by Tomblin and his colleagues from the University of Iowa was first published in 1994 and then again in 2000 (Tomblin, Morris, and Spriestersbach 1999, 2000). The editors include the following diagnostic categories in their coverage: language disorders, aphasia, speech sound disorders, motor speech disorders, stuttering, voice disorders, disorders associated with head and neck cancer, traumatic brain injury (omitted from the 2000 version), cleft palate, disordered swallowing, adults with mental retardation, children who are hard of hearing, and children who are deaf.

This list has only a trace of the terminology used at the beginning of the century (aphasia). Some of the diagnostic categories used at the beginning of the century reappear here, under more common names (paralalia⇒speech sound disorders; paralytic alalia⇒motor speech disorders; dyslalia or dysrhythmia⇒stuttering; dysphonia⇒voice disorders). Other disorders in the early taxonomies are not in the current one (dyslogia, dysphemia). And there are categories in the Tomblin et al. text (Tomblin, Morris, and Spriestersbach 1994, 2000) that are not in the original taxonomies (traumatic brain injury, disordered swallowing).

There are other diagnostic categories, originating in the last 30 years, that are treated as subcategories in the Tomblin text or are not mentioned there at all. These more recent diagnostic arrivals are guaranteed to have a shelf life, at least in the short run, because they have been promoted world wide by the World Health Organization for purposes of achieving international uniformity in diagnosis. The new diagnoses are commonly referred to as the ICD categories, an acronym for International Classification of Disorders. An overlapping and equally sanctioned set of categories are provided in a manual by the American Psychiatric Association called the Diagnostic and Statistical Manual (DSM). Included in both the World Health Organization and the American Psychiatric Association lists are at least three diagnostic clusters that have impacted the diagnostic practices of speech-language pathologists.

One cluster includes a list of five types of communication disorders (expressive language disorder, missed receptive-expressive language disorder, phonological disorder, stuttering, and communication disorder not otherwise specified).[2] This list is one that is being used as a way to code speech and language services to children and adults with communication disorders.

A second set of categories provided in the 2000 version of the DSM list (DSM-IV-TR) are ones that fall under the rubric of Pervasive Developmental Disorders. Included in this set are: autistic disorder, Rett's disorder, childhood disintegrative disorder, Asperger's disorder, and pervasive developmental disorder not otherwise specified (PDD NOS).[3] These disabilities are seen as primary etiologies that have communication disorders as a secondary or concomitant problem. The cluster as a whole is sometimes referred to as "autism spectrum disorders" (Wetherby and Prizant 2000).

And a third cluster of categories in DSM IV-TR affecting diagnosis in speech-language pathology are those that fall under Attention-Deficit and disruptive Behavior Disorders. This list includes: attention-deficit/hyperactivity disorder, attention-deficit/hyperactivity disorder not otherwise specified, conduct disorder, oppositional defiant disorder, and disruptive behavior disorder not otherwise specified. Children with attention-deficit hyperactivity disorder are sometimes diagnosed as having central auditory processing disorders, or as being learning disabled, or as language disordered, depending upon the predilections of the diagnostician and the results of tests used to evaluate them.

An interesting diagnostic category that does not make the DSM or ICD lists is one that has been called Specific Language Impairment. The use of this diagnostic category depends upon whether the diagnostician is a researcher or not. A huge research industry has evolved in recent years involving the study of children with this diagnosis.[4] The aim of the research is to discover whether language operates in the human mind as a separable module, as would be suggested by the presence of children whose only difficulty is learning language. But the researchers are not the ones who ordinarily diagnose the children. The same children who are diagnosed with specific language impairment for research purposes are not likely to be so diagnosed in the clinic or school where they are receiving therapy (Kamhi 1998).

## 3. Conclusion

This excursion through the last century has shown a number of ways that diagnosis in speech-language pathology is culturally grounded. In the 19th century, before the medicalization of the profession, elocutionists were the ones who worked with individuals with communication disabilities. They offered "courses" or regimens to their "pupils" without diagnosing their problems.

Later, with the influence of scientific and medical models, the field became a clinical one, adopting diagnostic practices and thinking that continue to this day. The medical view of diagnosis, which locates the problem within the individual, preferably within the person's biological system, provided the centerpiece around which revolved other aspects of service provision.

The diagnosis has long provided a common ground for speech language pathologists and their "patients" or "clients." A primary part of the clinician's job has involved diagnosing what is wrong with the client – what is causing their communication difficulty. Diagnosis has also served clinicians as a guide for planning assessment and therapies – to lessen the symptoms, or to eliminate, minimize or circumvent the conditions causing the symptoms.

Other cultural factors that influenced diagnostic practices in the 20th century were: (1) the testing movement that began in the 1920s that provided normative and quantifiable measures for evaluating children's speech and language performance; (2) the second world that led to the development of the field of audiology, the creation of new diagnostic categories, and the immigration to the US of outstanding European "speech doctors"; (3) the civil rights movement that revealed to clinicians that they had been misdiagnosing individuals with dialect differences; and (4) the recent managed care and international health care systems that have attempted to standardize diagnostic terminology.

The diagnostic handbooks written during the 20th century also provide a picture of the changes in diagnostic categories and understandings of speech-language pathologists working during different periods in the century. Table 4 summarizes the contributions of some of the most influential of the handbooks and what they contributed.

The table shows that diagnostic names have changed and diagnostic categories have been added. But even more informative is the understanding from this historical picture that the very notion of diagnosis gets construed differently depending upon the cultural ethos. The center stage that diagnosis has played over the years is fading. There is evidence that current practitioners in speech-language pathology are depending more on soft diagnostic categories spending and less time looking for a physical etiology. Today's diagnostic emphasis is based on assessment practices that identify areas of competence and incompetence. Yesterday's was on classifying their clients into an etiological category.

The main lesson to be learned from this history of the American practices in the field of speech-language pathology is that diagnosis has not been an activity that exists in limbo outside of the context of the times or outside the frameworks used by the diagnosticians. Rather it is a constructed out of the social and professional milieu affecting the diagnosticians of the period.

*Table 4.* Chronological summary of diagnostic contributions of authors of 20th century American handbooks and texts

| | | | |
|---|---|---|---|
| *Potter (1882)* | *Robbins and Stinchfield (1931)* | *West et al. (1937–1960, 4 editions)* | *Berry and Eisenson (1942)* |
| 1. Biological categories | 1. Added psychological to biological categories;<br>2. Said some causes were unknown<br>3. Described causal chain | 1. Deafness added<br>2. Diagnosis vs. description<br>3. Physiogenic vs. psychogenic distinction | 1. Translated terms from Greek and Latin to English<br>2. Minimized organic vs. functional distinction |
| *Myklebust (1954)* | *Johnson, Darley Spriestersbach (1963–1978, 3 editions)* | *Nation and Aram (1977, 1984)* | *Lass et al. (1988)* |
| 1. Auditory disorders<br>2. New emphasis on perception<br>3. Differential diagnosis focus | 1. Associated diagnosis with etiology<br>2. Added diagnostic category of language disorders | 1. Used an information processing model to guide diagnosis<br>2. Broad view of diagnosis, including assessment and intervention plan | 1. Deemphasized causality<br>2. Deemphasized primary and secondary causes<br>3. Increased emphasis on assessment as diagnosis (soft diagnosis) |
| *Tomblin, Morris, Spriestersbach (1994, 2000)* | *DSM (2000) and ICD (2001)* | | |
| 1. Added traumatic brain syndrome<br>2. Added swallowing problems | 1. Clusters of diagnostic categories<br>2. PDD cluster<br>3. ADD cluster | | |

## Notes

1. The first residential schools for "idiots" were established in the late 1800s.
2. An example of "not otherwise specified" would be a voice disorder, since it does not fit the other specified categories.
3. See Galasso's chapter in this volume for the impact of the diagnosis of PDD NOS on her family.
4. For an outstanding review of this literature and the defining characteristics of SLI see Leonard (1998).

## *References*

American Psychiatric Association
2000 *Diagnostic and Statistical Manual IV-TR.* Washington DC: American Psychiatric Association.
Aram, Dorothy and James Nation
1982 *Child Language Disorders.* St Louis: The C. V. Mosby Company.
Aronson, Arnold
1980 *Clinical Voice Disorders.* New York: Thieme-Stratton.
Bell, Alexander Graham
1872 *Establishment for the Study of Vocal Physiology: for the Correction of Stammering, etc., and for the Practical Instruction in "Visible Speech".* Boston: Rand Avery.
Berry, Mildred
1969 *Language Disorders of Children: The Bases and Diagnoses.* New York: Appleton Century Crofts.
Berry, Mildred and Jon Eisenson
1942 *The Defective in Speech.* New York: Appleton-Century-Crofts.
Bishop, Dorothy
1997 *Uncommon Understanding: Development and Disorders of Language Comprehension in Children.* East Sussex, UK: Psychology Press.
Bloodstein, Oliver
1969/1981/1995 *A Handbook on Stuttering.* Chicago, Il: National Easter Seal Society for Crippled Children and Adults.
Bloom, Lois and Margaret Lahey
1978 *Language Development and Language Disorders.* New York: John Wiley.
Bonner, T.
1963 *American Doctors and German Universities.* Lincoln, Nebraska: University of Nebraska Press.
Bradbury, D.
1937 The contribution of the child study movement to child psychology. *Psychological Bulletin* 34, 21–38.
Cremin, L.
1988 *American Education: The Metropolitan Experience (1876–1980).* New York: Harper and Row.
Darley, Frederick, Arnold Aronson, and Joe Brown
1975 *Motor Speech Disorders.* Philadelphia: W. B. Saunders.
Darley, Frederick and Duane Spriestersbach
1978 *Diagnostic Methods in Speech Pathology* (2nd ed.). New York: Harper and Row.
Duchan, Judith
1984 Language assessment: The pragmatics revolution. In Naremore, R. (ed.), *Language Science: Recent Advances.* San Diego, CA: College-Hill Press, 147–180.
2004 *Frame Work in Language and Literacy.* New York: Guilford Press.

2005 The phonetically-based speech therapy methods of Alexander Graham Bell. *Journal of Speech Language Pathology and Audiology* 29, 70–72.
Dunglison, R.
1798–1869 *A Dictionary of Medical Science* (2nd ed., 1874). Philadelphia, PA: Henry C. Lea.
Froeschels, Emil
1943 Survey of the early literature on stuttering, chiefly European. *Nervous Child* 2, 86–95.
1946 Cluttering. *Journal of Speech Disorders* 11, 31.
Froeschels, Emil (ed.)
1948 *Twentieth Century Speech and Voice Correction.* New York: Philosophical Library.
Gesell, Arnold
1925 *The Mental Growth of the Pre-School Child: A Psychological Outline Of Normal Development from Birth to the Sixth Year, Including a System of Developmental Diagnosis.* New York: Macmillan.
1928 *Infancy and Human Growth.* New York: Macmillan.
1929 Maturation and infant behavior pattern. *Psychological Review* 36, 307–319.
1949 *Gesell Developmental Scales.* New York: Psychological Corporation.
Goldstein, Kurt
1942 *Aftereffects of Brain Injuries in War: Their Evaluation and Treatment.* New York: Grune and Stratton.
1948 *Language and Language Disturbances.* New York: Grune and Stratton.
Groher, Michael (ed.)
1984 *Dysphagia: Diagnosis and Management.* Boston, MA: Butterworths.
Hanson, F. Allen
1993 *Testing Testing: Social Consequences of the Examined Life.* Berkeley, CA: University of California Press.
Ingram, David
1976 *Phonological Disability in Children.* London: Edward Arnold.
Johns, D. F. (ed.)
1978 *Clinical Management of Neurogenic Communication Disorders.* Boston, MA: Little Brown.
Johnson, H.
1928 *Children in "The Nursery School".* New York: Agathon Press.
Johnson, Wendell, Frederick Darley, and Duane Spriestersbach
1952 *Diagnostic Manual in Speech Correction.* New York: Harper and Brothers.
1963 *Diagnostic Methods of Speech Pathology.* New York: Harper and Row.
Kamhi, Alan
1998 Trying to make sense of developmental language disorders. *Language Speech and Hearing Services in Schools* 29, 35–44.
Keith, Robert (ed.)
1977 *Central Auditory Dysfunction.* New York, NY: Grune and Stratton.
Lahey, Margaret
1988 *Language Disorders and Language Development.* New York: Macmillan.

Lass, Norman, Leila McReynolds, Jerry Northern, and David Yoder
1988 *Handbook of Speech-Language Pathology and Audiology.* Philadelphia, PA: B. C. Decker.
Leonard, Laurence
1998 *Children with Specific Language Impairment.* Boston, MA: MIT Press.
Logemann, Jeri
1983 *Evaluation and Treatment of Swallowing Disorders.* Austin, TX: Pro-Ed.
Lund, Nancy and Judith Duchan
1988 *Assessing Children's Language in Naturalistic Contexts.* Englewood Cliffs, NJ: Prentice Hall.
McCarthy, Dorothea
1946 Language development in children. In Carmichael, L. (ed.), *Manual of Child Psychology.* New York: John Wiley, 476–581.
Miller, Jon
1981 *Assessing Language Production in Children.* Boston, MA: Allyn and Bacon.
Moore, Paul
1971 *Organic Voice Disorders.* Englewood Cliffs, NJ: Prentice Hall.
Moores, Donald
1978 *Educating the Deaf: Psychology, Principles, and Practices.* Boston, MA: Houghton Mifflin.
Morley, Atkinson
1941 The function of the speech clinic in the national emergency. *Journal of Speech Disorders* 6, 141–142.
Myklebust, Helmut
1954 *Auditory Disorders in Children: A Manual for Differential Diagnosis.* New York: Grune and Stratton.
Nation, James and Dorothy Aram
1977 *Diagnosis of Speech and Language Disorders.* St Louis, MO: C. V. Mosby.
Nation, James and Dorothy Aram
1984 *Diagnosis of Speech and Language Disorders* (2nd ed.). San Diego, CA: College Hill Press.
Osgood, Charles and Murray Miron
1963 *Approaches to the Study of Aphasia: A Report of an Interdisciplinary Conference on Aphasia.* Urbana, IL: University of Illinois Press.
Owens, Robert
1999 *Language Disorders: A Functional Approach to Assessment and Intervention.* Needham Heights, MA: Allyn and Bacon.
Paul, Rhea
2001 *Language Disorders from Infancy through Adolescence: Assessment and Intervention* (2nd ed.). St. Louis, MI: Mosby.
Peacher, W. G.
1948 Disorders of articulation due to gunshot wounds of the head and neck in World War II. In Froeschels, E. (ed.), *Twentieth Century Speech and Voice Correction.* New York: Philosophical Library, 236–248.

Philips, B. J. and D. Ruscello (eds.)
1998 *Differential Diagnosis in Speech-Language Pathology.* Boston, MA: Butterworth-Heinemann.
Potter, Samuel
1882 *Speech and Its Defects.* Philadelphia: P. Blakiston.
Rees, Norma
1973 Auditory processing factors in language disorders: A view from Procrustes' bed. *Journal of Speech and Hearing Disorders* 38, 304–315.
Robbins, Samuel D. and Sara Stinchfield
1931 *Dictionary of Speech Terminology.* American Speech Correction Association.
Ross, Mark
n.d. A retrospective look at the future of aural rehabilitation. http://www.hearingresearch.org/a_retrospective_look_at_the_futu.htm
Simon, Clarence
1953 Development of education in speech and hearing to 1920. In Wallace, K. (ed), *History of Speech Education in America.* New York: Appleton-Century-Crofts, 389–421.
Stinchfield, Sara
1933 *Speech Disorders: A Psychological Study of the Various Defects of Speech.* New York: Harcourt Brace.
Taylor, Orlando
1986 *Nature of Communication Disorders in Culturally and Linguistically Diverse Populations.* San Diego: College Hill Press.
Templin, Mildred
1957 *Certain Language Skills in Children: Their Development and Interrelationships.* Minneapolis: The University of Minnesota Press.
Thagard, Paul
1999 *How Scientists Explain Disease.* Princeton, NJ: Princeton University Press.
Tomblin, J. Bruce (eds.)
1994 *Diagnosis in Speech-language Pathology.* San Diego, CA: Singular Publishing Group.
Tomblin, J. Bruce, Hugh Morris, and Duane Spriestersbach (eds.)
2000 *Diagnosis in Speech-language Pathology.* San Diego, CA: Singular Publishing Group.
Travis, Lee Edward (ed.)
1971 *Handbook of Speech Pathology and Audiology.* New York: Appleton-Century-Crofts.
Travis, Lee Edward
1931 *Speech Pathology.* New York: D. Appleton.
1957 *Handbook of Speech Pathology.* New York: Appleton-Century-Crofts.
Trent, James W.
1994 *Inventing the Feeble Mind: A History of Mental Retardation in the United States.* Berkeley, CA: University of California Press.
Weiss, Deso
1964 *Cluttering.* Englewood Cliffs, NJ: Prentice Hall.

Wepman, Joseph, L. Jones, D. Bock, and D. VanPelt
1960 Studies in aphasia: Background and theoretical formulations. *Journal of Speech and Hearing Disorders* 25, 323–332.
West, Robert
1936 *Diagnosis of Disorders of Speech: A Clinical Manual of Methods and Apparatus.* Madison, WI: College Typing Company.
West, Robert and Merle Ansberry
1968 *The Rehabilitation of Speech; A Textbook of Diagnostic and Corrective Procedures Based upon a Critical Study of Speech Disorders* (4th ed.). New York: Harper and Row.
West, Robert, Merle Ansberry, and Anna Carr
1957 *The Rehabilitation of Speech; A Textbook of Diagnostic and Corrective Procedures Based upon a Critical Study of Speech Disorders* (3rd ed.). New York: Harper.
West, Robert, Lee Kennedy, and Anna Carr
1937 *The Rehabilitation of Speech: A Textbook of Diagnostic and Corrective Procedures.* New York: Harper.
West, Robert, Lee Kennedy, Anna Carr, and Ollie Backus
1947 *The Rehabilitation of Speech: A Textbook of Diagnostic and Corrective Procedures Based upon a Critical Study of Speech Disorders* (revised ed.). New York: Harper.
Wetherby, Amy and Barry Prizant (eds.)
2000 *Autism Spectrum Disorders: A Transactional Developmental Perspective.* Baltimore, MD: Paul H. Brookes Publishing.
World Health Organization
2001 *International Classification of Disease* (Vol. 10th revision, clinical modification). Albany, NY: World Health Organization.

# Chapter 11
# The diagnosis of deafness in Nicaragua

*Laura Polich*

*In this chapter Laura Polich examines how the diagnosis of deafness is construed by Nicaraguans. Her description vividly illustrates the cultural embeddedness of a diagnosis. She finds in her ethnographic study that many Nicaraguans define deafness as an inability to speak rather than a hearing problem. They see it as a divine retribution inflicted on family members of the deaf person because of a sin that someone in the family committed. In stark contrast to this stigmatized, hopeless view of deafness is the perspective of members of the National Nicaraguan Association for the Deaf. Those associated with this recently formed group of people who are deaf treat their diagnosis as a positive characteristic – it has to do with people "like us." This group carefully distinguishes the diagnosis of "deaf" related to hearing loss and "deafmute" related to the inability to speak. It is being a "deafmute" and unable to talk that is stigmatizing. Deafness as hearing loss, on the other hand, is not.*

In Nicaragua, deafness is a disease, but its diagnosis is typically made without reference to the ear. All attention is focused upon the mouth. A person who is deaf is one who does not talk. Such a label is not given lightly, because deafness is among the diseases that for many years was considered to have no cure and to be an insuperable obstacle to participation in society.

In a country with historically low levels of school achievement and high rates of illiteracy (Merrill 1994; Smith 1993), the inability to communicate orally is a serious detriment. Nicaragua is a country in which news and information are passed more by oral than through written means. *Trends in Latin American Networking* (TILAN), a resource of the Latin American Network Information Center (LANIC) at the University of Texas at Austin, notes that while newspapers reach 30 of every 1,000 inhabitants, there are 26 telephones per 1,000 and 170 television sets per 1,000 people (TILAN 2001). No figures were given for radio sets. In a 1995 poll, residents of the capital, Managua, reported that 49.9% considered radio to be their major source of news and information, while 38.5% turned to television, and only 10.1% to newspapers (Norsworthy 1997). These results, no doubt, are linked to the fact that the illiteracy rate recognized by the government is 34% (TILAN 2001), while unofficially it is known to be much higher (Arrién, De Castilla, and Lucío 1999; Vargas 1999).

Trucks mounted with public address systems wend their way daily through the towns and cities of Nicaragua advertising goods for sale, funeral announcements or political party propaganda, at high decibel levels in order to reach inhabitants both inside and outside of their houses. The garbage collectors have very erratic schedules, and their presence in a neighborhood is announced by the pealing of a handbell at the end of each block. (On one occasion, the garbage truck rang the bell for the block where I lived at 10 p.m. Someone in every household dutifully ran outside to submit their garbage bags for the weekly collection.) The inability to respond well to acoustic stimuli isolates individuals not only from national or international happenings, but also from the interchange of daily goods, services, and announcements.

Even at a familiar level, oral communication is highly valued. The ability to carry on extended "small talk," or tell jokes or stories is what allows people to weave themselves into the society of a particular section of town (*barrio)* or neighborhood (*vecindad*) in a country where (due to the tropical climate) more time is spent outside on a porch adjacent to the street than ensconced within a house's four cinderblock walls. Leaving a person alone in a house (i.e., with no one to talk with) is considered a "very sad [*muy triste*]" situation, and friendly neighbors offer to send an unoccupied child over to provide the solo person someone with whom to converse (personal observations 1994–2001). With the average number of occupants per house at 5.8 (INEC 1995), compared to 2.63 in the United States (U.S. Bureau of the Census 1990), lack of conversational partners is rarely a problem.

In 1997, I conducted a survey of 225 deaf adults that included questions about communicative modality and communication with family members (Polich 1998). Since the actual number of deaf adults present in the country at the time was unknown, and is, in fact, unknowable (INEC 1995; personal communication with spokesperson at The Nicaraguan Institute of Statistics and Census (INEC) 1997), it is not possible to say with certainty whether those surveyed constituted a representative sample of the actual adult deaf population in Nicaragua. But, because the National Nicaraguan Association of the Deaf (ANSNIC) [the only organization of deaf adults in the country] had only 385 registered members in 1997, certainly a large percentage of the members of ANSNIC, as well as non-member deaf adults known to members of ANSNIC were questioned.

The results in regard to communication were disheartening. Twenty percent (45) of those surveyed were non-ANSNIC members who did not use sign language (Polich 1998). Their surveys were completed through homesign, gestures or information provided by other family members. In all of those cases, communication by the deaf person was profoundly limited in the larger society, and severely limited even within the immediate family. Of the remaining 180 persons surveyed, approximately 10 could carry on an oral conversation with persons familiar with speech patterns of the deaf (e.g., their immediate family members) but were basically unintelligible to typical members of the greater Nicaraguan society. Sixteen percent (36) of those surveyed stated that in spite of being unable to use oral communication, they were the only signers in their homes (Polich 1998). They communicated with immediate family members only through mime and gesture. Fifty-two percent (117) replied that there was one other immediate family member with whom they could communicate, by using sign language (the family members' sign language skills ranged from rudimentary to fluent), and that all communication with their other family members had to be channeled through that one designated interpreter. Only 26 percent of those surveyed had two or more family members with whom they could communicate directly (Polich 1998). Perhaps the saddest result of the survey [noting that 98% of those surveyed lived with relatives; only 2 percent had established their own homes (Polich 1998)] is the fact that when asked the question, "With which [hearing] person living in your home do you communicate most easily?" a full 40 percent (90) of the respondents replied "No one."

This survey was conducted in 1997, eleven years after ANSNIC was founded, and only included deaf adults known to members of ANSNIC. One would expect that deaf adults unknown to ANSNIC (the organization has received wide-spread public exposure) would be even more isolated, and have even more limited communication networks. The situation prior to the organization of the Association in the early 1980s (Polich 1998) could only have been more communicatively restrictive than it is at present. In short, today, deaf adults have little communicative interaction with society, or even their immediate families, and, in earlier times, were probably even more isolated.

Deafness is classified by typical Nicaraguans as a permanent disease, and grouped with such other "illnesses" as blindness, mental retardation, and cerebral palsy. These are the diseases against which doctors have traditionally been helpless, and it is common to attribute their occurrence to the "will of God" (*la voluntad de Díos*). Nicaragua, like the rest of the Spanish and Portuguese colonies from the fifteenth to the nineteenth centuries, inherited a Roman Catholic world view which placed great emphasis upon sin, the role of sin in influencing "God's will" and the necessity of expiating or atoning for one's sins to calm God's wrath. In Medieval Europe plagues were commonly attributed to communal sin, with the ensuing need for communal penitence. Later, the work of the Inquisition escalated to extreme levels in the quest to root out sinners and assure the expiation of their sins, even if the atonement were gained only through the torture applied by the Inquisition itself.

This religious worldview has influenced how deaf children, who are so communicatively shut out of an oral world, were (and are) seen by society: most likely the result of God's wrath brought on by some sin. This makes the identification of causality problematical. Deafness as a just divine punishment is, with difficulty, assigned to an innocent creature, who obviously had done nothing to merit such a "vile destiny" (*destino vilo*). Blame, then, fell on the child's progenitors or family. One or more of them must have done something so serious that divine punishment visited directly upon their own persons could not be enough. It was retribution that hurt the perpetrator even more forcefully than personal pain. Deafness was a punishment visited upon that which was most precious, a son or a daughter.

While performing ethnographic fieldwork in Nicaragua from 1994 to the present, I have heard many stories expressing this attitude toward the diagnosis of deafness. Some were told by persons who recounted how their parents or grandparents had reacted to the deafness of a sibling, or an aunt or uncle, but I have also heard similar tales from parents who had searched, or were in the midst of searching, their own or their spouse's past behavior to explain the present deafness of a son or daughter.

In Nicaragua, the diagnosis of deafness is a lay decision, made first by family members. One of my research assistants, Luis Gonzáles, interviewed the mother of a deaf son (who, at the time was 16 years old) in a northern Nicaraguan town. He asked her what had caused Eduardo's hearing loss.

> She told me that it was a punishment from God *(un castigo de Diós)* to have a deaf child. It was God's punishment for her. That was why it was so difficult to understand Eduardo at first, when no one could understand what he was trying to communicate. She thinks that someone in her family must have done something very bad or acted wrongly, or maybe it was because her husband has a "roving eye" and goes around with other women *(es muy mujeriego)*. She says it must have been something like that for God to have sent them this punishment.

And while it is now no longer common to hide deaf persons from society, some cases unfortunately still come to light. Milagros Galo, the principal of one of the Department of Special Education's schools in northern Nicaragua described such a situation to me:

> Three years ago I went to the house of a child who is now in our school named Juanito. At the time he was six years old and deaf. Others had reported his existence to us, and we wanted the mother to send him to school so I went to the house to talk with her personally. Finally, she literally brought him out from underneath the bed. His mother was ashamed of him because he was six years old and couldn't talk. He was dirty, stuck under the bed, with no clothes on. He was given food, but simply the leftovers because he was seen as a "useless being" *(inútil)* and therefore not worth wasting good food on.

Deafness in Nicaragua has traditionally been characterized as primarily the lack of intelligible speech and inability to understand spoken language. By its nature, deafness cut an individual off from social contact, and prohibited social participation. In Nicaragua, a society where one's identity is based upon active social membership in large extended families, and where verbal fluency in repartee and poetry are highly admired, deafness is an ominous diagnosis.

Family members often suspect nothing until, when the child becomes mobile, the lack of attention to oral commands becomes noticeable. But family members usually only put all symptoms in perspective and come to a diagnosis when the child fails to use speech at an age in which older siblings or contemporary neighbor children are happily chattering away. The recriminations can become quite hostile at this point, and many households have shattered over the causation of a child's deafness.

Nor is hearing status necessarily linked to the observed lack of speech. In 1995, an older rural woman, who lived so far from a major town that a four-hour bus trip was necessary to reach the clinic in which I was doing voluntary hearing testing, brought me her five-year-old granddaughter. I tested the child, who co-operated excellently with play audiometry, and told the grandmother that her granddaughter had a severe-to-profound hearing loss in both ears. With the air of someone who has gone to very much trouble for very little gain, the grandmother replied: "I *know* that she is deaf. Why I brought her *here* was to find out why she doesn't *talk!*"

Nicaraguan parents continue, as before, to refer to their deaf children as *enfermos* ('ill'). But during the last fifty years, the hope of a remediation, a treatment that could "cure" the child, has slowly appeared on the Nicaraguan scene. Perhaps these children could be *taught* to speak, thus dissolving their disease. The first Nicaraguan school accepting children with deafness, blindness, developmental delay or motoric problems opened in January 1946 (*La Gaceta* 1946a) in the country's capital, Managua. It was small, and the personnel were all *empiricos* (persons with no formal training, but who learned on the job).

Its existence, however, implies that at some point in the first half of the 1940s, influential persons in Nicaragua must have become convinced that while deaf children may be *enfermos,* that the disease did have some hope of a cure, or they would not have spent the time and energy to set up the school. In other words, a shift in the thinking of some Nicaraguans before 1946 convinced them that a diagnosis of deafness did not have to be the irrevocable judgment it once was. If deaf children could learn to talk, they could be cured and no longer considered *enfermos*. Importantly, the cure was not one to be administered at home by family members. It necessitated specialized treatment provided by a school.

Why this change in attitude occurred in the early 1940s is not clear. Mexico had a school for deaf children in the 1800s, but its history in the 1900s is not well documented, and there is no evidence (to date) that any Nicaraguan children ever attended that school. The most well known school for the education of deaf children in Mexico, the *Instituto Mexicano de la Audición y del Lenguaje (IMAL),* which some Nicaraguan children *did* later attend, did not open until 1949, three years after Nicaragua's first school. The first Guatemalan school that accepted deaf children began in 1949, and it was not until 1956 that a school accepting deaf children was founded in El Salvador.

In Costa Rica, however, Dr. Fernando Centeno Guell, a Central American leader in education for the developmentally delayed, set up a school which accepted deaf children in Costa Rica in 1939. News of his successes in teaching special education students must have reached Nicaragua, because when the first Special Education school opened in Managua in January 1946, Dr. Centeno Guell was invited to give the inaugural address, and he remained in the capital another month, helping to choose the pupils, and give advice to the personnel of the new school (personal communication, Olga Tenorio Hernandez, July 24, 1997).

The history of education for the deaf in neighboring Honduras is far from clear. María Cristina Valentine wrote a book published in 1949 in which she referred to her school for the deaf in Tegucigalpa, but she provides no date at which the school began. Its founding is likely to have been contemporary to Dr. Centeno Guell's school in Costa Rica. Two Nicaraguan deaf sisters had government-funded scholarships (*La Gaceta 1946*b) to the Honduran school, which were officially cancelled in March 1946 (indicating that the Honduran school must have predated the Nicaraguan school) when the two returned home after finishing their course of study at the school for the deaf in Honduras. Soon after, they both accepted regular positions as Home Economics teachers in two different girls' high schools (*La Gaceta* 1946c). Perhaps the progress in speaking that those two exhibited on visits home in the early 1940s during their Honduran education impressed other Nicaraguans to lobby for schooling for deaf children. There is no evidence (to date), however, that the deaf sisters had any contact with the deaf students at the new Special Education school.

From interviews conducted in 1997 with three teachers who had worked in the Nicaraguan special education school in the 1950s and 1960s, it appears that, while remediation for deafness through the teaching of speech was now considered possible, success was not just around the corner. None of the teachers could remember a deaf student from those early years (approximately 1948–1970) who had learned to speak well enough to be characterized as "cured." When I asked for specific names of speaking deaf Nicaraguans, I was always given the names of the two sisters (but they were not educated in Nicaragua, and it is not clear whether they were actually deaf or hard-of-hearing), and sometimes a few other female students were mentioned as being "successful" because they had married hearing husbands (personal communication, Olga Tenorio Hernandez, July 24, 1997).

Although the first otolaryngologist set up a practice in Managua in the late 1950s, he did not have an audiometer (personal communication, Dr. Alma Acuna de Isaba, May 26, 1994). "Whisper tests," and tuning forks were the tools available to test hearing then, but the severe-to-profound hearing losses which characterize deafness and the lack of oral communication are apparent without those rudimentary tools. Deafness continued to be a lay diagnosis made by the family on the basis of the lack of speech.

In 1961, Dr. Pedro Berruecos Téllez (the founder of *IMAL* in Mexico in 1949) was in Nicaragua to present a series of lectures on the possibilities for teaching deaf children to speak (personal communication, Sylvia Ayon, May 19, 1997). In the audience were Antonio and Sílvia Ayón, parents of a child born in 1959 who was deaf. Dr. Berruecos told Mrs. Ayón that the best way she could help her son was to move with him to Mexico, and enroll herself in the education for the deaf curriculum while her son could attend the *IMAL*'s demonstration school. Mr. Ayón, at first only accompanying his wife to Mexico City, soon decided to enroll himself in the program. They were later joined by a third Nicaraguan, Olga Tenorio Hernandez, a teacher since 1948 at the Special Education School in Managua. In 1963 when they all returned after completing their certificates in Voice and Speech Development, Ms. Tenorio went back to the Special Education School, while the Ayónes opened a small private school in their home to teach speech and language to deaf children.

The first audiometer to be used in Nicaragua was introduced in 1966 by Claire Cooper, an audiologist, aboard the U.S.S. "Hope," a floating hospital that traveled as part of the Alliance for Progress throughout Latin American ports providing medical attention otherwise unavailable in those countries (personal communication, Dr. Alma Acuna de Isaba, May 26, 1994; Sylvia Ayon, May 19, 1997). The "Hope" was docked at the Pacific port of Corinto for at least six months. All of the children at the Special Education School in Managua were bussed there for audiometric evaluations, and most received donated hearing aids. All the schoolchildren of the areas near Corinto (Chinandega, León, etc.) were bussed to the ship for hearing screenings, and follow-up diagnostic testing, if needed. This effort marked the first shift in the diagnosis of deafness, from a lay decision based upon speech toward one focusing upon hearing ability and conducted by professionals with calibrated machines. Although underway, that shift has not yet, even today, become general in Nicaragua.

Prior to the use of audiometers, hearing ability could not be defined on an objective scale, so the diagnosis of deafness, of necessity, depended on whether or not a person talked. An audiometer, however, can measure precisely what level of sound an individual can perceive. These measurements can be compared to national and international norms, thus categorizing an individual's abilities as "normal" or "abnormal." Audiometric results clarified the correlation between a lack of speech and a lack of lack of hearing ability. Diagnosing the cause of not speaking as due to a certain level of not hearing meant that an underlying cause could be separated from a surface-level symptom, which, it was hoped, would lead to a more effective treatment.

While audiometers were known to improve the precision of a diagnosis of deafness by a professional (and, therefore, represented an advance in medical care), it was not until 1969 that Dr. Alma Acuña de Isabá (trained in Speech and Audiometry at the *IMAL)* brought an audiometer and sound booth permanently to Nicaragua, installing them in the office she shared with her husband, who had trained as an otolaryngologist (personal communication, Dr. Alma Acuna de Isaba, May 26, 1994).

Although the deafness of most children continued to be diagnosed by their families, those with more financial resources began to seek a professional confirmation of the decisions they had already made. Children were tested audiometrically by Dr. Isabá, the audiologist, and then examined medically by Dr. Isabá, the otolaryngologist, who pronounced the diagnosis. If the loss was considered remediable (i.e., there was potential that speech could be taught), the children were sent back to Dr. Isabá, the audiologist, to be fitted with a hearing aid, and enrolled in her nursery school program which emphasized speech stimulation.

When the extent of the loss was too severe to expect any improvement by remediation, parents were simply told to take their children home, and plan to care for them for the rest of their lives, because they were *enfermitos* who would never be cured. The bluntness of Dr. Isabá, the otolaryngologist, when pronouncing the diagnosis is legendary. Among the many stories I heard from parents about this decisive moment for them, was that of the mother of a deaf child born in the early 1980s (Personal communication, Jacqueline Aburto, September 12, 1997). She described the interview in which she received the professional diagnosis (although she and her family members had already made a lay diagnosis):

> Although I knew in my heart that he [the child] was deaf, I still took him to Dr. Isabá in hope that there might be some way to cure him. My child was tested [audiometrically] and examined [medically], and then I was told to dress him while the doctor went out of the room. When the doctor returned, he sat down, looked at me, and said, "He's deaf. See that knob on the door over there. He hears just about as much as that knob does. Just take him home and don't waste anyone else's time. He is going to be a burden to you for the rest of your life."

The same advances that led to building audiometers that could diagnose hearing ability on a fine scale, also led to improvements in hearing aids or personal amplifiers that could amplify sound more efficiently into the ear. Thus, persons with severe or profound hearing losses could experience the fact that the jaw-wagging routinely performed by hearing persons was accompanied by an added component, sound, which determined the majority of its meaning. Unfortunately, the type of hearing loss (sensory) that causes most deafness results from damaged hair cells in the cochlea of the ear. Amplification levels necessary for deaf persons to perceive sound also introduce inherent distortion into the acoustic signal (Alpiner and McCarthy 2000).

The sound a deaf person gains from hearing aid use is not, by itself, a "cure," or sufficient for natural speech development. Use of hearing aids is only the beginning. Intensive individual training must be combined with the inherently distorted sound made possible by the hearing aids if any progress toward speech is to be made. Mr. and Mrs. Ayón, and Dr. Isabá set up two small schools in which selected deaf children were accepted for individual and small group lessons in learning to speak. It is difficult to find their "successfully remediated" pupils today. When I asked Dr. Isaba and Mrs. Ayon for a list, most of those cited had emigrated to the United States (inferring that their families were well-off) in the 1980s, so I could not interview them. The other names they cited are persons now active in the Nicaraguan National Deaf Association, and who use sign language as their major (and preferred) form of communication.

The "remediationists" were strengthened in the early 1970s, when a young, dynamic teacher of the deaf from Moscow, Natalia Popova, came to live in the country after marrying a Nicaraguan national. Popova would become the most vocal advocate for the oral remediation of the deaf, and a dominant figure in the history of deaf education in Nicaragua. After the Sandinista Revolution in 1979, the existing special education schools were absorbed into the national educational system run by the Ministry of Education (MED), curricula were standardized, and many new special education schools were built. The number of schools accepting deaf pupils rose from five in 1979 to twenty in 1981. Natalia Popova was named Coordinator of Deaf Education at the Ministry of Education (MED), and thus her approach, in which "making the students talk" (personal communication, Yadira Miranda, September 27, 1997) was fundamental, became the required methodology.

Only a miniscule minority of deaf children had access to amplification. (Even today no hearing aids or batteries are manufactured in Nicaragua. All are imported. Prices are competitive with those charged in the country of origin [U.S.A., Germany, Denmark, etc.]). In spite of the lack of amplification, all forms of manual communication (except finger spelling of Spanish words) were strictly prohibited in the elementary schools.

During this time deafness continued to be a lay diagnosis, occasionally confirmed by a professional. The vast majority of deaf children enrolled in the special education schools were brought to and enrolled in the schools because they did not talk (personal communication, Dr. Natalia Popova, July 15, 1997). The Ministry of Education did not acquire an audiometrist until 1987, and throughout the ten years she was employed by the Ministry of Education (she transferred to *Los Pipitos'* Audiological Counseling Center in 1998, and was never replaced), she did not have access to a sound-treated testing booth. Although various teachers of the deaf, at times, were trained in "logopedagogy" with an eye to working on speech perception and production in small groups, no speech pathologists or therapists have been employed in the public school system since 1980, and during this time no individual speech training has ever been offered in any of the public schools. The overwhelming majority of the deaf pupils who graduate from the Ministry of Education's Special Education program do not talk, or at least not intelligibly.

In the late 1980s, upon her return from a period of study in the then-Soviet Union, Natalia Popova went to work for *Los Pipitos*, the commonly-used name for an advocacy group of parents of handicapped children organized in 1987, and now the largest such group in the country. She began an early language stimulation program for deaf children, focusing upon pre-schoolers, and was instrumental in founding the Audiological Counseling Center (ACC) in 1992 where speech therapy for deaf children was combined with audiological testing and parent training modules.

The ACC, which receives the majority of its support from foreign donors, presently represents the bastion of the oral remediationist philosophy in Nicaragua. It is also the only site known to teachers of the deaf where (affordable) audiometry is done (personal communications with fifty teachers of the deaf in Special Education schools throughout Nicaragua, January–November, 1997). The audiological services offered by the center outrun speech services by a wide margin (personal communication, Dr. Natalia Popova, July 15, 1997; confirmed in subsequent years through personal visits to the ACC).

Dr. Popova stated that her major goal in founding the AAC was earlier identification of deaf children so that professional speech stimulation could be initiated immediately after the diagnosis, which should improve the abilities of those children to learn speech (personal communication, Dr. Natalia Popova, July 15, 1997). Dr. Popova has been the major, and a most vocal, spokesperson for the view that the diagnosis of deafness is the province of professionals, and that immediate professional intervention is imperative if the child is to learn to talk, or in other words, if the disease is to be "cured."

Nevertheless, the majority of children entering deaf classrooms in the Special Education schools have never been evaluated audiologically (personal communications with fifty teachers of the deaf in Special Education schools throughout Nicaragua, January–November, 1997). They simply do not talk. Thus, while Dr. Popova has been vigorously advocating professional diagnosis of deafness for the past thirteen years, it is clear that her opinion is not yet shared by the majority of Nicaraguans.

There is one group, the National Nicaraguan Association for the Deaf, for whom the diagnosis of deafness is not considered a negative stigma or disease, but just another characteristic. This group appeared only within the past twenty years, and it definitely represents a minority opinion. To members of the Deaf Association, a diagnosis of deafness simply describes a person as "like us." It is simply one more characteristic that will be listed on one's identity card, noted in the same way as having dark hair or a particular birthmark. To members of the Deaf Association, a diagnosis of deafness describes another potential member, another person who will prefer to communicate visually rather than auditorially.

I once asked a Nicaraguan woman what it was like to be deaf. She told me that she was content with being deaf. She felt happy to be a deaf person. I then asked her what she would change if she could change anything at all about herself. She responded:

> I am deaf, that's all. I want to be this way, to be deaf. It feels right to me. I don't know why, but even if I could be born again, I would choose to be deaf. It is a blessing. To me it has the same meaning that being a hearing person has for you.

The hearing world's preoccupation with speaking or not speaking is unintelligible to deaf persons in Nicaragua. It is, to them, a surface feature, and one that can be compensated for very well by using sign language. Their experience of the word *mudo* ('mute') is one of derision and humiliation, and a term they reject and abhor. When I asked Oscar Sequeira (1997) (whom I have never heard utter a sound, although I have seen him engaged in intense conversations in sign language) about the term he preferred to be called, he responded [in sign language]:

> I don't get it. I am deaf, but they call me mute. My family doesn't make fun of me. They respect me, and I don't have any problems with them. In the neighborhood, I try to be friendly with other hearing guys, but they're always laughing at me, calling me "mute," especially if they see me and some of my friends using sign language. I ask them not to say "mute." I tell them, "I'm deaf, not mute. Don't call me mute." But they don't pay any attention. It makes me really mad at hearing people. I don't care if they call me deaf. But mute, that is something else.

The importance of passing from being a non-talker to at least being a marginal talker was emphasized for me when I went looking, accompanied by another deaf person, for the home of a child enrolled in a classroom for the deaf at the special education school in Managua. His teacher had provided the address, and once we arrived approximately where we believed the house should have been, I inquired for the boy. *Andamos buscando la casa de un niño sordo que vive por aquí. Nos puede indicar la casa?* ('We're looking for the house of a deaf boy who lives around here. Could you point out which house it is?') A man in his 30s was sitting on the porch, and he shook his head: *No, por aquí no vive ningún sordomudo* ('No, no deafmute lives around here'). I checked the directions again, and then added: *La maestra de la escuela nos ha dicho que por aquí vive un niño que no oye bien y no habla claramente. No lo conoce?* ('The teacher at the school told us that a boy who doesn't hear well and doesn't talk clearly lives around here. Don't you know him?') *Ahhhh! Sí, sí, sí. Está hablando de mi hijo. Es cierto que era sordomudo, pero ya se superó. Ya habla* ('Ohhh! Yes, yes, yes! You're talking about my son. It's true that he used to be a deafmute, but he has overcome that. He talks now'). The father invited us in.

The eight-year-old boy was out playing, and the father sent a sibling to fetch him. When he arrived, the father urged him to talk to me to display his hard-earned speech, which had saved him from the category of "deafmute." The boy was barely intelligible, and from the father's description, had an oral vocabulary of perhaps thirty words, mostly the names of relatives and food and clothing items. He lip read a similar amount. What was salient, as his father's words indicate, however, was that he could, at least, talk.

Some deaf people do speak. One man in Managua, in his late-30s, who, through intensive speech training and excellent hearing aids (his family had the means to send him to Germany to be fitted with new hearing aids) is able to communicate orally. His voice has a quality typical of "deaf speech" and a conversation with him is a laborious dialogue in which he tries to guess what the speaker is saying, and the speaker tries to guess what his response means. But he does talk.

In 1997 at every conference or meeting advocating oral training that I attended (about five altogether), this man was singled out as an excellent example of someone who had "overcome his destiny." The audience was triumphantly told that he knew no sign language because he chose not to learn it. He could not be counted among the deaf, Popova said, because he had learned to speak. He was cured.

Yet, when I talked with him personally later towards the end of that year, he told me he had never been allowed to associate with other deaf people until he was an adult. His inability to understand any conversation at the Deaf Association was the reason he was not a member, and why he relied only upon speech. He had no aversion to sign language; he simply had never learned it.

A few years have passed now. On my latest visit to Nicaragua I learn that the same man who had conquered deafness by learning to speak now socializes regularly at the meeting-house of the Deaf Association, and although his signing skills are still rudimentary, he is participating. According to Popova he is a recidivist. He has thrown away all the benefits that his excellent oral education gave him. Popova says that because he has chosen to participate in the deaf community and learn sign language, he has opted to become deaf and not speak.

His case baffles most Nicaraguans. His hearing ability is unchanged; he has, and always has had, a severe-to-profound hearing loss. His expensive hearing aids have not disappeared. He has the option of turning back to speech whenever he chooses. But the question they cannot answer is: If he was cured, and able to talk, why could he possibly want to give that up? To Nicaraguans it is very perplexing: he talked, he was one of us, so why didn't that satisfy him?

Anyone familiar with deafness knows why. The oral ability he had did not make him an *active* member of the majority society. Although pointed out as a wonderful example of how a deaf person could be "integrated" into hearing society, he had no friends and he rarely understood what was happening in anything larger than one-on-one encounters: he was lost in workshops, at group lunches, or staff meetings. Even conversations with one other person were ordeals of trial-and-error because he hadn't heard any of the context surrounding the portion of speech he could understand. He lived within an oral society, but his participation was minimal.

Now he is voluntarily learning sign language, and choosing to socialize where he has full access to the visual message. As he gains skill in the language (which will be difficult, because he is starting at a very late point) he will be able to become an active member of the society of the deaf community, even if his social action is limited to making friends or enemies. But the society of the deaf community is open and accessible to him, whereas in oral society, his participation is marginal, at best. And he is one of the few who can choose his memberships. Because speech is the prerequisite, the overwhelming majority of the members of the Deaf Association have no entry to an oral society.

When deafness was considered a divine punishment, and thus, an unchangeable condition, most Nicaraguan families reacted to their speechless children with shame. Deaf persons were typically kept at home, unmentioned to neighbors, and cared for until they died. The lack of communication made it unthinkable that such a person would one day be a functioning member of society – they would always need a guardian. These are the "Eternal Children." This perspective on deafness was predominant in all of Nicaraguan society until the middle of this century, and it continues in some sectors even now.

When deafness was reformulated as a medical condition, an illness that could have a cure if speech could be taught, then the potential for social participation became a possibility. If one could speak, one could be integrated into society, and thus be normalized. This image of the deaf I call the "Remediated Subject." It is predominant now, even in the schools where sign language is used on a daily basis.

Only a very small number of people have rejected both of these models in favor of an alternative conceptualization of deaf persons. To do this, they had to reject the fundamental assumption that only speech could be language. Language remains essential for societal participation, but when the definition of language is expanded to include a manual mode – sign language – then the crucial obstacle to societal participation is removed. A portion of society could run on manual language alone and provide a place for social structures to be woven and re-woven. Furthermore, through bilingual individuals, that community could participate in the wider society. Thus, individual deaf persons could function actively within the deaf community, but also have access to the larger society. This paradigm can be called the "Social Agent" model. It is a rather new conceptualization in Nicaragua, with its beginnings less than twenty years ago. Ill-formed even up to the early 1990s, it is a model that is still developing. But its presence in the Nicaraguan collective mind means that independent social functioning is now a possibility for a non-oral deaf person.

These three models co-exist. They did not follow each other as discrete events, but are layered one atop another. In present-day Nicaragua, in some places, deaf children are still considered "useless" and are fed last, while at the same time other parents make exorbitant sacrifices to buy a precious hearing aid with the hope that it will transform their child into a talker. And other parents allow their sons and daughters to visit the clubhouse of the Deaf Association so that they may become part of the deaf community (usually, unfortunately, without bothering to learn any sign language themselves).

## *References*


Alpiner, Jerry and Patricia McCarthy

2000 *Rehabilitative Audiology: Children and Adults* (3rd ed.). Philadelphia: Lippincott Williams and Wilkins.

Arrién, Juan, Miguel De Castilla, and Rafael Lucio

1999 *Nicaragua: la educación en los noventa.* Programa de Promoción de la Reforma de la Educación en America Latina (PREAL). Available at: http://www.uca.edu.ni/biblioteca/PREAL/preal.html.

Instituto Nicaraguense de Estadísticas y Censos (INEC)

1995 *Censos Nacionales 1995: Cifras Oficiales Finales, Republica de Nicaragua.* Managua: INEC.

*La Gaceta* (official newspaper of record for Nicaragua)

1946a "Decreto No. 11," Ano L, NO. 24, 4 de febrero de 1946, 300–301.

1946b "Cancelese la pension," Ano L, No. 61, 19 marzo de 1946, 748.

1946c "Nombramiento," Ano L, No. 155, 22 de julio de 1946.

Merrill, Tim

1994 *Nicaragua: A Country Study.* Washington, D.C.: United States Department of Defense.

Norsworthy, Kent

1997 The mass media. In Walker, Thomas (ed.), *Nicaragua without Illusions.* Wilmington, DE: Scholarly Resources, 281–295.

Polich, Laura
1998 *Social Agency and Deaf Communities: A Nicaraguan Case-Study.* Unpublished Ph.D. dissertation, University of Texas at Austin.
Smith, Hazel
1993 *Nicaragua: Self-Determination and Survival.* London: Pluto Press.
TILAN
2001 Trends in Latin American Networking. A resource of the Latin American Network Information Center at the University of Texas at Austin, available via Internet at: http://lanic.utexas.edu/project/tilan/countries/nic.html. Last updated.
United States of America Bureau of the Census
1990 *General Social and Economic Characteristics, PC80-1-C1, Table 237, 1990 Census.* Washington, D.C.: Government Printing Office.
Vargas, Oscar-Rene
1999 *Nicaragua después del Mitch...que?* Managua: Imprimatur Artes Graficas.

# Section 3. Reasoning diagnostically

# Chapter 12

# Documenting awareness of the cultural process of diagnosis: Letters of recommendation for medical school faculty

*Frances Trix*

*Frances Trix takes us along a new path, veering away from how an expert's diagnosis impacts on individuals, to show us how diagnosis pervades the thinking of those engaged in everyday problem solving activities. Here she illustrates how diagnoses can be situated culturally as a type of gatekeeping discourse where the signs and symptoms of individuals are to be explained and evaluated with respect to their suitability for employment. As an authoritative naming practice and a form of social reasoning, diagnosis operates both positively and negatively for the evaluated candidates.*

Letters of recommendation for applicants seeking positions or advancement in institutions of higher learning are a colloquial form of expert discourse. That is, the letters are most commonly written by senior faculty to similarly placed faculty in other institutions, and while the letters often include scientific parlance, their purpose is more general and their structure that of letters. These letters are at the same time a form of gatekeeping discourse in that they are required for consideration for positions in the institutions. While the usefulness of such letters in predicting future success is highly contested (Friedman 1983), at least in medical schools, such letters continue to be considered among the most important criteria in screening candidates (DeLisa, Jain, and Campagnolo 1994; Ross and Leichner 1984). Indeed there has been considerable research on letters of recommendation for medical schools, but it has focused primarily on the efficacy of such letters in selecting and placing students in residency training programs (Greenburg, Doyle, and McClure 1994). This study differs from earlier studies in that it considers letters of recommendation for medical school faculty, not people in training. It also differs in that it attempts to relate such letters of recommendation to awareness of the broader cultural practice of diagnosis.

Diagnosis in the strictly medical sense is not a common element of letters of recommendation for medical school faculty. Indeed, where clinical medical diagnosis does appear in such letters, as in the following excerpt from a letter for an associate professor position in a medical school, it is certainly unwise and potentially actionable:

> ... Her last years in my laboratory were impacted by serious health problems that have fortunately gone away – she had really debilitating problems with a herniated disk that apparently was a paraneoplastic phenomenon that went away once an early carcinoma of the left ovary was identified and removed.

In contrast, diagnosis understood as a cultural practice draws its model from the inquisitive stance of clinical medical learning, but is more pervasive in that it is a form of social reasoning, an authoritative naming practice, an evaluative discourse with consequences. Some of the features of the evaluative discourse of diagnosis are also present in the weighing, selecting, and supporting of qualifications that the letters of recommendation embody. One could argue that the familiarity of the recommenders and readers of these letters of recommendation, all largely physicians by training and practice, accounts for the affinity of features of the cultural practice of diagnosis in the letters. However, I see the larger cultural context as equally a source of this practice. Indeed, anyone who reads mystery stories, and these are read by a wide spectrum of people, or watches thrillers on television, movies, or video is affected by this cultural practice. It is interesting to note that a prominent author of early books of the mystery genre, Sir Arthur Conan Doyle, was himself a 19th century British physician, and the methods of deduction of his famous detective, Sherlock Holmes,[1] can be traced to methods of medical inference.

Diagnosis as a process in the medical context is understood to be based on two sorts of data: signs and symptoms. Signs, like a skin rash or temperature, may be objectively observed while symptoms, as in "I have a dull pain in my neck," are what the patient subjectively reports (Atkinson 1997: 164). Similarly, with letters of recommendation, a recommender has the objective data of the curriculum vita including numbers of publications, papers presented, and grants, as well as the more subjective data of his or her own experience with the applicant. And just as a competent medical diagnosis depends on the perception and integration of both signs and symptoms, so a good letter of recommendation includes the careful selection and integration of both objective data and subjective data on the applicant.

Further, in the process of medical diagnosis, there is the comparing of signs and symptoms to the "normal disease" posited. There may be aspects of the patient's condition that do not square with what has been documented regarding the disease. Here the physician must either discount the aspects as unrelated to the underlying pathology, or if part of the pathology, see them as a newly discovered part of the pathology or a reason to rethink the entire diagnosis. Similarly, in terms of a letter of recommendation, when some of the applicant's data does not square with what would be expected of a person in the desired position, then the recommender has the options of ignoring the data, or explaining it in such a way that the applicant can still be considered, or suggesting to the applicant that the position is not appropriate.

The danger of explaining a problem in an applicant's data in a letter of recommendation is that this calls attention to the problem. The "taint" of the problem may be what stays in the mind of the readers, not the explanation. In contrast, the excerpt below from a letter for a research assistant professor position is one of the more successful of "explanation of problem" letters.

> Because Bill has continuously worked on some very difficult problems regarding spinal cord injury, the number of his publications or amount of grant funding does not adequately reflect the amount of hard work he has put into his research.

This discussion of "problems" in an applicant's data should not be confused with the pathology of diagnosis. Rather, the analogy to the "pathology," or what is wrong, in terms of letters of recommendation, is actually the need to fill a particular position. Thus the more appropriate analogy to the physician trying to diagnose a disease would be to the representative of the medical school trying to fill a position with the best possible candidate. However with letters of recommendation, we do not have the words of the representative of the medical school, but rather the words of multiple recommenders of multiple applicants for the position. What the astute recommender tries to do in the letter is to prefigure and model the process of reasoning and consideration for the medical school decision makers.

Here, though, I would emphasize an important difference between diagnosis as it is generally understood and letters of recommendation. Diagnosis generally deals with situations that began at some time in the past, whose trajectory and cause or causes people seek to define, label, and understand. Similarly, after a candidate has been chosen for a position, one could analyze and even diagnose the process of selection, seeking to understand key factors in that decision process, and even label the overall procedure. Indeed, there is a cultural propensity to seek causes as a means of understanding in various realms. However, letters of recommendation are written before the fact, that is, before the actual selection. Thus such letters prefigure the selection process. It is through these letters that recommenders seek to influence the final labeling, to support future arguments by defining boundaries of the yet to be made decision. And as many of those who write letters are also involved in making decisions on new hires and promotions in their own institutions, they know this process. Their letters reflect this process, as a sort of yin to the yang of future selection.

Further, diagnosis can be understood as both process and product. As previously noted, the process of selecting, weighing, presenting, and supporting qualifications by a recommender can be seen as similar to the medical diagnostic process of weighing signs and symptoms. In terms of product, however, the diagnosis is the labeling that provides a coherent understanding. In letters of recommendation, the analogy is to the choice of appropriate applicant. Through the letter, the recommender can be seen as trying to prefigure, to model the choice to be taken by the medical school. Indeed, in particularly well written letters, the recommender works to convince the medical school that the applicant is so superior that its need should be framed according to the qualifications of the particular applicant.

As it is not common to think of the practice of diagnosis in the broader cultural and prefigurative sense, I will work to make this clearer with memorable examples from letters. But first I will present background on the data of the study, followed by a section on the structure of letters of recommendation and the assumptions underlying such letters for medical faculty. With the context thereby clarified, I will then bring out issues of presentation in letters of recommendation through carefully chosen excerpts from contrasting letters. I will conclude with the thought that one of the reasons medical schools continue to rely on letters of recommendation is that the particularism and epistemological individualism of clinical diagnosis, that is such a core value in medical training, is also particularly congenial with the ethos of letters of recommendation.

## 1. Data and previous studies

The data for this study is three years of letters of recommendation of all the successful applicants for faculty positions at a large medical school in the United States. This is 312 letters for applicants for 103 faculty positions (approximately three letters per applicant). It is naturalistic data in that the letters were for all faculty hires over the period from 1992–1995. For obvious legal reasons the letters are only those of the successful applicants. My assumption is that if I had had the letters for all the applicants, including the unsuccessful ones, the patterns of contrast that I found would have been even more pronounced.

The positions applied for were both clinical and research, largely at the assistant professor level, but also including adjunct positions, as well as eight associate professor level positions and one full professorship. A problem here, corroborated by the Personnel Office, was that recommenders did not always use the correct title of the position in the letter. Having multiple letters helped determine the correct position. The medical specialties included thirty-seven different ones, from surgery, oncology, and neurology to internal medicine, obstetrics-gynecology, and urology; from radiology, pathology, and psychiatry to pediatrics, family medicine, and anatomy. We[2] attempted to categorize these specialties but in the end gave up. Apart from gross differences of surgery, medicine, and basic science, physicians could not agree on the categories. Suffice it to say it was a broad spectrum of specialties.

The gender of the successful applicants was 29% female and 71% male. The medical school in question had slightly higher than national percentages of female faculty at the different ranks: 10% at the full professor level (national average 9%), 26% at the associate level (national average 21%), and 37% at the assistant professor level (national average 32%), with the national figures calculated from the national data for 1995 (Jolly and Hudley 1996: Table C5). So the assumption is that the gender variance in the relative percentages of successful applicants is not unusual for the times. The recommenders were 85% male, 12% female, and 3% unknown (probably foreign names that could not be easily categorized by the office charged with blacking out the names). This high proportion of male recommenders certainly reflects the convention of having department heads write letters of recommendation and the preponderance of males in such senior positions.

The institutions from which recommenders wrote letters were largely university teaching hospitals and major urban hospitals from all over the United States, Canada, and overseas. We attempted to categorize these institutions of origin for we felt that there could easily be cultural differences in how letters of recommendation are written. We grouped the places of origin into four categories: United States-local (215 letters), United States-not local (79 letters), Canada, England, Australia, South Africa, or Israel (abbreviated CEASI) (12 letters), and Europe but not Britain (5 letters). By "local" we refer to the geographic region surrounding the medical school in question, comprised of areas of three adjoining states. We assumed that physicians in this proximity in the same specialties would know each other and their letters might differ from those who didn't know each other. The CEASI group is a largely English and American oriented group. The problem with this sort of classification, however, is that physicians from different cultural backgrounds could be in any of these locations, and we did not know how long people had been in the locations.

Nevertheless, we did notice that letters from Europe tended to be shorter. Even letters from Canada were less hyperbolic than those from the United States. But we did not have enough letters to make more than general observations. Anecdotally we have been told that in Germany, for example, the stature of the recommender matters more than carefully constructed content. This may also have been true earlier in America when physicians knew all the main people in their fields and there were many fewer hospitals and medical schools. We were told by older physicians that in the 1940's, phone calls alone were often sufficient for providing recommendations. This suggests a more unitary and informal structure of decision making, one fraught with potential misuse by today's standards. We would imagine that these more informal recommendations were less diagnostic in evaluation and explanation, but we cannot know for sure.

In analyzing the data we used a qualitative research instrument (Nud*ist, "non-numerical unstructured data indexing, searching, and theorizing"). The advantages of this instrument were that the coding could be changed throughout the research process and that the texts were always available for easy viewing and annotating.[3] I also used software from the Summer Institute of Linguistics (Conc: a Concordance Generator) to do simple concordance studies. The most time-consuming part of the research was the initial scanning of over 300 letters with various ornate letterheads and long side column lists of associates, and the standardizing of format and basic gender information.

After we had conducted the initial analysis of the letters, we took sets of nine letters that we had rated high (three), average (three), and deficient (three) and showed them to physicians of different specialties. We asked the physicians to rank the letters and comment on them. Their rankings were in line with ours; a few also commented on subtexts that we had not noticed. For example, one physician noted after reading the closing paragraph of a letter we had all ranked high, that the recommender had also implied the candidate was good enough for the proposed institution but not for his own. Interviews with physicians reinforced our understanding of the strong hierarchical consciousness of the American medical profession.

Overall, it should be noted that it is not easy for researchers outside medical schools to obtain such extensive data. In this particular case, a highly placed female staff person in a medical school, who had served several terms on the Executive Committee for Hiring and Promotion, asked me as an anthropological linguist to examine letters of recommendation to see if there were systematic differences between letters written for female and male faculty applicants. She offered me fifty letters to examine with names blacked out. When I recognized how relatively fewer in number the female applicants were, I requested six times the number of letters for statistical reasons. I conducted the research looking for systematic differences across gender lines (Trix 1998). I also gave three workshops to medical faculty at the medical school to report my findings and to alert them to common ways that such letters of recommendation might be gendered and unintentionally affect an applicant's chances of being hired. But the data is culturally richer than just questions of gender difference. Indeed, I like to think of the letters as multiple views of how a profession sees its junior members, as a privileged post for observing how a profession interacts and replicates itself.

This study contrasts with other studies of letters of recommendation in the amount of data, in the naturalistic and longitudinal nature of the data, and in the more anthropological questions asked. Previous studies of letters of recommendation outside medicine have come largely from the disciplines of Education (Morrisett 1935; Raber 1985), Psychology (Cowan and Kasen 1984; Hatcher 1983), English (Doyle 1993; Eger 1991), Applied Linguistics (Bouton 1995), and Anthropology (Watson 1987). Of these, Eger's non-published dissertation (1991) is the most theoretically interesting, but his methodology of paying women who work in real estate and unemployed professional men to write letters of recommendation for fictional candidates with similar and contrasting personalities to the writer's own is the most problematic. Some of the other studies were written before there was widespread use of computers, thus making analysis of larger sets of data more difficult.

As for studies of letters of recommendation in medicine, as mentioned earlier, they have been largely concerned with choice and placement of applicants in residency programs (DeLisa, Jain, and Campagnolo 1994; Gayed 1991; O'Halloran et al. 1993). One of the finest of these studies is Greenburg, Doyle, and McClure's "Letters of recommendation for surgical residencies: What they say and what they mean" (1994). This is based on three years of data of letters of recommendation for successful applicants to a surgical residency program (approximately six accepted from a pool of over 300 applicants per year). These letters were combined with letters for applicants to the program for one year that were ranked at the bottom (nine applicants), ranked at midlevel (seven applicants), and ranked at the top as potentially acceptable (ten applicants), for a total of 42 applicants and 80 letters. The strength of the methodology of this study was that these letters were sent in packets of 10, half with full letter-head and names, and half with only text and no names, to surgeons in programs around the country to be ranked and a questionnaire filled out. One finding was that school of origin did not turn out to be statistically significant, although surgeons had thought it would be (Greenburg, Doyle, and McClure 1994: 194). Thus researchers were able to compare what surgeons said they valued with what they actually valued in ranking the letters. Another finding was that junior level surgeons and senior level ones disagreed on the importance of personalization of the letters (Greenburg et al.: 197). Most interesting, while the rankings largely coincided, the researchers acknowledged that there may be "code phrases" or understandings that as of yet have not been specified and yet affected the rankings, especially those between the mediocre and acceptable groups (op. cit.).

None of these earlier studies of medical letters of recommendation considered other cultural forms that could be related to the letters, let alone questions of the cultural practice of diagnosis. What does relate to diagnosis in these studies, however, is the importance accorded what was not said, referred to more generally as "knowledge gaps" (LaCroix 1985: 25). I will refer to this later in the contrastive analysis of the good and the weak letters, including those with less than effective explanations of problems. But first I will describe the structure of letters of recommendation within which recommenders work to define boundaries they hope will influence decision makers in their diagnoses of the most appropriate candidate.

## 2. Structure of letters and underlying assumptions of medical faculty

In the context of institutions of higher learning, medical schools and the medical profession appear to require letters of recommendation to a greater extent than other graduate programs at universities or law schools. This reflects the length and multiple stage process of current medical education. It is estimated that a physician requires four to five sets of letters of recommendation in his or her career (medical school, residency, fellowship, diplomate check, hospital staff privileges), while an academic physician requires an additional three to five more sets of letters (specialty or graduate school, medical school junior faculty, associate professorship, full professorship, administrative position). Indeed one academic physician interviewed for this study reported that he wrote an average of two letters of recommendation a week for medical students and junior faculty. As might be expected with this level of letter writing, letters of recommendation of medical school faculty on the whole tend to be less elaborated than many current letters for university faculty positions in the Liberal Arts.[4] The structure of the letters is, however, very similar.

A study of the structure and content of letters of recommendation, based on 130 letters for a graduate program in Liberal Arts, identified the simple tripartite structure of such letters as introduction, body, and closing (Bouton 1995: 214). In this study, Bouton also identified four basic concepts in the content of such letters, namely: the relationship of referee and candidate that provides credibility for what is written, academic traits and achievements, personality traits, and the recommendation (Bouton 1995: 221). He then proceeded to specify what was found in the three parts of the letter and to distinguish between direct and indirect comments as potential sources of ambiguity.[5]

My preference is to take a more functional and interactive approach to structure. Thus I define the main elements in the structure of letters of recommendation for medical faculty as: establishment of the authority of the recommender, acknowledgement of the addressee, description of the abilities and performance of the applicant, and recommendation for a course of action. Inclusion of the acknowledgement of the addressee comes from understanding that the letters represent discourse between professional colleagues, often equals. This is indicated in the tone of the letters, in the fairly common practice in the salutation of typing the title and name of addressee, but then drawing a line through the formal name and writing above it a first name or a nick name, and in particular, comments often in the last paragraph. The stronger the letter, often the stronger the interactive nature of the prose, as if to say, "This is an applicant for your institution, if you should be so fortunate to hire him or her."

The establishment of the authority of the recommender includes the explicit mention of the capacity and the length of time that the recommender has known the applicant, usually in the first paragraph. But the establishment of authority is not limited to this. Rather, establishment of the authority of the recommender resides as well in the elaborate letterhead, in the long list of associates that often cascade down one side of the page, and in the formal titles and many initials presenting medical achievement that follow the recommender's typed name after the signature. I am especially aware of the issue of these initials, for example, Dr. Alfred Hood, M.D., F.A.C.O.G., F.R.C.O.G., followed modestly by three full titles. In the first presentation of the results of my study to medical faculty of the university medical center that had asked me to do the research, I playfully disguised the identity of a recommender as Dr. Alfred Hood, M.D. H.O. T.S. T.U. F.F. The doctors were not amused and I removed these initials for future presentations. The hierarchical nature of medical institutions and especially of academic ones, like that of the military, is not something to play with, at least not by outsiders in the context of public presentations. The authority of the recommender is also evidenced in the use of the scientific description of the applicant's research, in reference to important national organizations, and the way the recommendations are made in the final paragraphs, never as requests, but in a range from formal to colloquial banter.

Authority is also an important part of diagnosis in the medical context where the distinctive clothing, title, neckwear, and prerogatives of the physician all continually work to assert this authority. The assumption is that these symbolize the distinctive status, knowledge, and experience base of the physician that give him or her the right to make medical diagnoses.

The third element in the structure of letters of recommendation is the description of the abilities, achievements, and qualities of applicants. As Bouton (1995) also found, this is the part of the letters that showed the most variation. Indeed, I would like to classify some letters whose discourse on abilities, achievement, and qualities is so brief as "letters of minimal assurance," rather than as letters of recommendation. It is true that the letters for adjunct faculty tend to be shorter, but there are even letters for associate professor positions that are of this ilk as well. For example:

> Dear Dr. Koop:
>
> Dr. Harvey is a superb clinician and there is no reason that he should not be appointed to the Centvingtcinq faculty for clinical and hospital staff. He has been a superior member of Northsouth University Junior Faculty during his fellowship.
>
> With best regards,

To preserve anonymity, I have standardized the names of all the addressees to "Dr. Koop" for our former Surgeon General. I refer to the institution where the applicants are seeking appointment as "Centvingtcinq" since there were one hundred and twenty-five schools of medicine at the time the letters were written in the mid-1990s. Other universities are all referred to as "Northsouth University" while institutes all referred to as the "Carnafellar Institute." Similarly all male applicants are referred to "William Harvey," who first described circulation of the blood in the 16th century, while all female applicants are referred to "Sarah Gray," a relative of mine who, in the 19th century, was the first woman to study surgery at the University of Edinburgh. Another example of a letter of minimal assurance is the following:

> Dear Dr. Koop:
>
> Re: Sarah Gray, M.D.
>
> It is a pleasure to write a letter of recommendation for Sarah Gray, M.D. I have known Dr. Gray since the time of her residency here at Northsouth University. She is an outstanding neurologist and an extremely hardworking and conscientious physician. I recommend her without reservation.
>
> Yours truly,

However, most of letters of recommendation are significantly longer and more detailed. The average length of letters for full-time faculty is 319 words, whereas the two above letters of minimal assurance are 47 and 55 words respectively.

There are various organizational ways of presenting abilities, achievements, and qualities of applicants that can be categorized broadly as chronological or thematic. Since the training of a physician is long and multi-stage (medical school and/or graduate studies, residency, fellowship, clinical or research work), some accounts of these abilities, achievements, and qualities follow this training trajectory. An especially common structure is for recommenders to make clear at what stage in the applicant's training they came to know the person, and then to summarize earlier stages and comment on later ones from their vantage of continued contact at conventions or through publications or personal contact. The other main way of organizing information on the applicant is thematically, which generally includes paragraphs on teaching, research, service, and/or administration. Or a simpler thematic organization is to have separate paragraphs on professional achievements and personal qualities.

A main division in medical school positions is between those that are primarily for clinical work and those that are principally for research. In reading the letters of recommendation it became clear that recommenders were able to write more persuasively about research than about clinical work. It appears easier to quantify the results of research in numbers of publications, presentations, or research grants and then to elaborate on these. As for clinical work, rarely, except for transplants, is there enumeration of operations. Instead, the usual references to clinical work are general and not memorable. Perhaps with changing conditions in medical education and the greater need of medical schools for clinical revenues, this too will become more quantified and better elaborated.

Within the descriptions of abilities and achievements, there are also references that are unique to letters of recommendation for medical positions. These generally occur at the end of the description of abilities and achievements. For example, in one letter the following was written, immediately following a statement of how helpful the applicant had been with children with spina bifida:

> ... To my knowledge she has never had problems with alcohol, drugs, medical malpractice, and she has never had her hospital privilege suspended.

Or the closing of a letter of recommendation for an anesthesiologist read:

> I would not hesitate to recommend him for a position in your group. As far as I know he has no health problems or history of drug or alcohol abuse. Please contact me if you have any questions.

These reflect the potential legal actions that a hospital might take were a recommender not to be forthcoming about certain problems an applicant might have. Such references are most common in letters for anesthesiologists and obstetricians, I was told, since these are the areas that have the most malpractice cases. These references are regarded as procedural and not suggestive. Even the last sentence about possible contact is common to the level of being procedural, although combined with other clues it could become a red flag.

The final element of the structure of letters of recommendation for medical school faculty is the recommendation itself. This is most often found in the last paragraph or last sentences of the letter, although more general recommendations are sometimes found in introductory portions as well. The following examples of closings show the general form:

> She is a competent physician who will make an excellent addition to the medical staff. *I support her nomination fully.*

> In summary, *I strongly recommend Dr. Harvey for the available position.* He has the background, energy, skills and imagination to become an independent, contributing investigator who, in time, will add to the stature of your group.

> I believe sincerely that Dr. Gray will be an excellent addition to your Department and Division and recommend her highly without the slightest reservation.

As Bouton noted (1995: 240), the form of the actual recommendation involves a movement from description of the applicant, to the first person of the recommender with common performative verbal phrases such as "I support," "I recommend," and "I believe that ..." The recommendation is also often in the immediate context of a summary of the person's qualities. In a sense the whole preceding letter, imbued with the authority and persuasiveness of the recommender, leads to the recommendation which is to prefigure the choice of the decision makers at the medical school that is seeking to hire or promote. A strong favorable diagnosis so modeled is "this applicant is the most appropriate," while the suggested action, for one of the qualities of diagnoses is that they imply consequences, is "hire this applicant."

## 3. Issues of diagnosis in contrasting letters

What constitutes a good diagnosis? Building on Atkinson's insightful discussion of "reproducing disease" in his ethnography of the clinical experience (1997: 164–188) I consider a good diagnosis as the integration of appropriate signs and symptoms in a coherent analysis, preferably one that coincides with a documented pathology for which there is treatment. As noted previously, in the case of letters of recommendation the pathology is the need to fill the vacancy with the most appropriate applicant. The qualifications for filling a medical faculty vacancy are not mysterious. Indeed, they are largely agreed upon and include: documented training, skills, and experience in the specific field, combined with productivity and efficiency. If the position is for research, the applicant should show evidence of independent research; if for clinical work, the applicant should show competence and a non-problematic record. Overall, applicants are also expected to be team players or at the very least not antagonize elder players.

But recall that letters of recommendation are second-tier affairs in terms of determining the final outcome. That is, they can influence, and hopefully model this final choice, but they do not officially determine it. Thus they must be persuasive in spelling out why their applicant is the most appropriate – in the aptness of the signs and symptoms and the coherence of their message. The challenge is to present their applicant in the best possible light for the position, although some recommenders may have the lower expectation of an honest account, it should be recognized that such an account is never neutral. After discussing letters of recommendation with physicians, it is clear to me that some are not aware of the implications of their language. Further, a problem with all letters of recommendation is that whatever the strengths and weaknesses of the recommender in selecting data and in writing, these tend to be read as attributes of the applicant.

In this section I will outline good and weak presentations – to shape future diagnosis – as they appear in letters of recommendation. By my above definition, a good presentation is an integration of appropriate objective and subjective qualifications, organized into a coherent analysis that projects the applicant as most appropriate for the position. I will give examples of paragraphs from letters that exemplify this. (To maintain anonymity, I cannot reproduce entire letters.) It is, however, easier to talk about negative features. This is not just perversity. Research on medical letters of recommendation supports that there is more knowledge and unanimity of what constitutes a bad letter than what distinguishes a mediocre one from an excellent one (Greenburg, Doyle, and McClure 1994: 195–196).

Another feature that researchers on letters of recommendation agree upon is the importance of the "unspoken," what is not stated, that is, what is not addressed in a letter. LaCroix refers to these as "knowledge gaps" (1985: 25), again supporting the notion that appropriate criteria are known and shared. Medical researchers comment on this repeatedly – "letters suggest more by what they don't say than by what they do" (ibid.: 197). What this leads to is a strong propensity to "read between the lines." This can often lead to over-interpretation of what may have been merely lack of fortuitous phrasing by the recommender, Therefore, I will organize the discussion of issues of good and weak presentations according to what is said – the positive and the negative, and subsequently, according to what is left unsaid – the obvious and the medical field specific.

Beginning with what is said and with examples of good presentations, the following paragraphs demonstrate integration of appropriate objective and subjective qualifications for each applicant. In the first paragraph, the signs or objective qualifications are more explicit, with numbers of manuscripts and the actual title of the position presented as if the applicant already had the job. This paragraph is the fourth in a seven paragraph letter:

> Dr. Harvey's research endeavors at Northsouth University have been particularly fruitful. He is the first author on five full manuscripts and eight abstracts. Dr. Harvey's research has provided important insights into the pathophysiology of ischemic stroke and the clinical sequelae of upper extremity paralysis, facial paresis and speech dysfunction. He is an eager, young investigator who is not afraid of tackling tough clinical questions. In his position as the director of cranial computerized axial tomography at University Hospital, he should have the opportunity to significantly advance our understanding of cerebrovascular disease using this quantitative imaging modality. Thus I expect that Dr. Harvey will continue to make impressive contributions to the cranial ct scan literature, and that his reputation within the stroke community will continue to grow as we all benefit from his research endeavors.

The following paragraph may appear stronger on the symptom or subjective side. However, the way the recommender compares or ranks the applicant's productivity with other researchers in his lab, leads this to be seen as a sign as well. This is the fourth paragraph in a five paragraph letter:

> Overall, I would say that Sarah is one of the most productive molecular geneticists and chemists among scientists that I would identify as being in a comparable stage of their careers. Her capacity for organizing experimental work and carrying it out efficiently approaches the phenomenal. In fact I can think of no one who has worked in my laboratory over the years who has been more efficient and effective in producing a large body of critical and definitive information. Her level of productivity is a legend in my research group and in the field of mutational genetic research. In addition, she is extremely easy to work with and has highly productive interactions with large numbers of people in the department.

Note also the repetition of the word "productive" in the above paragraph. It is a key term that is highly appreciated in the medical research community.

Turning to the problematic in what is said, the first example is one where the recommender undercuts her own authority. In this case the recommender is writing from Canada and doesn't know the addressee, but still her words about herself weaken subsequent claims she may make regarding the applicant. In this second paragraph in an eight paragraph letter, the recommender states the obvious and elaborates the extraneous:

> First, just a few notes about my background as someone able to assess another's faculty potential. As the above letterhead indicates, I have both university and hospital service and teaching responsibilities. Starting as an undergraduate, I have been teaching in one capacity or another for 34 years and am tenured faculty. Also I have been on the faculty of our Effective Teaching Techniques program for 10 years. I would be pleased to provide a detailed curriculum vitae if you wish.

The following is another example of a letter that is problematic due to what is said, and one that also calls into question the judgement of the recommender as well as the qualifications of the applicant. The three paragraph letter builds through a series of backhanded comments and negative references (in italics) to a conclusion that the recommender is giving a "solid recommendation." If it was intended as a positive presentation, it is not coherent. My experience with physicians has shown me that some see this as clever and careful and are not aware of the negative implications that hit others in the face:

> *1st paragraph*: William Harvey has asked me to write in support of his application for an Assistant Professorship in your unit, and I am pleased to do so.
>
> 2nd paragraph: William has communicated to me his interest in applying for the R01-type research support, *for which he believes he is competitive* ... as I read it (in an ad for the position) *his area of expertise is not excluded.*

> 3rd paragraph: ... He was a very good *student although not the best I saw in my 33 years there*. ... Although his interest in computers will serve him well for years to come, it obviously took some time away from his basic laboratory pursuits. While I believe *he could have finished his doctoral work sooner than he did*, the time he spent on the doctorate was about par for Professor Livingood's laboratory. ... On the basis of all I know about him, I can give him a very solid recommendation for the position he seeks.

The following and last grouping of negative implications from what is said relate to problems in the applicant's data for which the recommender gives explanation. Unfortunately this explaining (shown in italics) may lead instead to the foregrounding of the problem and the possible inference that the problem is not over. The following two examples come from the same nine paragraph letter, from the seventh and ninth paragraph, respectively:

> *Sarah's personal life was in turmoil* during the time I worked with her, and in view of the difficulties she was experiencing in that arena, her performance was especially impressive ...

> ... While she has not been able to accomplish a lot in academic pathology during the past few years *due to career changes and other personal issues*, she has continued to grow and mature, and I am sure she would be an even stronger and more effective member of your department than she was in New Orleans.

An even shorter letter, of barely two paragraphs, also had two problem explanations (in italics) that took center stage in the first paragraph. In this letter the recommender was recommending two people, a couple, both for research jobs at Centvingtcinq University in the same short letter. I feel the second explanation is superior to the first, but the combination in such a short letter is problematic:

> ... More recently they initiated an independent line of research aimed at testing the hypothesis that a DNA transcriptional error might be responsible for common forms of myotonic dystrophy. After significant effort, this postulate was unfortunately proven to be wrong. *The unsuccessful outcome of the project does not however detract from the strength of these skillful investigators.*

> ... A point of concern may be the relatively poor record of independent research, particularly at such a relatively late stage in their careers. *I believe that this reflects a particular kind of academic environment that is mostly preoccupied with the productivity of the group as a whole, rather than the independence of its individual members.*

Another letter for the husband of this couple dealt with the problem of his limited record of independent research differently. I am not sure it is an improvement. This is found in the seventh paragraph of an eight paragraph letter:

> The one deficiency that is apparent about William's career as a scientist is that he has not yet generated his own independent research support. *This is in part due to the fact that he spent considerable time and effort helping his wife Sarah Gray develop her own NIH sponsored studies on myotonic dystrophy..*

As for the unsaid, the most obvious examples are what I referred to earlier as "letters of minimal assurance." A problem with short letters is that their brevity can have various interpretations, none of which are particularly good. A brief letter can reflect the recommender's lack of knowledge of the applicant. It can reflect laziness on the part of the recommender. Worse, it can suggest that the applicant has no positive achievements to document. Or it can be a way of dodging substantive problems that the applicant does have. Indeed length of letters is one of the most common features analyzed in letters of recommendation. And a common finding is that the better letters are longer. Greenburg, Doyle, and McClure found that the letters ranked the highest by all groups of surgeons were twice as long as those ranked at the bottom, and the high ranked letters contained much more substantive information (1994: 197). Letters like the following one paragraph letter are lacking in such substantive information. In fact it is only through reading other letters that I found out that the applicant had been the Director of Pediatric Cardiology for several years. The recommender had not bothered to include her title in the letter, among other things:

> Dear Dr. Koop:
>
> Re: Sarah Gray M.D.
>
> I am writing in support of Sarah Gray, M.D.'s application for the position of Associate Professor of Cardiology in your department. I have worked closely with Dr. Gray both as her chairman and fellow faculty member doing pediatric cardiology for the past three years. She is a superb clinician and academician. I truly enjoyed working with her. Your gain is my loss. I believe that you will find that she will (sic) a genuine adjunct to your faculty. If you require more specific information, please do not hesitate to notify me.
>
> Sincerely,

Another way unsaids appear or are inferred are when recommenders include what looks like faint praise or irrelevancies. The reason I include these written examples in the section on unsaids is that they are usually interpreted to suggest that the recommender had nothing better to say about the applicant and so was forced to fall back on these. That is, they indicate a lack of positive qualifications. The examples below come from the third paragraph of a four paragraph letter for an applicant for an associate professor position:

> ... If he is going to be late to a research meeting or planning session he will be considerate enough to inform members ahead of time.
>
> ... William has always been friendly, cooperative and void of mood swings or temper tantrums.

The final one sentence paragraph sums up the lack of enthusiasm of the recommender for the above applicant:

> I highly recommend William Harvey to any position for which his training qualifies him.

An example of an unsaid is implied by the following paragraph that constitutes the third paragraph of a four paragraph recommendation. Most academics would see this as a most positive recommendation. However, in the medical field it is clear that there is something missing from this paragraph and from the recommendation overall:

> Dr. Gray is also developing into a fine basic scientist. She has had many years of experience in collaborative research and is well known and held in high regard by many physicians and scientists locally, nationally and internationally. In fact, if it were not for the demands of the clinical laboratory and her doctoral studies, she could have been actively involved in research with laboratories in South Africa, Texas and St. Louis. It is my hope, with adequate support from the department until external funding is available, Dr. Gray will be able to bring many of the opportunities presented to fruition.

What is missing, and this is deemed most important for medical faculty, is evidence of independent research and of having secured support for this.

Finally, and this relates to both what is said and what is left unsaid, I would like to demonstrate variation in the way a potentially but not necessarily negative piece of information is portrayed across three letters of recommendation for the same applicant. I will begin with the most negative portrayal in that the information is not explained. It doesn't help that it is noted at the end of the first paragraph of a four paragraph letter in which there are also irrelevancies, one of which I include as well:

> ... Sarah is quite close to my wife, and they frequently seek each other's company out. ... I get the sense that she is looking to develop a clinical program now that she has chosen to leave the laboratory and concentrate exclusively on clinical medicine.

In a second letter for the same applicant, the same piece of information is portrayed differently. This occurs in the second paragraph of a four paragraph letter:

> Although she has recently focused her research interests on clinical projects, she also has a background of successful microbiology research.

While in the third letter for the same applicant, this information is portrayed in the following manner in the second and third paragraphs of a three paragraph letter:

> Sarah is establishing herself in the cystic fibrosis arena nationally. She received a three-year Physician/Scientist Award from the National Diabetes Foundation in 1990, and for the past several years she has been asked by the Juvenile Diabetes Foundation to moderate sessions at the annual meetings. Her pancreatic transplant research has resulted in publications and abstracts. In December, 1993, I asked Sarah to assume my role and responsibilities as the Director of the Cystic Fibrosis Care, Teaching and Resource Center at Northsouth University.
>
> For the past year Dr. Gray has devoted her major effort to clinical care of children with cystic fibrosis and other lung diseases, and in running our diabetes program ...

It is fascinating to see how a piece of information can be given such different spins. Thus, not only do multiple letters provide information on an applicant, like titles, that might be ignored were there only a single letter, multiple letters also provide different perspectives from which a fuller understanding of the applicant can be known. With the vagaries of recommenders' writing abilities and the variation in their willingness to spend the requisite time to construct a truly persuasive letter of recommendation, the importance of multiple letters cannot be overstated. In the Greenburg, Doyle, and McClure study of letters for surgical residents, they found that "two of the letters rated the lowest within their group were on behalf of the same students whose other letters were rated at the top of their group" (1994: 197). They therefore concluded that reliable pictures of applicants can only come from multiple letters. In this they present the view of the decision makers. To continue our analogy, similarly, multiple data and perspectives, combined with requisite knowledge, lead to more reliable diagnoses.

## 4. Societal implications

In a society like modern America where diagnosis is an authoritative and pervasive cultural practice, it should come as no surprise that people prepare for diagnoses in advance. The most obvious such preparation is where a patient prepares for consultation with an expensive specialist, making sure to recount systematically symptoms he or she has noticed. At a simpler level in terms of outcome, a skater prepares him or herself for competition by carefully noting scoring practices and preferences of particular judges and competitions and then incorporating moves for these effects in the skating program. At one remove, the skating coach also seeks to second guess the preferences of particular judges and competitions and have the skater incorporate moves for these effects. Also at this level an attorney prepares a defendant to testify in court before a particular judge and jury. Stepping back from direct participation by the defendant, an attorney also prepares a witness to testify on behalf of the defendant in court before a particular judge and jury. Or the attorney works to assemble a jury most positive to his or her case during the initial stages of a jury trial by dismissing on various bases other potential jurors.

Thus there is a range of directness of participation from the patient whose very body is responding to some infection or trauma, to the attorney who tries to manage jury selection and presentation of evidence on behalf of a defendant at a much more distanced participation. The letters of recommendation fall within this range although closer to the attorney's side. There is also a range in complexity of final labeling with the medical diagnosis having a potential of many category labels, the defendant more restricted in possible legal categories in which the case falls, while the labeling of the skater is along a grid of top scorer down. Here the final labeling of candidates for a medical faculty position parallels that of the skater's ranking. As for final outcomes there is a simplicity in all of them, from terminal or not terminal for diseases and medical conditions; to winner, almost winner, or loser among the skaters; to guilty or innocent as charged in the legal arena. As for the letter of recommendation writers, either their candidate is selected or not.

All the above examples involve determination of what is deemed relevant on the part of the authority, be it medical, sport, legal, or personnel, and then a careful weighing of subjective and objective data before the final labeling. Still some would divide these examples with the medical diagnoses and legal case on one side as situations where cause or truth is sought, and the skater and letter writer on the other where the best among candidates is sought. But there is nonetheless similarity of process in the choosing of relevant evidence and the weighing of subjective and objective particulars. It is awareness and influencing of this process that I have sought to present in this chapter.

Returning to the letters themselves, in research on letters of recommendation for medical positions, there have been multiple calls for different ways of collecting data from recommenders (Doutre et al. 1993; O'Halloran et al. 1993). Most of these involve some sort of improved check list of qualities in place of letters, in attempt to structure the recommendations and make them more comparable. But none of these new forms have been put into practice systematically. And while I expect these discussions to continue, I think the reason that medical schools will continue to use letters of recommendation, largely structured by the recommender, is that there is a cultural affinity of these letters with the particularism and epistemological individualism that so characterize medical learning and the medical profession. This affinity between letters of recommendation and clinical medical learning asserts the overriding value of individual professional experience as the source of knowledge for evaluating applicants and for evaluating signs and symptoms of disease.

## *Acknowledgment*

I gratefully acknowledge the assistance of Dr. Suzanne S. Toce, Medical Director of the Neonatal Intensive Care Unit, Gundersen Lutheran Medical Center, Lacrosse, Wisconsin, in preparing the manuscript.

## *Notes*

1. The Baker's Street Irregulars are international organizations of people who enjoy gathering to share their knowledge and pleasure in Holmes' exploits and ways of solving puzzles or mysteries. In my community the group is reportedly largely made up of physicians.
2. Graduate student in Anthropology, Carolyn Psenka, worked with me at different stages in this project, in early literature review, in interviewing physicians, and at the first national presentation of the data to the American Anthropological Association in Washington DC in 1997.
3. Gabrielle Singleton, computer consultant extraordinaire, has worked with me on this project since its inception. Her software knowledge saved many hours and her fine design sense permeates the tables and graphs with which I summarized my data for various local, national, and international presentations as well as for this chapter.
4. Currently I am in the process of conducting a joint study on letters of recommendation with fellow linguist Helen Aristar-Dry, based on a contrastive data pool of the letters of this study for medical school faculty, and letters for positions in an English Department at a large state university. It is on the basis of this data pool as well as experience with hiring in my own Anthropology Department that I judge the medical letters to be somewhat less elaborated. When the research is complete, the analysis will of course be more precise.
5. Bouton describes the purpose of his study as the identification and delineation of cross-cultural differences in the construction of text as exemplified in the letter of recommendation. Unfortunately, the weakest part of his research is the cultural part. For example, he lists half the letters as coming from Asia, as if Asia were one cultural variable, and no consideration is taken for what might prove to be models of such

letters in different countries in Asia – probably British in some instances. In contrast, the strongest part of his article was the structural analysis which I refer to repeatedly. Still the importance of studies of cross-cultural communication is incontestable. In one medical school study, 73% of directors of American residency programs reported that they considered letters of recommendation from a foreign country to be useless (Gayed 1991: 700). However, what constitutes "foreign" wasn't made clear. I would assume it is a euphemism for "third world" and does not include letters from what we termed "CEASI" (Canada, England, Australia, South Africa, Israel).

## *References*


Atkinson, Paul A.
1997 *The Clinical Experience: The Construction and Reconstruction of Medical Reality*. Aldershot UK/Brookfield, USA: Ashgate.

Bouton, Lawrence F.
1995 A cross-cultural analysis of the structure and content of letters of reference. *Studies in Second Language Acquisition* 17, 122–144.

Cowan, Gloria and Jill H. Kasen
1984 Form of reference: Sex differences in letters of recommendation. *Journal of Personality and Social Psychology* 46(3), 636–645.

DeLisa, J. A., S. S. Jain, and D. I. Campagnolo
1994 Factors used by physical medicine and rehabilitation residency training directors to select their residents. *American Journal of Physical Medicine and Rehabilitation* 73(3), 152–156.

Doutre, W. H., A. S. Buesing, N. B. Ingrim, B. G. Guernsey, J. A. Hokanson, and E. Galvan
1993 Behaviorally anchored ranking scale versus letters of recommendation for evaluating residency candidates. *American Journal of Hospital Pharmacy* 41(11), 2367–2370.

Doyle, Anne E.
1993 Genre conventions as rhetorical decisions in book reviews and letters of recommendation. Unpublished dissertation, University of Illinois, Chicago.

Eger, Henrik
1991 Writer perception, writer projection: The influence of personality, ideology, and gender on letters of recommendation. Unpublished dissertation, University of Illinois, Chicago.

Friedman, Richard B.
1983 Fantasy land (on problems of letters of recommendation). *New England Journal of Medicine* 308, 651–653.

Gayed, N. M.
1991 Residency directors assessments of which selection criteria best predict the performances of foreign-born medical graduates during internal medicine residencies. *Academic Medicine* 66(11), 699–701.

Greenburg, A. Gerson, Jennifer Doyle, and D. K. McClure
1994 Letters of recommendation for surgical residencies: What they say and what they mean. *Journal of Surgical Research* 56(2), 192–198.
Hatcher, Larry L.
1983 Letters of recommendation: Validity and contribution to variance in judgments about applicants. Unpublished dissertation, Bowling Green State University, Ohio.
Jolly, Paul and Dorothea Hudley (eds.)
1996 *Association of American Medical Colleges Data Book: Statistical Information Related to Medical Education.* Washington DC: AAMC (Association of American Medical Colleges).
LaCroix, Patricia P.
1985 Sex in recs. *The Journal of College Admission* Fall, 24–26.
Morrisett, Lloyd, N.
1935 *Letters of Recommendation: A Study of Letters of Recommendation as an Instrument in the Selection of Secondary School Teachers.* New York: Teachers College, Columbia University.
O'Halloran, B. A., Elizabeth Altmaier, Wilbur Smith, and Edmund Franken
1993 Evaluation of resident applicants by letters of recommendation: A comparison of traditional and behavior-based-formats. *Investigative Radiology* 28, 274–277.
Raber, Gloria and Ann Beers
1985 Source of letters of recommendation and subsequent teaching performance of first-year teachers. Unpublished dissertation, University of Georgia.
Ross, C. A. and P. Leichner
1984 Criteria for selecting residents: A reassessment. *Journal of Psychiatry* 29(8), 681–686.
Trix, Frances
1998 Beyond he and she M.D.: Pronouns, gender, and maintenance of hierarchy in letters of recommendation for medical school faculty. Paper presented to the International Pragmatics Association, Reims, France.
Watson, Carol
1987 Sex-linked differences in letters of recommendation. *Women and Language* X, 2, Spring, 26–28.

## *Software*

Conc: a Concordance Generator, version 1.70 beta (developed by John Thomson)
1992 Dallas, Texas: Summer Institute of Linguistics.
QSR (qualitative data analysis) Nud*ist (non-numerical unstructured data for indexing, searching and theorizing) 4
1997 Sage: Thousand Oaks, CA.

# Chapter 13
# Speaking about menopause: Possibilities for a cultural discourse analysis

*Cindy Suopis and Donal Carbaugh*

*Cindy Suopis and Donal Carbaugh follow the lead of Francis Trix in examining non-medical discourse talk about diagnosis. In this case the discourse relates to lay talk about menopause. These authors first describe some features of diagnostic discourse found in their data and then they consider the cultural premises and values associated with the use of those features. They find that women treat menopause both as a developmental stage in life (they are "in menopause") and as an illness that has symptoms that require treating. They conclude with a cogent discussion of the problems associated with medicalizing life stages where people treat naturally occurring events as unnatural problems in need of remedies.*

This chapter responds to three basic questions: Through what communicative forms do women diagnose themselves as menopausal? Within these, how do they assess treatments for menopause? And what cultural premises are presumed and created in this talk about menopause? In our response to these questions, we are exploring one principal communicative phenomenon, women's ways of speaking about menopause, which itself is composed of a communication event including two prominent acts of "lay diagnosis" and treatment talk. It is important that we emphasize at the outset that the questions we are raising here are not questions we posed for interviews and thus were not asked by us of women. The discursive phenomena we report about here were produced as a routine yet contingent part of these women's lives, a local achievement of a way of speaking about menopause. Through our study, then, we seek to highlight the communicative forms and acts of this talk and some of its cultural features.

In his influential studies of medical interviews, Elliott Mishler (1984: 104) has distinguished a "voice of the lifeworld" from a "voice of medicine." In his words:

> the voice of the lifeworld refers to the patient's contextually grounded experiences of events and problems in her life. These are reports and descriptions of the world of everyday life expressed from the perspective of a natural "attitude." The timing of events and their significance are dependent on the patient's biographical situation and position in the social world. In contrast, the voice of medicine reflects a "technical" interest and expresses a "scientific attitude." The meaning

> of events is provided through abstract rules that serve to decontextualize events, to remove them from particular personal and social contexts.

We find Mishler's distinction helpful for it helps us draw attention to our main focus, the "voice of the lifeworld," at least as an initial way of orienting to the discourse produced by women who are discussing menopause. What we seek to understand is just how women speak about this stage of life in their own, non-medical, scenes. Yet also, what we find in this talk is a kind of medical voice, a way of speaking about physical conditions, symptoms, and treatments. While this talk is not being produced, for the most part, by medical specialists, it does import into its terms and propositions a medical vocabulary and thus at times weaves into the voice a lifeworld, "medical concerns." It is this voice, crafted outside medical contexts yet manufactured in part as a result of them, that we find our main focal concern.

Our study follows in the wake of a recent scholarly discussion concerning "lay diagnosis" (e.g., Beach 2001; Drew 2001; Sarangi 2001; ten Have 2001). Parts of this discussion have emphasized the importance of investigating lay medical theories and lay belief systems about physicality and its treatment (see Sarangi 2001: 5), self-assessments and self-diagnosis (Frankel 2001), the "phase structure of medical consultations" (see Robinson 2001, as well as ten Have 2001: 254), including the larger sequential, event structures relating prior diagnostic talk at home to that of medical consultations (e.g., Beach 1996, 2001). Our hope is to contribute to studies such as these as we focus upon a kind of "lay diagnosis of menopause," beliefs about it and its treatment, and a larger sequence of communication in which these communicative acts find their place.

The perspective we adopt in what follows is a cultural and pragmatic approach to conversation and discourse (Carbaugh 1996; Carbaugh, Gibson, and Milburn 1997; Philipsen 1997; Suopis 2002). In particular, we seek to understand, for example, the ways cultural sequences provide a symbolic context for specific communicative acts, like self-assessment, or self-diagnosis. We seek further, in our analyses, to understand how communicative acts such as these create and presume cultural premises about menopause and the identity of a woman at this life stage, that is, "being a woman" at menopause, thus hearing in these very communicative acts, culture at work.

The primary data for this study were collected as part of a larger project on how women talk about and generate support during menopause (Suopis 2002). Two field sites, public informational meetings about menopause, and an online chat group, supplied the primary data for this study. We discovered, by perusing these data through the above perspective, a kind of self-assessment talk. Our analyses endeavor to show the larger sequential context of that talk, ingredients in self-diagnostic talk including assessments of possible treatments for menopause, and some of its prominent cultural premises about being a female at this life stage.

## 1. Diagnosing menopause as a stage of life: Like puberty yet unlike illness and pregnancy

One kind of diagnostic discourse can be understood through the following form:[1]

- X (a disease, illness or condition) is something P (a person or organism) gets at point Z.
- X is caused by agent C.
- X is known because of symptoms (1,2,3,n).
- P exhibits symptoms (1,2,3,n).
- Therefore, P HAS X.
- Given that P has X, treatment T is given.

Through this form, a disease or illness carries with it specific and particular beliefs about existence, about the body, the natural world, and ways organisms are linked to minds and spirits. Presumptions about how the body normally works and relates to its physical and non-material surroundings are active in such a form. Further, these conceptions of the disease are also linked to values, to what is deemed good and pleasing, or bad, abnormal, and not pleasing. In particular, conceptions of diseases presume not only what exists, but what is deemed normal and good, including ways of treating that disease in order to return the body to its normal and good condition. In this sense, a conception of a disease rests upon particular beliefs and values, these being expressions of a presumably shared understanding.

The "voice of medicine" Mishler describes rests upon a common sense premise, generally, that diseases are localized in persons such that: P HAS X, and that you know X because of symptoms (1,2,3,n). As a result, if person P exhibits symptoms (1,2,3,n), P is said to HAVE disease X. Typically, we believe we know what can cause X, an agent, or agents, of C. We present this raw bone logic here as a way of introducing a common form of logic which is presumed for a lay diagnosis, and to make the point that lay diagnosis rests upon some shared premises of belief and value which are active through this form, or one like it.

One case study which superbly demonstrates cultural differences in diagnostic discourse is Anne Fadiman's (1997) popular book, *The Spirit Catches You and Then You Fall Down*. In this book, a disease, X, which is known to western medicine as epilepsy, is believed to be caused by a neurological or brain disorder (or the cause is unknown), is noticeable because of symptomatic seizures which a person exhibits, and is treated through various chemical means. For Hmong people, however, X is known as "qaug dab keg" ("the spirit catches you and you fall down"), is caused by having one's soul stolen ("dab"), is noticeable through a person's symptoms of shivering and pain but moreover through their "intuitive sympathy" (p. 21), and is treated through, among other ways, "neeb," or a ceremony of sacrifice. For Hmong, "qaug dab keg" is also attached to a social position which is conceived less as an illness and more on the order of a "calling" or "vocation" in which one may have special access to things unseen. As such, the condition (X) is not simply a physical affliction but rather a social vocation which can have considerable cultural value (e.g., equipping one for the role of a doctor or shaman).

Our brief cross-cultural comparison is offered here simply as a way of demonstrating how deeply diagnostic discourses invoke and create cultural premises. Note how these create conceptions of X, its possible causes, symptoms, and treatments. As a result, discourses about X bring forth a complex belief system about identities or social positions (e.g., as one with X, as one who treats X), about actions (e.g., regarding treatments, what one can do as a P with X), about feelings (e.g., whether one is sad, pleased, or both with X), and nature (e.g., what exists for X to be as it is, from souls to syringes). And so with menopause.

The women in our study talk about menopause as something they are **in**. A woman does not ***have*** menopause. The condition is expressed as: "I am ***in*** menopause" or "I **am** menopausal." Consider the following utterances:

(1) Gerry: I'm Gerry and I'm in menopause ...
(2) Phyllis: I'm Phyllis. I am 49 and three quarters and I guess you could say I am in perimenopause ...
(3) Pam: Hi, I'm Pam. I'm 44 and I am perimenopausal ...
(4) Sally: I'm Sally. I'm 57. I've been menopausal for about I think a year and a half ...

Speaking about menopause in this way, then, draws attention to it as something, a physical condition one is *in*, a stage of life, in some ways unlike a disease one *has*. In this sense, menopause is distinguished from a disease. It is deemed more similar to *being* pregnant, yet it is also different; it is similar in the sense that it is a period of life one is in, and it lasts for a finite period of time; it is different in that menopause marks the end, rather than the realization of one's reproductive abilities. Further, while menopause is expressed as a stage one is *in*, pregnancy is something that you *are* (e.g., you *are* pregnant, you don't *have* pregnancy, you *have* a baby). Like *being in* puberty (e.g., you are *in* puberty or you are *coming out of* puberty, you don't *have* puberty), menopause is a stage of life one moves in and out of, this being coded into the women's talk. Thus, menopause is unlike a disease, like yet unlike being pregnant, and most like puberty.

Menopause is also talked of like an illness, with causes, and symptoms which can be treated, as we will see below. Yet the phrasing used is different from a medical diagnosis that says: You *have* cancer. You *have* heart disease. You *have* diabetes. In sum, then, menopause stands at the juncture of two discourses: through a life stage discourse it marks a stage of life, the end of one's reproductive years; through a medical discourse, it is deemed a symptomatic and treatable condition which is like yet unlike an illness. We can clarify the difference between menopausal and disease based discourses by reformulating the above form to suit the shape and meanings of menopausal talk:

- Y (menopause) is something P (a person or organism) goes through at point Z.
- Y is caused by agent C (C meaning a depletion of estrogen).
- Y is known because of symptoms (1,2,3,n).
- P exhibits symptoms (1,2,3,n).
- P is *in* Y.
- Given that P is going through Y, treatment T (a,b,c ...) is possible.

## 2. Menopause as a life stage malady: A sequencing of communicative acts

In a review of literature on lay diagnosis, Paul ten Have remarks that most research has focused upon medical consultations themselves, and given relatively less attention both to lay diagnosis as an "essential precondition" for "first visits," and to post-visit discussions (ten Have 2001: 252). One exception is Wayne Beach's research, which focuses on pre-clinical talk (1996) and upon post-clinical concerns (2001).

These remarks and studies prompt us to report an overall event sequence of talk concerning menopause. Within our corpus of data, we can distinguish at least four phases or stages of talk in this sequence. We summarize the stages or phases as a decision-making process which is the outcome of a complex sequencing of communicative acts:

(1) A preliminary diagnosis or curiosity
(2) A medical consultation, formal or informal
(3) Peer support and review of the doctor's views about symptoms and treatments
(4) A decision about what to do

The sequence can be initiated in one of two general ways. Onc involves a woman's noticing a physical, psychological, or social trait in herself which she considers possibly symptomatic of menopause. We will analyze how this is discursively constructed below. The second way the sequence can be initiated is by curiosity, as when a woman simply wonders about menopause and what to expect from it.

A second stage in the sequence occurs when the noticing of symptoms attributed to menopause is deemed considerable enough, or the curiosity about menopause is deemed sufficient enough, from the woman's view, to warrant a medical consultation. At times this decision was made as the result of discussions with peers. In most cases, in our corpus, this decision to seek medical information was made, apparently, privately without engaging in any discussions.

The result of the decision to become more informed about menopause was to engage in one or more of a set of communicative activities. These included scheduling an appointment with a doctor, attending a public informational session on menopause, and/or logging onto an online chat room where menopause is discussed such as Dr. Koop, MD, Power Surge, alt.menopause, or Ivillage. In these activities, the woman heard and discussed the nature of menopause, possible treatments, and the advantages and disadvantages of the treatments.

A third phase in this larger sequence constitutes the bulk of our data, women talking together about menopause. We note here that the diagnoses proffered by medical professionals, and the advice given concerning treatments, were subjected through this talk to the discussion of the woman's peers. The chain of information has thus, up to this point, in its fullest version, moved from the woman's initial self-diagnosis, to medical consultations, to a peer review. It is this peer review of symptoms and treatments that is the most elaborate form of talk in our corpus, and which we turn to below. We note here, initially, how this phase of talk assumes an authoritative air in our corpus. As doctors' and experts' recommendations are presented in and subjected to this discourse and to subsequent reactions and commentaries from other women, the symptoms and treatments of menopause themselves become shaped and molded to the circumstances of the woman's life. While the qualities and extent of this talk may be unique to menopause, the phase itself may be active more generally for other "physical conditions."

A final stage, the outcome of the above sequence, is the woman's decision about what to do about menopause.

## 3. Personal impact statements: Speaking about the speaker and symptoms

Let's listen to several women who have come together to talk about menopause.

(5) Segment 1:
Phyllis: I'm Phyllis. I am 49 and three quarters
and I guess you could say I am in perimenopause. I am
having some hot flashes that are worse at different

times at night and when they are I find that I am extremely tired and do not feel like myself.

(6) Segment 2:

Pam: Hi, I'm Pam. I'm 44 and I am perimenopausal. *Struggling in some ways, in other ways, not.*

Sally: I'm Sally. I'm 57. I've been menopausal for about I think a year and a half. I am not on HRT but I have started black cohosh and it does work on the vaginal dryness – it corrected that and I know its working cuz my breasts were very tender and I've been sleeping but I don't know if it's because I'm tired from the trip or whatever. I didn't sleep over there because I just had a hard time sleeping, but in general I do think I'm sleeping better. And the hot flashes I have noticed, they're not so much.

Kim: I'm 49 and taking HRT and have done some shuffling around on it and finding the right place to be and decided to go on it because I had a lot of hot flashes at night, not sleeping well, and those emotional moody things, and disease in the family so there was a lot of reason why I chose to do this and it will remain to be seen with the new research coming out whether I will remain on it or I won't.

(7) Segment 3:

Sherry: My name is Sherry and I am in perimenopause. I am concerned about osteoporosis and I have horrible hot flashes … so my doctor said I should be on HRT and I love it.

Bette: Are you worried about breast cancer?

Sherry: There's no breast cancer in my family and the studies say you should be concerned about heart disease and weak bones.

Bette: That's what you want to do … It makes sense to you.

What we notice in these and similar utterances is a form of "lay diagnosis," a way in which these women "assess and accomplish their health-related belief systems on a contingent basis" (Sarangi 2001: 4). This communicative act involves, for these women, several possible ingredients. We will discuss these under the general title of a self-assessment of their physical condition. This involves commentary along the following lines: a) the stage of menopause; b) the name, and age of the woman; c) the woman's family situation; d) the woman's medical history; and e) the woman as a bearer of symptoms.

The stage of menopause: In the above and similar excerpts, the women identify themselves as *in* one of three general stages of menopause, perimenopause, menopausal, and postmenopausal. The stage of "perimenopause," as identified by Phyllis, Pam, and Sherry, refers specifically to being around the point when symptoms are anticipated or beginning to appear. The stage of being "menopausal," as mentioned by Sally, refers to a woman in the "heat" of menopause, experiencing its symptoms. And postmenopausal refers to women having moved "out of" menopause.

Name, age, family situation: Most often a woman identifies herself through her name and age, with there being quite great variability in our data regarding age, ranging from the twenties (typically from women who had a hysterectomy) to the fifties. Also, women sometimes mention, as Kim did, a history of "disease in the family," or much less frequently, their partners and/or children.

The woman as symptom-bearer: By far the most elaborate discourse and discussion in our data focused upon the nature, intensity, and status of symptoms which a woman considered (possibly) associated with menopause. The most frequently discussed of these were "hot flashes," "difficulty in sleeping," "being tired," and "mood swings." Also mentioned were "vaginal dryness," "tender breasts," "difficulty in working," "being forgetful," "heart palpitations," "anxiety attacks," "periods gone haywire," and "swollen ankles," among many others.

We have come to identify this kind of menopausal talk as a "personal impact statement" or PIS (Suopis 2002). The PIS is a two-part statement where the woman accomplishes a considerable amount of interactional work. She identifies herself possibly by name, by age and/or by the particular phase of menopause she is *in*. She further can specify her physical condition through a discussion of her symptoms and perhaps her medical history. Then she explains how she experiences her symptoms. In these rather brief segments, we can then hear how a menopausal woman identifies herself as such, as at a symptomatic stage of life which might warrant some kind of treatment.

Three unspoken features are being presumed by and created in this very discourse. We will introduce these here, and return to them below. In particular, age is being linked to menopause as a strong causal agent, such that progressing age creates symptoms at this later stage of life, yet also that the age at which symptoms may appear can vary greatly. Second, when in this life stage, expectations for living are being established for a woman's life such as anticipating and living with symptoms, something like those being discussed above. Third, there is the belief that this condition can be treated, as is mentioned in the comments of Sally, Kim, and Sherry. So, what about this treatment?

## 4. Treatment talk

The expressed need for treatment is sometimes accompanied by a tremendous sense of urgency. Consider the following:

(8) Segment 4:

Meg: I'm Meg and I am definitely in perimenopause. My hot flashes are terrible! I simply cannot live with these any longer. Is anyone else experiencing this? I need to do something about this and this is why I am here. I can't work and I can't sleep because I feel like I am in a hot oven.

We mention this datum because treatment talk can be deemed urgent, at times responding to an immediate and serious situation. A woman might feel any symptom intensely and thus search for remedies by talking and engaging in a deliberative discourse about treatments. One woman called for "help!" and wondered if she was "going crazy." Such intense reactions can be addressed perhaps initially through a Personal Impact Statement, but sometimes by participating directly in treatment talk.

In segment two above, Sally mentions she is "not on HRT" (Hormone Replacement Therapy) but has "started black cohosh" (an herbal remedy). The latter treatment she has found to be a successful way of treating a variety of symptoms from "vaginal dryness," to "tender breasts," and "hot flashes," and perhaps this will even help her difficulties in sleeping. Kim mentions, on the other hand, that she is "taking HRT," and with it hopes to alleviate her symptoms including hot flashes, sleep deprivation, mood swings, and other diseases such as heart disease and osteoporosis?

Through this kind of "treatment talk," we find women deliberating about various ways of treating menopause, discussing various objectives in these treatments, as well as debating various effects of these treatments. Let us treat each in turn.

One kind of treatment, HRT, is synthetic and chemical and is deemed "unnatural" by some women, yet greatly effective by others, as alluded to by Sally and Kim above, and by Beth, below. We also see in what follows how various treatments are mentioned as possible treatments, from "hormones" to herbs to "vitamin E":

(9) Segment 5:

Lesley: I really need some help with these hot flashes.

Carrie: Have you tried black cohosh?

Lesley: Well, I've heard of it, but I'm not sure…

Beth: Ever since I started on HRT, my hot flashes are not as bad.

Lesley: I know, my doctor says I should take hormones but I am worried about…

Meg: I don't blame you. Have you tried Vitamin E? It works most of the time.

Similarly, the following posting demonstrates how "estrogen replacement therapy" is deemed at times as a "drug" or "chemicals," and thus as less "natural" than other treatments such as "de-fatted soy flour." This distinction between "natural" and "unnatural" treatments appears throughout our data:

(10) Segment 6:
Message Board Posting 23: I had some very negative side effects to estrogen replacement therapy so I had to find a natural alternative. I checked several hundred medical research studies and concluded that de-fatted soy flour was the best alternative available as a natural way to replace my estrogen. I have a summary of the research reasons on my homepage (homepage given). I also have a series of recipes using de-fatted soy flour on that page. De-fatted soy tastes great when it's used in good recipes, and costs very little. I hope this helps you as it has me.

One of the problems mentioned repeatedly, concerning treatment, is the way it effects one's body. Further complicating the effects are interactions among natural remedies, as in the following segment, and interactions among various natural and unnatural remedies in others.

(11) Segment 7:

Pam: So that you find if you're taking something there might be the possibility that they're interacting. I was thinking of flaxseed, soy – those kinds of things – have you ever heard of interacting with them?

Mary: Just like fiber it takes time for your body to get used to it. The point that I I'm trying to say is that if you tried soy at one point and you didn't care for it – it may just have been the brand. And they've just come on the market with some of these newer ones that are in the refrigerator section and you may find that they're more palatable to you. You might want to try that.

The expressed objectives in treating menopause are both to address the symptoms, and to enhance one's "quality of life." Consensus about increasing one's "quality of life" is reached below by Pam and Leslie.

(12) Segment 8:

Lesley: Well, I am going to continue with the vitex.
I just want to control my period and I want
to prolong [prevent?] menopause as long as possible.

Cheryl: How long do you think you can avoid it?

Lesley: Probably only a few more years, but I am
going to stay with it.

Pam: It's a quality of life thing.

Lesley: Yes, it is…it is what I want to do.

Difficulties and complications, however, also can arise. Consider, for example, the discussion below where HRT and its positive and negative side effects are being discussed.

(13) Segment 9
Message Board Post 1: I'm staying on the HRT. I don't want to fall and break my hip because my mother ended up that way … when you break your hip, it is almost over.

(14) Segment 10
Message Board Post 2: It's your quality of life. That's why you take HRT.

(15) Segment 11
Message Board Post 3: I'm more concerned about breast cancer.

(16) Segment 12
Message Board Post 4: Then you probably shouldn't take HRT.

This discussion and the ones above help make the point that there are a variety of treatments for menopause, any one might work for some but not others, and each one has possible side effects which can be positive and/or negative. In any case, each is discussed as alleviating some symptoms for some (e.g., hot flashes, sleep deprivation, mood swings, control of menstrual periods), having some expressed positive side effects (e.g., helps prevent osteoporosis), but may also be risky (e.g., can increase the risk of breast cancer).

In sum, then, treatment talk is a complex kind of talk: 1) it can be sought in response to urgent needs; 2) it provides a variety of treatments deemed natural (e.g., black cohosh, flaxseed, soy, vitamin E) and unnatural (HRT, vitex, provera, prempro, premphase); 3) each treatment has its own benefits and disadvantages; 4) in an effort to alleviate symptoms, treatment talk is designed to reach decisions which enhance one's quality of life; and 5) further, there is no one treatment that helps all women. As a result, women feel that they must engage in this talk as a way of taking the initiative for their own health concerns, sorting through all of its possibilities, and doing something about this stage of life. While advice may be given by a doctor or medical counselor, the ultimate authority in the these matters is placed squarely on the shoulders of the woman. While this choice can be empowering, it can also be a heavy burden to bear. There is, as a result, an urgency and frustration heard in the talk that illustrates how physicians and medical science have left the decision of whether to treat menopause, and if so how so, up to the patient, suggesting that the patient is now somehow responsible for her own healthcare. This unique position can be veiled in the popular theme of patient empowerment, but in reality, there is a practical cry from the women for guidance on what to "do" about the choices being offered to them.

## 5. Menopausal discourse: Problems and the personhood of "baby boomer"

In the above discourse is a complex of communication practices. These embody a folk logic of menopause, a discourse of a woman's life world that is given voice through the idioms of a life stage *and* a medical condition. This discourse is given a particular form as it flows through a specific sequence of communicative acts and phases, and can be understood more particularly as active in "personal impact statements" and treatment talk. In our concluding discussion, we want to sketch a system of cultural premises we hear as both created in and a condition for this discourse.

Any physical condition is experienced and expressed as a realization of particular beliefs and values. For example, in Japan, we are told that women do not use the phrase, "hot flashes," as symptomatic during menopause (Lock 1991). We wonder, then, do Japanese women experience these symptoms, and menopause in the ways the women in our study do? Similarly, in Argentina today (Berti 2001), we understand women do not discuss (nor experience?) menopause in the ways presented here, but express it as a natural part of life which is not worthy of much comment, like the passing of another day. Yet in Nova Scotia, there is a similar entitlement of menopausal symptoms as "blood and nerves," as a way of encapsulating psychological and physical changes during this stage of life (Davis 1983). One can only wonder what the Hmong have to say about menopause. Each such comment from elsewhere suggests its own cultural discourse, its own idioms, its own sequences and system of communication practices.

One set of premises we want to highlight regarding menopausal talk is the result of combining a life stage and medical idiom. We have come to think of the result as the "medicalization of a life stage." In effect, this has created a mounting sense of dis-ease concerning this life stage, and an urgency that something be done about it. In short, menopause has been transformed from a natural stage of life to a *problem in need of a remedy.* This transformative quality of this discourse includes the following features: 1) as a medicalized condition, this life stage is deemed "unnatural," sub-optimal, or in some sense flawed or abnormal; 2) as a result, a diagnosis is possible, although in any one case this diagnosis may be inexact and uncertain; 3) possible treatments are varied and of variable use; 4) there are various opinions from medical experts concerning any one treatment, thus many treatments carry a controversial "air" about them.

In addition to the above features, an economic dimension serves to precipitate a diagnosis to ensure reimbursement for an office visit. In short, menopause must be diagnosed before its symptoms can be treated from a medical and economic perspective.

Menopause, then, unlike a natural stage of life, is talked here through a discourse which envisions it largely as a problem. And it is not only expressed as a problem, but moreover what can and should be done about it is problematic.

Coupled with the above conception of menopause is an identity of women who, throughout this discourse, collectively avow a *"baby boomer" identity*. They have said things like, "my mother didn't talk about it" (see Suopis 2002). Through this and related sayings, the women invoke a set of premises regarding problems generally, and menopause in particular. Some of these can be made explicit. For example, we are a generation unlike our mothers. They did not talk about menopause, we do. They did nothing about menopause, but we are going to do something about it. They did not support each other by talking this through, but we are. Through these premises about the social identity of a "baby boomer," we can hear a generational stance to problems like menopause. Problems are to be talked about, solutions sought, support given. In the process, we become informed and empowered to "do something!"

The combination of the premises casting menopause as a problem, and crafting the woman as a boomer, creates a cultural scene in which menopause becomes not only a physical but a cultural condition, one more problem to be "worked through" in an informed and assertive way. This way involves coming together in support and informational sessions, getting all necessary information, and consulting with medical experts. Through a personal impact statement, women inform each other about who each is, and what one is going through. Through treatment talk, they wrestle with what exactly can and should be done, given their unique circumstances. And so we notice in this way of speaking, as in all such ways, cultural premises in its production, for these are the ways people in various places know who they are, physically and culturally, and what to do about their life's circumstances.

## Notes

1. The following form is constructed with the benefit of Pietro Barbetta's comments on "diagnosis as a colonial practice," University of Massachusetts, April 25, 2001.

## *References*

Beach, Wayne A.
1996 *Conversations about Illness: Family Preoccupations with Bulimia*. Mahwah, NJ: Erlbaum.
2001 Introduction: Diagnosing "lay diagnosis". *Text* 21(1/2), 13–18.
Carbaugh, Donal
1996 *Situating Selves*. Albany: State University of New York Press.
Carbaugh, Donal, T. Gibson, and T. Milburn
1997 A view of communication and culture: Scenes in an ethnic cultural center and a private college. In Kovacic, B. (ed.), *Emerging Theories of Human Communication*. Albany, NY: SUNY Press, 1–24.
Drew, Paul
2001 Spotlight on the patient. *Text* 21(1/2), 261–268.
Fadiman, A.
1997 *The Spirit Catches You and You Fall Down*. New York: Farrar, Straus, and Giroux.
Frankel, Richard M.
2001 Clinical care and conversational contingencies: The role of patients' self-diagnosis in medical encounters. *Text* 21(1/2), 83–111.
Lock, M.
1991 Contested meaning of the menopause. *The Lancet* 337(8752), 1270–1272.
Mishler, Eliot G.
1984 *The Discourse of Medicine: Dialectics of Medical Interviews*. Norwood, NJ: Ablex.
Robinson, J. D.
2001 Asymmetry in action: Sequential resources in the negotiation of a prescription request. *Text* 21(1/2), 19–54.
Sarangi, S.
2001 Editorial. On demarcating the space between 'lay expertise' and 'expert laity'. *Text* 21(1/2), 3–11.
Suopis, Cindy A.
2002 Women speaking about menopause and Hormone Replacement Therapy: An ethnographic exploration in communicating personhood. Unpublished doctoral dissertation, University of Massachusetts, Amherst.
ten Have, Paul
2001 Lay diagnosis in interaction. *Text* 21(1), 251–260.

# Chapter 14
# The diagnosis of the constituents of communication in everyday discourse: Some functions, enabling conditions, consequences, and remedies

*Christian Nelson*

*Christian Nelson offers another poignant illustration of how diagnostic thinking is embedded in everyday reasoning and action. Nelson shows how a disease metaphor is commonly used to depict communication such as when the media is diagnosed as being "sick" or "viral." He finds this disease metaphor depicting communication in a variety of discourse contexts, discusses its function and its potential negative impact, and ends by making a plea for minimizing its use.*

Diagnosis is not the purview of professionals alone; laypeople also offer up diagnoses of themselves, others, and a variety of other social phenomena. Some of these diagnoses are manifestations of a particular metaphor about communication commonly utilized in everyday discourse – the COMMUNICATION IS THE TRANSMISSION OF A DISEASE metaphor. Because diagnosis is an action associated with the occurrence of disease, and because metaphors are the articulation of more elaborate schemas (Johnson 1987), speaking of the transmission of messages as the transmission of disease gives rise to acts of diagnosis. Thus, in our everyday communication about communication we quite commonly diagnose communication recipients including ourselves (e.g., *I'm sick of the media's conservative slant* or *I'm sickened by the coverage of Columbine*). In addition, we commonly diagnose communication sources. For instance, it is not unusual to hear complaints like *I think the recent spate of school shootings is a result of a sick media*. Further, we commonly diagnose communication messages themselves (e.g., *That was a sick show* or *That was a sick joke*).

In what follows, I will examine this metaphorically motivated practice of diagnosing communicators and communicative messages not only because of its pervasiveness in our everyday talk, but also because of its significant potential consequences. More specifically, I will examine the function of this practice and the sociolinguistic conditions that support the underlying metaphor's use. Following this, I will briefly consider the possible detrimental consequences of metaphorically diagnosing communication and its constituents, after which I will discuss some means for preventing these consequences.

Before producing any of the above, I will provide a more elaborate description of the metaphor in question through an examination of its manifestation in a variety of discursive contexts. This description will not only enable presentation of further examples of the resulting diagnostic discourse but also provide necessary groundwork for understanding some of that discourse's functions.

## 1. The underlying metaphor

The first manifestation of the COMMUNICATION IS THE TRANSMISSION OF A DISEASE metaphor that I will describe occurs in everyday discourse about the media. The cultural significance of this discourse is demonstrated by a graphic rendering of British culture by the artist Gerald Scarfe. Scarfe's sculpture, entitled *British Culture*, depicts a television spewing out what appears to be a sickening, mucus-like liquid onto a horrified viewer who cannot escape the growing sea surrounding him because his forearms and hands have begun to fuse with his armchair (see http://www.turnoffyourtv.com/international/thedome.html for a picture).

As suggested, this disease metaphor is manifested by characterizations of mass communication's source ("sick media"), as well as by characterizations of mass communication recipients ("sick viewers") and messages ("sick program"). In addition, it is manifested by references to "contagious" or "infectious" ideas presumably contained within such messages.

Unelaborated references to a "sick" media, to "sick" messages, or "sickened" audience members seem to be far and away the most prevalent manifestations of the COMMUNICATION IS THE TRANSMISSION OF A DISEASE metaphor in discourse about the mass media. (One can confirm this through Internet or Lexis-Nexis searches of keywords like *sick media*.) The metaphor's manifestation is therefore rather limited. Seldom are there references to the more technical synonyms for these terms or references to having or spreading any of a variety of specific illnesses.

Nevertheless, people do occasionally speak of more specific media-induced illnesses. For instance, one crusader against television viewing argues on his web site (http://www.turnoffyourtv.com/) that television viewing causes what he terms *beautiful people syndrome* – a disease which causes people to think they should look like what are popularly referred to as the "beautiful people" – those who star in television programs, advertisements, and the like. According to this lay commentator, beautiful people syndrome itself leads to *post-traumatic-television* [sic] *depression*, which "can set in after you realize that your life isn't as wonderful as it TV [sic] says it should be" (Kaufman 2000). Further, one visitor to the site in question left the following commentary:

> Television is nothing but a spiritual parasite. It sucks the very life of it's [sic] victims. I know some people who LITERALLY are 'dead' as they live. They live in front of their televisions. I feel nothing but pity, shame, and disgust for these people. (Luke n.d.)

Also, everyday discussions of the mass media often involve reference to "exposure" to TV just as one might reference exposure to a disease. Indeed, this practice carries over to many academic studies of mass communication, as does reference to "inoculations" against mass mediated messages (see Lumsdaine and Janis 1953; McGuire 1961).

With regard to mass communication message production, everyday discourse also contains frequent reference to how media "spreads" an idea, and, more infrequently, contains reference to the creation of "epidemics" of certain ideas. A much less common manifestation of the COMMUNICATION IS THE TRANSMISSION OF A DISEASE metaphor, though hardly a surprising one given talk of the epidemic spread of certain (communicated) ideas, is its use in the following obituary:

> Paul Klite was trained at the Duke University Medical School and became a public health professional. That was the concern that motivated him to move into media work, first as a radio producer for "Terra Infirma" (Sick Earth) ... After 100 shows, "Terra Infirma" gave way in 1992 to "Media Infirma," another term for the sick media climate in public broadcasting that rarely sustains hard-hitting programming. It was then that he brought his public-health concerns to mainstream broadcasting by taking a close look at local news programs in his hometown. (Schechter 2000)

Here, the disease metaphor of communication manifests itself in metaphorical references to the media as a public health issue and to media critics as public health practitioners.

The second manifestation of the COMMUNICATION IS THE TRANSMISSION OF A DISEASE metaphor is in the popular discourse about memes. In his book *The Selfish Gene*, Dawkins (1976) defines a meme as an idea, thought or belief that, like both genes and computer viruses, replicates itself. Of course, genes are biological entities that replicate within the cells of an organism due to sex or viral infection, while memes are mostly treated as the contents of brains (hence Lynch's 1996 title *Thought Contagion* and Brodie's 1996 title *Virus of the Mind*; though see Gatherer 1998) that replicate due to humans' genetic disposition toward imitation (Blackmore 1999). Most memeticians also suggest that memes evolve as genes do by succumbing to variation during replication from organism to organism with only certain variants surviving. They also compare memes to computer viruses, which do not vary during transmission.

As Dawkins (1993) puts it, cells are the sites of genetic replication regardless of whether the genetic material being replicated is that of the cell's organism (due to sexual reproduction) or due to viral infection. Further, just as there are two kinds of genetic material, one of which is usually benign while the other is usually not, Dawkins suggests that there are two kinds of memetic material – memes and viruses of the mind. Dawkins specifically identifies religious beliefs as mind viruses, arguing that they are such because they are irrational – i.e., developed and maintained by means other than scientific inquiry and unable to withstand scientific scrutiny.

So, in the memetics literature, the COMMUNICATION IS THE TRANSMISSION OF A DISEASE metaphor is principally manifested through the diagnosis of certain (communicated) ideas as viruses. Blackmore (1999: ch. 15) explicitly follows Dawkins in this practice of identifying negative memes as viruses. These two memeticians and their followers also talk of how such viruses "spread" in ways that make an "epidemiology" of them possible. However, aside from a few references to persons "infected" by viral memes, there is a paucity of references to "sick" persons who spread such memes, or persons who are sickened by them.

Of the few remaining manifestations of the COMMUNICATION IS THE TRANSMISSION OF A DISEASE metaphor, a notable one occurs in writings by Brodie (1996), Lynch (1996), and Rushkoff (1996), who share a tendency to blur the distinction between memes and mind viruses and even use the terms synonymously, to Blackmore's dismay (Blackmore 1999: 22). In doing so, they treat viruses as neutral rather than negative phenomena. Indeed, Brodie (1996) prominently counteracts the negativity of viruses on the back of his cover by making light of it. In what looks like a cigarette warning label box he states:

> Warning! This book contains a live mind virus. Do not read this book unless you are willing to be infected. The infection may affect the way you think in subtle or not-so-subtle ways, or even turn your current world view inside out.

Of course, no one would put such a warning on a book if that person thought the book would cause any harm. As for Rushkoff (1996), he even temporarily reverses the usual valuation of viruses by stating,

> Just as scientists use viruses to combat certain diseases within the human body or to tag dangerous cells for destruction by the person's own antibodies, media activists [whose work Rushkoff admires] use viruses to combat what they see as the enemies of our culture. (Rushkoff 1996: 15)

To close this discussion of memetics discourse, I should indicate two elaborations of the COMMUNICATION IS THE TRANSMISSION OF A DISEASE metaphor that Rushkoff (1996) introduces. First, he extends the metaphor by talking about the "husks," or "protein shells" of messages, much as virologists speak of such as components of biological viruses. That is, Rushkoff argues that certain messages slip into our minds just as a virus slips into a cell. Second, Rushkoff also speaks of society (or the social *datasphere*, which he identifies as the host within which mind viruses operate) as possessing an "immune system," operated by society's elite, which seeks to destroy viruses such as those produced by media activists.

Another manifestation of the COMMUNICATION IS THE TRANSMISSION OF A DISEASE metaphor occurs in popular marketing discourse. In that discourse field it has become extremely popular to speak of *viral marketing*; indeed, the term was named "buzzword of the year" (Tchong 1998) just one year after its introduction. According to the marketing professionals who coined the term (Jurvetson and Draper, n.d.), viral marketing is a popular marketing message that is rapidly communicated through a network of people via word of mouth. For these authors, the prime example of viral marketing was that conducted by Hotmail subscribers themselves through their use of that free E-mail service. When sending E-mail messages through that service, users also unwittingly sent the message "Get your free E-mail at Hotmail," since that message was automatically appended by Hotmail's software. Because of most Hotmail message recipients' interest in free E-mailing, and their trust in what appeared to be the recommendation of a friend, many readily adopted Hotmail, and thus began to send out Hotmail's marketing messages themselves, snowballing Hotmail adoption. As a result Hotmail gained 10 million subscribers within a year, 3 times quicker than what it took Netscape to get that many users, and 15 times quicker than it took TV (Godin 2000: 16–17) to acquire similar numbers of viewers. This occurred despite the fact that Hotmail reportedly spent only $500 in advertising.

In an influential book, Godin (2000) elaborates the idea virus and MARKETING COMMUNICATION IS THE TRANSMISSION OF A DISEASE metaphors in a way that makes viral communication seem unthreatening. He does so by calling persons who pass viral marketing messages on to others as "sneezers," rather than using more foreboding terms like "carriers." This is predictable, since no one wants to be perceived as advocating the distribution of something negative or harmful.

## 2. Functions of diagnosing communication constituents

In what follows I will suggest some different functions of the different types of metaphorical diagnoses that stem from the metaphorical speech described above, particularly as they are found in popular writings. This analysis partly relies on unaided recollection of everyday talk – a resource that is not without its problems. However, my speculations of the functions of everyday messages are also partly grounded by an examination of written messages.

To begin this functional analysis, I will consider the diagnoses of communication producers or sources, receivers, and messages that occur in popular discourse regarding the mass media. As noted, all of these mass communication constituents are commonly labeled "sick" and messages are also referred to as "contagious," "infectious," and the like. In what follows, I will argue that the diagnoses of most mass mediated messages and their producers or sources are self-consciously produced to negatively evaluate the diagnosed communication constituents.

To support this argument, I will first note that the diagnoses in question are unspecific. This means that effective therapies are impossible to prescribe and thus these diagnoses are not produced for the reasons motivating a literal diagnosis (cf. Beach 2001; Sarangi 2001). Additionally, these diagnoses are made of media sources or messages that are frequently regarded as having negative social influences. This is in keeping with social members' inclination to regard television viewing and some Internet use as a guilty pleasure (e.g., Gauntlett and Hill 1999), and their mostly negative treatments of television – e.g., the popular display of bumper stickers advocating "kill your television," and popular references to television as the "boob tube." Media programs are also often labeled "sick" if they portray what is popularly viewed as negative – e.g., violence or sex.

Finally, synonyms for sickness in the discourse context under consideration – words like "twisted" (e.g., The media is sick and twisted), "disgusting" (e.g., That was a sick and disgusting video), or "excessive" (e.g., The excessive news coverage of Elian Gonzalez was sick) – underscore that the diagnoses of mass mediated messages and their producers create the stigma that frequently accompanies diagnoses of illness. (This can also be achieved through another metaphor by suggesting one has become unwittingly addicted to TV – the "plug-in drug" according to Winn 1985.)

But what of the function of the metaphorical diagnoses of media audience members? I believe such diagnoses are produced to characterize media audience members as passive victims when produced as self-diagnoses, which they often are. Of course, the *effect* of such diagnoses is to characterize persons sickened by the media or its messages as victims, for illness-causing agents commonly find us rather than the reverse. However, is such self-characterization of audience members the *function* of such diagnoses?

Evidence that such self-characterization is a function of metaphorical diagnosis comes from consideration of the *felicity conditions* (Austin 1975) of such diagnoses. People cannot make statements such as "*The Jerry Springer Show* makes me sick" or "TV makes me sick" in a sensible fashion without also admitting that they have viewed or listened to a stigmatized communication source. Moreover, both personal experience and polling results indicate that many who make such metaphorical self-diagnoses are quite familiar with the media sources they claim to be sickening them; as the press frequently notes, high ratings are associated with shows that people claim to find perverse, disgusting, and sick. The only way to avoid self-incrimination in complaints about media sources or messages (particularly popular ones) is to suggest that one is a passive victim, a suggestion made all the more possible and even likely given the common suggestion that the media "surrounds" us. Thus, it hardly seems coincidental that people make complaints about the media via the portrayal of themselves as passive recipients of disease that diagnosis affords.

Much of what I have just argued regarding diagnoses of messages or message sources in the popular media discourse also applies to much of the memetics discourse. In particular, the diagnoses of messages or message sources in Dawkins' (1976) and Blackmore's (1999) memetics discourse serve to stigmatize those messages or message sources. For example, memeticians have predominantly targeted religious messages and message sources in their popular writings, just as popular science enthusiasts have predominantly targeted these at least since Lucretius' *De Rerum Natura*. Notably, these diagnoses in the memetics discourse are quite limited – messages and their sources are labeled either viral or not, with no attempt to identify types of viruses in a manner that would lead to treatments. So, it would seem that they have no other purpose but to stigmatize. Further, this stigmatizing function is similar to diagnoses people make of hated personal opponents – e.g., the diagnosis "he's sick" which one spouse makes of the other during divorce. It is hardly surprising, then, that Dawkins (1993: 13 and 26) stigmatizes religion and its "carriers" at the same time that he stigmatizes his ex-wife in print for sending his "sweet, trusting, gullible six-year-old ... for weekly instruction ... to a Roman Catholic nun" (Dawkins 1993: 13) without his consent.

Other memeticians appear to diagnose messages in a more neutral fashion by diagnosing messages as "viral" or "thought contagion" without stigmatizing their contents or calling for "inoculation" or the like against such messages. I believe that these neutral diagnoses perform the less obvious function of enabling their producers (e.g., Brodie 1996; Lynch 1996; Rushkoff 1996) to appear scientific – an appearance as important to sincere pursuers and legitimated holders of the title "scientist" as it is to pretenders (cf. Goffman 1959), since neutrality is equated with objectivity and thus with scientificity in most circles. Regardless of their motives for wishing to appear so, it seems clear that the memeticians in question are concerned with diagnosing in a neutral fashion so as to be seen as producing scientific diagnoses. Thus, despite their obvious use of metaphor, Lynch (n.d.) and Rushkoff (1999) deny that their reference to viral messages and thought contagion is metaphorical, for metaphorical language is widely regarded as unscientific or a crutch any scientist can and should be rid of (e.g., Brown 1977: 91–99; Gross 1990: 80–81; Maasen 1995; Maasen et al. 1995; cf. Green 1983: 71–78).

True, Lynch (n.d.: para. 3), for example, denies that his term *thought contagion* is metaphorical because it can be defined using mathematical formula, but that claim is made without benefit of the literature demonstrating that models of any kind (including mathematical ones) are metaphors (e.g., McCloskey 1995). Whatever the case, Brodie (1996) demonstrates his concern for appearing scientific by including a positive review on his book's back cover by "Elan Moritz, Ph.D., Director, Institute of Memetic Research," even though Moritz's Institute apparently folded some years earlier and may never have received institutional funding – a hallmark of scientific legitimacy (Lynch 1998). (Indeed, it is not clear that the Institute had any funders or personnel aside from Moritz.) Lynch further exhibits great concern for scientificity on his website and elsewhere (Lynch, n.d.; Lynch 1998; see also further messages by Lynch posted on June 15, 1998 and May 16, 1998 to the *Journal of Memetics* discussion list) by fretting over priority claims, proper citation practices, specific definitions, and mathematical formulae, all of which should concern proper scientists.

While Rushkoff (1996) does not engage in pursuing the appearance of scientificity as vigorously as Brodie (1996) and Lynch (n.d.), he does coin scientific-sounding terms like *datasphere* to identify his central phenomena. While his book is far more concerned with describing the contemporary media scene and culture jammers' role in it than it is concerned with articulating on the nature of viral idea transmission, he titles it "Media virus."

To conclude, I will address the function of metaphorical diagnoses found in popular marketing discourse. As suggested by my previous descriptions of this discourse, these metaphorical diagnoses serve to identify certain types of messages – viral messages – and persons – promiscuous and powerful sneezers – as types whose production or successful targeting will guarantee the success of a marketing campaign. Identifying messages as viral serves to suggest that they are unstoppable because viruses are so hard to stop. In this regard, it is notable that popular marketing writers fail to elaborate the COMMUNICATION IS THE TRANSMISSION OF A DISEASE metaphor by speaking of message inoculation, despite the fact that a well-developed theory of message inoculation has existed for quite some time (again, see Lumsdaine and Janis 1953; McGuire 1961). Of course, suggesting that a certain type of marketing message is guaranteed to spread and omitting mention of the possibility of counter-measures makes the producer of viral messages a marketing genius – an understandable goal for those who write about viral marketing.

## 3. Enabling conditions

How is it that metaphorical diagnoses of the kinds described above came about? And how is it that they are so subliminally metaphorical that their use can actually enhance the apparent expertise of their producers? These questions can be answered by considering several other metaphors for communicative messages that promote various aspects of the COMMUNICATION IS THE TRANSMISSION OF A DISEASE metaphor.

One of these metaphors portrays communication *qua* message transmission as the transmission of magically effective or impacting messages. This metaphor promotes the metaphorical diagnosis of communicative messages more particularly in that viruses are perceived to be at least as effective as magical incantations. A second relevant metaphor is that which portrays communication *qua* message transmission as the transmission of things with a physical impact. This metaphor promotes the COMMUNICATION IS THE TRANSMISSION OF A DISEASE metaphor by depicting viruses as physical entities that have a significant impact. A third relevant metaphor is that which portrays communication *qua* message transmission as the transmission of living things. Of course, this metaphor promotes the COMMUNICATION IS THE TRANSMISSION OF A DISEASE metaphor in that viruses are living things. A fourth relevant metaphor is that which portrays communication *qua* message transmission as the transmission of containers. This metaphor promotes the COMMUNICATION IS THE TRANSMISSION OF A DISEASE metaphor in that viruses are DNA, or genetic "instructions" contained within what are called "protein shells" or "husks." In what follows, I will briefly describe these four metaphors to clarify them, show their relationship to the disease metaphor, and demonstrate the cultural prominence of each.[1]

The metaphor of communicative messages as magically impacting things is clearly manifested in phrases such as *his words were bewitching*, *her story was spellbinding*, as well as in references to "god terms" and "devil terms." The significance of this metaphor for our thought about communicative messages is also registered by our belief in the existence of magical words; words such as "abracadabra," "presto change-o," "open sesame," and the like are regarded as having specific effects regardless of their utterer or context.

The existence of such magical beliefs about words is strikingly illustrated by the coverage of President Clinton's discourse during and after his publicly televised admission of an "inappropriate relationship" with Monica Lewinsky. The absence of the magic word "sorry" in that initial public admission was noted as a significant omission by a legion of commentators. Further, Clinton's first utterance of "sorry" following his admission received significant attention from reporters – indeed, it was the entire story in a number of news reports, despite the fact that the sentence in which it was uttered did not seem to express an attitude toward his offense any different from that expressed in the original admission.

Less dramatic, but more convincing evidence of the pervasiveness of this metaphor is provided by much of the self-help literature. While offering advice about personal and professional relationships and interactions, this literature purveys message formulas that purportedly avoid or resolve conflicts, regardless of context or utterer (e.g., the formulaic *three part assertion messages* in Bolton 1979:

141), much as the formulaic pronouncement "presto chang-o" is presumed to create certain effects, regardless of context.

Implicit belief in the COMMUNICATION IS THE TRANSMISSION OF A DISEASE metaphor is also manifested by our treatment of some words as taboo. We treat certain words as though they possessed a power either so sacred or profane that they cannot even be uttered, at least without causing shock or other emotional reactions. Thus, Jewish, Islamic, and Buddhist traditions forbid the use of at least certain names for their god (Oboler 1974: 21), and Confucianism forbids use of Confucius' real name (Rothwell 1982), and obscenity laws, so clearly linked to taboos and beliefs in the magical power of words (Oboler 1974: chaps. 2 and 3), forbid the use of a whole host of profane words on the public airwaves. When we feel that uttering such words is inescapable we often seek to attenuate their presumed force by whispering them, and when we cannot avoid hearing them we sometimes even belatedly cover our ears (or the ears of those whom we think are "virginal") to obviate their presumed impact.

Belief in taboo words' capacity to magically impact interactional participants is emphasized by the fact that their very sounds, regardless of how they might be incorporated into a word or interaction, are considered meaningful in themselves – an attitude apparently shared by many cultures (Dixon 1980).[2] Thus, a small town in Texas required that its administrative officers answer the phone "heaven-o" rather than "hello" (*TV Guide*, December 13–19, 1997: 25 as cited by Suzette Haden Elgin, personal communication) and certain groups of speakers utilizing non-English languages in the presence of English speakers avoid the use of syllables that sound like single-syllable, English taboo terms (Allan and Burridge 1991: 24–25).

Of course, the fact that we treat certain words as though they impact their receivers due solely to their own magical properties does not necessarily mean that we treat all messages as capable of impacting their receivers. However, such treatment is discernible in our conceptual grammar regarding communicative messages when it manifests the more general COMMUNICATIVE MESSAGES ARE PHYSICALLY IMPACTING OBJECTS metaphor. For instance, we can speak of any message (and by extension, any instrument for producing messages like pens or tongues) as though it were a physical entity capable of physically impacting someone else. Thus, we speak of "powerful messages" that are "penetrating," "piercing," "blistering," or "searing," or that "cut both ways" or are "cutting." Further, as we do with physical weapons, we speak of "targeted" messages, or messages that are "on target," and we talk about letting someone "have both barrels" with our language, which we further characterize as sometimes being "loaded" or a "loaded weapon" (e.g., Bolinger 1980).

Again, by extension, we also compare pens to swords ("the pen is mightier than the sword") and complain that some people are "sharp tongued." Indeed, we speak of many communicated messages as having a "point." Surely this and the earlier described variant of the magical powers of metaphor are behind the popular and even academic willingness to believe that "subliminal messages" can have some specific, even compelling, effect simply because of their receipt (pace Brannon and Brock 1994).

The COMMUNICATION IS THE TRANSMISSION OF LIVING THINGS metaphor is at least as pervasive and culturally significant as the magical and physical power metaphors just surveyed. This metaphor is manifested in such foundational cultural texts as the gospel of John, which states that "In the beginning was the word ... and the word became flesh" (John, 1:1 and 14). It is also manifested at length in Milton's (1644 [1927]) *Areopagitica*, a work which defends freedom of the press in part by comparing censorship to murder. Further, it can likely be traced at least back to the time during the earliest period of philosophy when both bodily symptoms and words were brought together under the category of signs (Eco 1984).

Given the significance of this metaphor to central cultural values and its instantiation in fundamental cultural texts, it should come as no surprise that it is variously reflected in our conceptual grammar about communication. For instance, we speak of messages whose meanings "escape" us, or of texts that "speak for themselves," and we speak of particularly meaningful utterances as "pregnant" with meaning or of silences that are themselves messages as "pregnant pauses." We also speak of messages as "bearing fruit" or being "fruitful." We frequently describe the production of texts in terms of child bearing (e.g., we speak of their "gestation periods" or of the "labor pains" in producing them). And journalists speak of putting their stories "to bed" when they are finished. With regard to old texts we speak of works which "speak to us still today" or "have a life of their own" – something we also say of rumors and other message types we more regularly encounter. We also state that stories, poems, or simply heartfelt utterances "touch" or "move" us. Moreover, we speak of having "command" of a language or "marshalling" our words, as if words or messages were beings to be ordered about.

To close, I wish to note the currency and power of this metaphor by noting its use in recent and significant political discourse – the discourse regarding the vote recount controversy following the 2000 U.S. Presidential election. To justify his lawsuit which sought continuation of the recount in a nationally televised message, the Democratic candidate, Al Gore stated on 17 November 2000, "A vote is not just a piece of paper, a punched card or a chad. It is a human voice and we must not let those voices be silenced – not for today, not for tomorrow, not for as long as this country stands for the principle that the people must be heard and heeded."

The fourth widespread metaphor identified above – the COMMUNICATION IS THE TRANSFER OF MEANING CONTAINERS metaphor was first identified by Reddy (1979).[3]

Reddy identifies it through phrases such as "It's difficult to unpack the meaning of that poem," "You obviously put a lot of thought into your paper," and "Your paper is overflowing with ideas." As Grady (1998) suggests, the meaning container metaphor seems to derive from the metaphor "TO MAKE ACCESSIBLE (by revealing, being revealed, being brought out of, etc.) IS TO MAKE UNDERSTANDABLE (because it is to make seeable)" (cf. pp. 214–5), via the correlative metaphor "TO REQUIRE DEDUCEMENT (as meanings do) IS TO BE HIDDEN (as in containers)" (cf. p. 214).[4] Whatever the case, it is not only evident in everyday discourse but also in academic discourse concerning communication. Indeed, not only is it manifest in Shannon and Weaver's (1949) discussion of communication (Reddy 1979), but also in the ethnomethodological and conversation analytic literature despite the fact that it contradicts certain of their fundamental theoretical precepts (Nelson 2001a).[5]

While the metaphors just considered provide fertile ground for the production of the COMMUNICATION IS THE TRANSMISSION OF A DISEASE metaphor and metaphorical diagnoses, I believe that the Western cultural preference for monosemism promotes the metaphor more directly and does so in such a way as to disguise its character as a metaphor. Monosemism is the belief that words have but one meaning or definition. The preference for monosemism in Western society is clear enough – Wittgenstein (1958) observed our "diseased craving for generality" (Pitkin 1972) regarding word meanings. This craving is perhaps most evident in the sciences, where traditional scientists explicitly insist on the rule "one word, one meaning" (Singleton and Straits 2005) as though that were possible. As I have shown elsewhere (Nelson 2001b), this monosemism leads people to conflate different senses of a term – to invoke one sense of a term when using it to refer to phenomena associated with a different sense.

Because the conflation of word meanings can result in a metaphor, and the conflation of the two senses of communication considered thus far naturally leads to the COMMUNICATION IS THE TRANSMISSION OF DISEASE metaphor, monosemism seems an obvious contributor to the phenomenon of metaphorical diagnosis. Further, given that monosemically created metaphors are created out of a confusion of already existent word meanings, their nature as metaphors is difficult to discern. Because of this, such metaphors should not threaten the appearance of scientificity. Notably, attributing the metaphor under discussion to monosemism also explains why communicated ideas are not only equated with biological viruses but also with computer viruses (e.g., Dawkins 1993). This is because computer viruses are communicated in yet another sense of the term *communicate* – i.e., they are communications *qua* transmissions of an electronic signal. Thus, the Western tendency toward monosemism sets the ground for a variety of the findings in the previous sections.

Finally, the metaphorical equation of communication *qua* message transmission and communication *qua* disease transmission is promoted by a fact easily overlooked but underscored by the tragic anthrax mailings in late 2001. The fact is that the transmission of a message often quite literally and more often at least potentially involves the transmission of a disease. The metaphor in question and the resulting metaphorical diagnoses could well be merely an over-extension of that sometimes tragic fact. However, the previous linguistic influences cannot help but provide fertile ground for such over-extension.

## 4. Consequences

The metaphorical diagnosis of communication's constituents and the metaphor this practice manifests may have a number of significantly negative consequences. It can lead to an impoverished understanding of the very grounds of our sociality – communication. In particular, it threatens to prevent or void recognition of the role of purpose in message production and the role of interpretive procedures in the process of message reception. Further, in the way that metaphorical diagnoses of communication are actually made in the contexts surveyed above, this practice also threatens to impede recognition of the agency of message sources and thus hamper recognition of those sources' responsibility for their messages. This is all the more worrisome at a time when very powerful message sources are very negatively affecting society.

Additionally, I believe metaphorical diagnosis of the constituents of communication can disable rigorous study by removing the study of communication from the context of past disciplined investigation. Diagnosis of this kind also aids biological determinism, which itself is quite an unfortunate perspective, at least as presently manifested. Finally, I will suggest that the metaphorical diagnosis of communication's constituents and the influence of its underlying metaphor may also be behind peoples' fears regarding the health risks of cell phone use despite little supportive evidence.

The metaphorical diagnosis of the constituents of communication as described above and the metaphor of communication this practice manifests threatens to prevent or void recognition of purpose and interpretation in communication because it portrays both communication production and reception as an involuntary activity. This is so because the passing of viruses is an involuntary process both on the part of virus carriers and those to whom viruses are spread. The metaphorical diagnosis of communicative messages thus suggests that the production and receipt of communicative signals is equally passive. This leads to an impoverished understanding of communication at a time when its importance to the constitution of society, is undeniable.

Further, characterizing message transmission as a passive process hampers recognition of the responsibility of powerful message sources when they negatively affect society. As numerous studies have indicated (see Comstock and Scharrer 1999 for a review), violence in the media encourages violence and fears of it among consumers, while desensitizing them to the effects of violence on others. However, given that we only hold those responsible who are seen as acting purposefully, the metaphorical diagnosis of messages makes it less likely that mass media producers will be held responsible for the consequences of their programming.

The COMMUNICATION IS THE TRANSMISSION OF A DISEASE metaphor can also easily suggest that the way to deal with producers of negatively perceived messages is not simply to "quarantine" them, though that is troubling enough, but to eradicate them through active counter-measures like censorship. Acts of censorship are not only negative by their very nature, but when portrayed as cures they are insidious since their negativity is masked. Much the same can be said of "idea disinfection," which the metaphor in question also suggests. Perhaps this is why Brodie (1996: ch. 12), who speaks of mind virus "disinfection," fails to consider the problems with the idea even in his chapter devoted to the "ethical questions" raised by virus disinfection.

The metaphorical diagnosis of communication's constituents and the metaphor that grounds it may also tend to disable rigorous study of communication. This disablement could occur due to the metaphor's discrediting of previous communication scholarship. That scholarship has been produced with little input from the field of biology; however, the metaphor in question suggests that the study of communication is properly the domain of biology and thus that the research on communication outside of biology is ancillary. While biologists are as rigorous as scholars in any other discipline, memeticians' ignorance of the anthropology literature has blunted the incisiveness of their work (cf. Bloch 2000; Kupper 2000) and there is no reason to suspect the loss of previous work in the communication discipline would be less problematic.

Another quite negative consequence of diagnosing communication's constituents is its encouragement of biological determinism. This is problematic for two reasons: first, there is little if any scientific support for biological determinism (see, e.g., Lewontin, Rose, and Kamin 1984); second, as both Lewontin and others (e.g., Lewontin et al. 1984; Lerner 1992) have shown, biological determinism lends itself to politically disastrous policies (e.g., the Nazis' genocidal policies toward Jews, gypsies, the mentally handicapped and others).

The metaphorical diagnosis of communication's constituents may also be behind peoples' fears regarding the health risks of cell phone. As Nicholson (2001) reports, this fear appears to be based on a very few anecdotes, and primarily one anecdote made public by David Reynard on *Larry King Live* in January 1993. Reynard's wife died of a brain tumor that he judged to have been just under the place where his wife's cell phone antenna would have been when the phone was in use, and further judged that it was in somewhat the same shape as the antenna. However, as Nicholson notes, there is little if any science in which to ground these judgments – a conclusion to which the courts also came. Nevertheless, Reynard's comments sparked a dramatic, albeit brief, plunge in cell phone company stock prices, and a decrease in cell phone use.

What caused, or at least enabled, this apparently groundless panic? Nicholson herself suggests via her observation of the various senses of the term *cell* that it may be due to the monosemic equation of communication *qua* message transmission with communication *qua* disease transmission instantiated in the practice of the metaphorical diagnosing of the constituents of communication. That is, if such an equation is made, it is not much of a leap for people to view communication technologies as disease bearing and causing.

## 5. Remedies

How do we remedy the unfortunate effects of the dis-easing discourse I have discussed above? One way might be to cease use of the disease metaphor of communication, but use of a metaphor is not a sufficient cause for the consequences above; as Turbayne (1970) and Maasen (1995) note, metaphors can be used for specific purposes without committing to their use in all circumstances. Further, it is nearly impossible to cease use of such deeply ingrained metaphors; in fact, I am sure I have utilized a number of the metaphors discussed above in writing about them. What needs to cease is the unwitting and unreflective use of the COMMUNICATION IS THE TRANSMISSION OF A DISEASE metaphor.

To that end, one might attempt to cancel the conditions that contribute to the unreflective use of it. For instance, one might point out the problematic nature of monosemism (e.g., Nelson 2001b), for monosemism necessarily prevents even awareness of the use of the metaphor in question.

Another tactic might be to underscore the limitations of metaphors (see, e.g., Nelson 2001a, for an example, and Maasen 1995, *inter alia*, for more general discussion of this). But many others have done this as well, and still metaphors are problematically utilized, even metaphors about communication by those who study it (again, Nelson 2001a). Within the sciences this is likely due to a particular philosophy of science, but in everyday talk it is likely because people are unaware of the existence of many dead metaphors much less the existence of such metaphors and their pervasiveness.

How can we counteract such obliviousness? Perhaps by studying them even more and making the results of such studies popularly accessible.

## 6. Conclusion

In the preceding I have described the COMMUNICATION IS THE TRANSMISSION OF A DISEASE metaphor, analyzed some of the functions of metaphorical diagnosis, and probed into the conditions enabling the metaphor's existence. I have also considered some of the possible unfortunate consequences of the metaphorical diagnosis of communication and other manifestations of the COMMUNICATION IS THE TRANSMISSION OF A DISEASE metaphor, and briefly considered remedies to counteract these consequences.

In doing all this, I hope to have made a number of contributions. First, I hope I have contributed to a growing body of knowledge about metaphors of communication (see Gozzi 1999; Krippendorff 1993; Lakoff and Johnson 1980: chap. 3; Nelson 2001a; Novek: 1992; Reddy 1979) – knowledge which communication researchers and other social scientists must have to be fully aware of what, besides empirical observations, shapes their thought.

I also hope that I have contributed to knowledge about metaphors in general, particularly as interactional phenomenon – that is, as phenomena that vary in articulation according to context of use and that serve multiple functions.

I also hope that I have contributed to an understanding of diagnosis as a cultural practice, and particularly to an understanding of that practice as it plays out in quite consequential ways in and across professional or academic and everyday contexts.

But besides contributing to the academy, I hope that I have contributed something that can serve as a foundation for making a wide range of social actors aware of an ordinary practice. The metaphorical diagnosing of communication constituents has important and dis-easing consequences that should be addressed.

### *Acknowledgments*

This chapter was conceived at a meeting of the Roundtable for Research on Language and Social Interaction in Communication Sciences and Disorders. I am indebted to the participants at that Roundtable, but I am especially indebted to its host, Dana Kovarsky, who invited me and made it such a pleasant and intellectually inspiring experience. Dana also provided valuable editorial assistance with my manuscript, as did Madeline Maxwell and, especially, Judith Duchan. Finally, I would like to note my debt to Michael Leff, with whom I studied rhetorical analysis in graduate school at the University of Wisconsin.

## Notes

1. The following four paragraphs are reprinted with revision from *Language and Communication* 21, Christian K. Nelson, "The haunting of communication research by dead metaphors: For reflexive analyses of the communication research literature", 245–272, 2001, with permission from Elsevier Science.
2. The author would like to thank Mark Donohue for this citation. Donohue also states that "This is widely reported in the Polynesian ... and African literature" as well (personal communication).
3. Actually, Reddy (1979) speaks of a *conduit metaphor* of communication rather than a container metaphor. However, so much of what he records and writes about suggests a container metaphor. Indeed, what he calls the conduit metaphor of communication is really a compound metaphor, made up of the container metaphor and the conduit metaphor; that is, what he describes is a way of talking about communication *qua* message transmission as though it were the transmission of containers of meaning through a conduit.
4. As indicated, my analysis of the metaphors related to COMMUNICATION IS THE TRANSFER OF MEANING and the CONTAINERS METAPHOR departs somewhat from Grady's (1998) analysis, but he himself notes that his analysis is incomplete. Further, I believe that Grady and I mostly differ with regard to our specific abstractive formulations of the metaphors in question, and that my formulations are in most ways just slightly more adequate renderings of his discussions of the metaphorical statements he presents for explanation.
5. Much of the preceding paragraph is reprinted from *Language and Communication*, 21, Christian K. Nelson, The haunting of communication research by dead metaphors: For reflexive analyses of the communication research literature, 245–272, 2001, with permission from Elsevier Science.

## References

Allan, Keith and Kate Burridge
1991 *Euphemism and Dysphemism.* New York: Oxford University Press.
Austin, John L.
1975 *How to Do Things with Words* (2nd ed., J. O. Urmson and M. Sbisa, eds.). Cambridge, MA: Harvard University Press.
Beach, Wayne A.
2001 Introduction: Diagnosing 'lay diagnosis.' *Text* 21, 13–18.
Blackmore, Susan
1999 *The Meme Machine.* Oxford: Oxford University Press.
Bloch, Maurice
2000 A well-disposed anthropologist's problems with memes. In Aunger, Robert

(ed.), *Darwinizing Culture: The Status of Memetics as a Science.* Oxford: Oxford University Press, 189–203.

Bolinger, Dwight
1980 *Language, the Loaded Weapon: The Use and Abuse of Language Today.* New York: Longman.

Bolton, Robert
1979 *People Skills: How To Assert Yourself, Listen to Others, and Resolve Conflicts.* New York: Simon and Schuster.

Brannon, Laura A. and Timothy C. Brock
1994 The subliminal persuasion controversy: Reality, enduring fable, and Polonius' weasel. In Shavitt, Sharon and Timothy C. Brock (eds.), *Persuasion: Psychological Insights and Perspectives.* Boston: Allyn and Bacon, 279–294.

Brodie, Richard
1996 *Virus of the Mind: The New Science of the Meme.* Seattle: Integral Press.

Brown, Richard H.
1977 *A Poetic for Sociology.* Cambridge: Cambridge University Press.

Comstock, George and Erica Scharrer
1999 *Television: What's On, Who's Watching, and What It Means.* San Diego: Academic Press.

Dawkins, Richard
1976 *The Selfish Gene.* New York: Oxford University Press.
1993 Viruses of the mind. In Dahlbom, Bo (ed.), *Dennett and His Critics: Demystifying Mind.* Oxford: Blackwell, 13–27.

Dixon, Robert M. W.
1980 *The Languages of Australia.* Cambridge: University of Cambridge Press.

Eco, Umberto
1984 *Semiotics and the Philosophy of Language.* Bloomington: Indiana University Press.

Gatherer, Derek
1998 Why the 'thought contagion' metaphor is retarding the progress of memetics. *Journal of Memetics: Evolutionary Models of Information Transmission* 2, Article 3. Retrieved July 23, 2001 from http://www.cpm.mmu.ac.uk/jom-emit/1998/vol2/gatherer_d.html

Gauntlett, David and Annette Hill
1999 *TV Living: Television, Culture and Everyday Life.* London: Routledge.

Godin, Seth
2000 *Unleashing the Ideavirus.* Do You Zoom, Inc. Retrieved July 23, 2001 from www.ideavirus.com

Goffman, Erving
1959 *The Presentation of Self in Everyday Life.* New York: Doubleday.

Gozzi, Raymond, Jr.
1999 *The Power of Metaphor in the Age of Electronic Media.* Cresskill, NJ: Hampton Press.

Grady, Joseph
1998 The 'conduit metaphor' revisited: A reassessment of metaphors for communication. In Koenig, Jean-Pierre (ed.), *Discourse and Cognition: Bridging the Gap.* Stanford: CSLI Publications, 205–218.

Green, Bryan S.
1983 *Knowing the Poor: A Case Study in Textual Reality Construction.* London: Routledge and Kegan Paul.

Gross, Alan G.
1990 *The Rhetoric of Science.* Cambridge, MA: Harvard University Press.

Hines, Stephen C.
1995 Referential skill or construct system development: Testing alternative explanations for role category questionnaire-based measures. *Communication Research Reports* 12, 15–24.

Johnson, Mark
1987 *The Body in the Mind.* Chicago: University of Chicago Press.

Jurvetson, Steve and Tim Draper
n.d. *Viral Marketing.* Retrieved July 23, 2001 http://www.dfj.com/files/viralmarketing.html

Kaufman, Ron
2000 *The Beautiful People Syndrome.* Retrieved July 23, 2001 from http://www.turnoffyourtv.com/commentary/syndrome.html

Krippendorff, Klaus
1993 Major metaphors of communication and some constructivist reflections on their use. *Cybernetics and Human Knowing* 2, 3–25.

Kupper, Adam
2000 If memes are the answer, what is the question? In Aunger, Robert (ed.), *Darwinizing Culture: The Status of Memetics as a Science.* Oxford: Oxford University Press, 175–188.

Lakoff, George and Mark Johnson
1980 *Metaphors We Live By.* Chicago: University of Chicago Press.

Lerner, Richard M.
1992 *Final Solutions: Biology, Prejudice, and Genocide.* University Park, PA: The Pennsylvania State University Press.

Lewontin, Richard C., Steven Rose, and Leon J. Kamin
1984 *Not in Our Genes: Biology, Ideology, and Human Nature.* New York: Pantheon.

Luke, Martin
n.d. [Message posted on web]. Retrieved July 23, 2001 from http://www.turnoffyourtv.com/public.opinions.html

Lumsdaine, Arthur A. and Irving L. Janis
1953 Resistance to "counterpropaganda" produced by one-sided and two-sided "propaganda" presentations. *Public Opinion Quarterly* 17, 311–318.

Lynch, Aaron
n.d. Thought contagion. Retrieved July 23, 2001 from http://www.thoughtcontagion.com/
1996 *Thought Contagion: How Belief Spreads through Society.* New York: Basic Books.
1998 [Message posted to the *Journal of Memetics* discussion list]. Retrieved July 23, 2001 from aldebaran.cpm.aca.mmu.ac.uk/~majordom/memetics/old/1269.html

Maasen, Sabine
1995 Who is afraid of metaphors? In Maasen, Sabine, Everett Mendelsohn, and Peter Weingart (eds.), *Biology as Society, Society as Biology: Metaphors*. Boston: Kluwer Academic, 11–35.
Maasen, Sabine, Everett Mendelsohn, and Peter Weingart
1995 Metaphors: Is there a bridge over troubled waters? In Maasen, Sabine, Everett Mendelsohn, and Peter Weingart (eds.), *Biology as Society, Society as Biology: Metaphors*. Boston: Kluwer Academic, 1–8.
McCloskey, Donald N.
1995 Metaphors economists live by. *Social Research* 62, 215–237.
McGuire, William J.
1961 The effectiveness of supportive and refutational defenses in immunizing and restoring beliefs against persuasion. *Sociometry* 24, 184–197.
Milton, John
1644[1927] *Areopagitica*. New York: Payson and Clarke.
Nelson, Christian K.
2001a The haunting of communication research by dead metaphors: For reflexive analyses of the communication research literature. *Language and Communication* 21, 245–272.
2001b If it sounds too good to be true, it is: A Wittgensteinian approach to the con flict literature. *Language and Society* 21, 1–22.
Nicholson, Judith
2001 Sick cell: Representations of cellular telephone use in North America. *M/C – A Journal of Media and Culture* 4, Article 6. Retrieved July 23, 2001 from http://moby.curtin.edu.au/~ausstud/mc/0106/cell.html
Novek, Eleanor M.
1992 Read it and weep: How metaphor limits views of literacy. *Discourse and Society* 3, 219–233.
Oboler, Eli M.
1974 *The Fear of the Word: Censorship and Sex*. Metuchen, NJ: The Scarecrow Press.
Pitkin, Hannah F.
1972 *Wittgenstein and Justice: On the Significance of Ludwig Wittgenstein for Social and Political Thought*. Berkeley: University of California Press.
Reddy, Michael J.
1979 The conduit metaphor: A case of frame in our language about language. In Ortony, Andrew (ed.), *Metaphor and Thought*. Cambridge: Cambridge University Press, 284–324.
Rothwell, J. Dan
1982. *Telling It Like It Isn't*. Englewood Cliffs, NJ: Prentice-Hall.
Rushkoff, Douglas
1996 *Media Virus: Hidden Agendas in Popular Culture*. New York: Ballantine Books.
Sarangi, Srikant
2001 Editorial: On demarcating the space between 'lay expertise' and 'expert laity.' *Text* 21, 3–12.

Schechter, Danny
2000 Honoring Paul Klite, media monitor extraordinaire. Retrieved July 23, 2001 from http://www.mediachannel.org/views/dissector/klite.shtml
Shannon, Claude E. and Warren Weaver
1949 *The Mathematical Theory of Communication.* Urbana: University of Illinois Press.
Singleton, Royce A., Jr. and Bruce C. Straits
2005 *Approaches to Social Research.* New York: Oxford University Press.
Tchong, Michael
1998, December 16 Macroview. *Iconocast*, para. 2. Retrieved July 23, 2001 from http://www.iconocast.com/issue/19981216.html#macroview
Turbayne, Collin M.
1970 *The Myth of Metaphor* (rev. ed.). Columbia: University of South Carolina Press.
Winn, Marie
1985 *The Plug-in Drug*, (rev. ed.). New York: Viking.
Wittgenstein, Ludwig
1958 *Philosophical Investigations* (3rd ed., G. E. M. Anscombe, trans.). New York: Macmillan.

# Author index

# Subject index

Bei Fragen zur Produktsicherheit wenden Sie sich bitte an:
If you have any questions regarding product safety,
please contact:

Walter de Gruyter GmbH
Genthiner Straße 13
10785 Berlin
productsafety@degruyterbrill.com